ADVANCE PRAISE
for

Abortion and America's Churches

"*Abortion and America's Churches* will be a go-to source for people wanting to understand the landscape of Christianity and abortion politics in the United States."

—Andrew R. Lewis, author of *The Rights Turn in Conservative Christian Politics*

"Meticulously researched and empathetic, *Abortion and America's Churches* fills an important gap in the history of the most divisive issue in the United States. Williams's even-handed, detailed account is a must-read for anyone trying to make sense of the role of faith in the American debate over reproduction."

—Mary Ziegler, author of *Roe: The History of a National Obsession*

"*Abortion and America's Churches* will be the definitive look at how Christians settled down on what is still unsettled."

—Marvin Olasky, co-author of *The Story of Abortion in America*

"This book is essential for anyone who wants to understand the debate over abortion in America. Williams's lucid, evenhanded account of this debate's twists, turns, and deep theological roots has forced me to revise the way I think about the history of sex, gender, and culture war in America."

—Molly Worthen, author of *Spellbound: How Charisma Shaped American History from the Puritans to Donald Trump*

"Daniel K. Williams provides an invaluable guide to the abortion debate as it has evolved since the 1960s, not simply in terms of national politics but also in terms of theological developments in the nation's Christian churches. Even readers who imagine themselves well-informed will learn from this accomplished and eminently readable book."

—Leslie Woodcock Tentler, author of *American Catholics*

"Thoroughly researched, theologically sophisticated, and politically astute, *Abortion and America's Churches* is a comprehensive account of the developing positions and shifting alliances of American Christian communities as they struggled with abortion before and after *Roe v. Wade*."

—Jerome E. Copulsky, author of *American Heretics*

"Daniel K. Williams reminds us that ideas have always mattered in politics. This thoroughly researched and masterfully crafted book should be essential reading for anyone interested in the subject."

—Mark Thomas Edwards, author of *Walter Lippmann*

ABORTION AND AMERICA'S CHURCHES

FAITH, GOVERNANCE, AND CIVIL SOCIETY
IN AMERICAN HISTORY

Series Editors:
Darryl G. Hart, Maura Jane Farrelly, and Samuel Goldman

The Faith, Governance, and Civil Society in American History series explores the nexus of the sacred and secular in American institutions. The series provides a platform to historians examining the two-way street of faith and public administration, church and state, parachurch agencies and nongovernmental organizations, political parties and faith-based nonprofits. The histories of specific and relevant institutions, prominent figures, and controversies will shed light not only on the ways that religious Americans negotiate secular society but also on the nature of the relationship between religious and political institutions in the United States. As such, Faith, Governance, and Civil Society in American History contributes to better understanding of the health and vitality of civil society in a liberal and democratic nation.

ABORTION AND AMERICA'S CHURCHES

A RELIGIOUS HISTORY
OF
ROE V. WADE

DANIEL K. WILLIAMS

University of Notre Dame Press
Notre Dame, Indiana

Copyright © 2025 by the University of Notre Dame

University of Notre Dame Press
Notre Dame, Indiana 46556
undpress.nd.edu

All Rights Reserved

Published in the United States of America

Library of Congress Control Number: 2025934556

ISBN: 978-0-268-21045-8 (Hardback)
ISBN: 978-0-268-21047-2 (WebPDF)
ISBN: 978-0-268-21048-9 (Epub3)

GPSR Compliance Inquiries:
Mare Nostrum Group B.V., Mauritskade 21D, 1091 GC Amsterdam, The Netherlands
gpsr@mare-nostrum.co.uk | Phone: +44 (0)1423 562232

To Nadya

CONTENTS

Acknowledgments ix

Introduction xi

CHAPTER 1	Liberal Protestants before *Roe*: Abortion as a Personal Moral Decision	1
CHAPTER 2	Catholics before *Roe*: A Theology of Unborn Life	43
CHAPTER 3	Evangelicals before *Roe*: A Moderate Conservatism on Abortion	93
CHAPTER 4	Catholics and Evangelicals after *Roe*: The Making of a Pro-Life Alliance	135
CHAPTER 5	The Rise and Fall of a Consistent Life Ethic	179
CHAPTER 6	Liberal Protestants after *Roe*: A Theology for a Pluralistic Nation	209
CHAPTER 7	The Conservative Christian Coalition That Overturned *Roe*	253

Notes 299

Index 343

ACKNOWLEDGMENTS

This book is the result of an invitation I received from Darryl Hart several years ago to write about the history of abortion politics for a series that he was editing, so I'd like to begin these acknowledgments by noting my debt of gratitude to Darryl, since without his invitation, this book would never have been written. I initially declined the invitation, protesting that I had too many other writing projects to take on an additional book, especially since I felt that I had said all I wanted to say about abortion politics in *Defenders of the Unborn* and some of my other books that touched on the subject. But when Darryl persisted—and when the Supreme Court overturned *Roe v. Wade* in 2022, thus changing the landscape of abortion politics—I decided that perhaps the time had come to return to this topic. I'm glad that I did. Thank you, Darryl, for encouraging me in this endeavor.

    I'm also grateful to Emily King, my editor at the University of Notre Dame Press, who expressed her enthusiasm for this project and did everything possible to streamline the publication process and facilitate the release of this book in as timely a manner as possible. Having worked with various editors in the past, I know the value of an editor's support for a project, and for this book I have had an editor whose belief in the project's value could not be surpassed.

    The archivists I have worked with in the course of researching this book—especially Ed Cade at the United Church of Christ Archives in Cleveland, Ohio, and Michelle Smith at the Archives of the Archdiocese of Cincinnati—have been consummately professional and enormously helpful, and I'm grateful for their assistance in locating material that would have been impossible to find otherwise. I am also grateful for the help my undergraduate research assistant Shira Hoffer gave me in locating and compiling sources at an early stage of this project.

It is impossible to list all of the supportive colleagues and friends who encouraged me in this undertaking, but I am especially grateful for Andy Lewis's suggestions and encouragement in the early stages of this project and for Mary Ziegler's unflagging support for my work, even when our historical or political interpretations have differed. Mary has put me in touch with numerous publications and media outlets for interviews about my research on abortion politics, and she has been a valuable conversation partner at various stages of my study. She also read through the entire manuscript and offered helpful feedback.

I completed most of the writing for this project while serving as a senior fellow at the Ashbrook Center at Ashland University, so I'm grateful to the center for giving me this opportunity. Because much of my thinking about the philosophical and theological framework for abortion debates can be traced back to my experiences in the James Madison Program at Princeton University more than a decade ago, I also want to express my appreciation to the administrators of the program for giving me an opportunity that facilitated not only my work on *Defenders of the Unborn* but also this book.

Finally, I am grateful to my wife, Nadya, for her encouragement throughout this project. As a mother and a writer, Nadya has a strong interest in the issues that are the focus of this book, and she has written on some of these topics herself. She believed in the importance of this book and encouraged me to write it. I'm grateful for the opportunity to make this journey with her, and I'm thankful for her love and support, which is why I am dedicating this book to Nadya.

INTRODUCTION

In 1967, Fr. Charles Carroll of California joined the pro-life movement. He was a civil rights advocate, an opponent of capital punishment, and a strong supporter of labor rights. He had marched with Cesar Chavez in support of the human dignity of agricultural migrant workers. For him, the abortion issue was just as much a human rights issue as civil rights for racial minorities, because it involved the life of the fetus. After having been an observer at the Nuremberg Trials, he could never forget the ease with which a seemingly civilized society could slip into the denial of the right to life. The defense of the unborn was for him a moral imperative.[1]

That same year, another priest, Robert Drinan, wrote an article declaring that "the law should withdraw from the area of regulating abortion." Although only two years before he had written strong denunciations of abortion, claiming it was the killing of an unborn human being, he decided in 1967 that abortion should be legalized up to the point of viability, a position from which he never wavered. As a Democratic congressional representative from Massachusetts in the late 1970s, he consistently voted pro-choice.[2]

Drinan was a Catholic priest and dean of the law school of Boston College. Carroll was an Episcopalian. That they both took positions on abortion that were contrary to the views their respective denominations eventually adopted was not unusual. There were Catholics in the 1960s and 1970s (and afterward) who thought that abortion should be legal, and there were liberal Protestants (including liberal Protestant clergy, such as Carroll) during the same period who thought that abortion was a moral evil that should be outlawed. The positions on abortion of nearly all major denominations during this period were in flux. Even when a religious organization took a clear theological stance against abortion, as the Catholic Church did, there was often a great deal of internal debate about how to apply that stance in the political sphere. And even when a church took a stance in favor of abortion rights, as many liberal Protestant denominations officially did, there were often numerous dissenters who joined the antiabortion cause, as Carroll did.

Abortion and the Churches is a historical study of that internal debate in the churches, but it is also more than that. It is the first comprehensive study of how each major Christian subgroup in the United States eventually arrived at a position on abortion that logically reflected its theological outlook about matters that often extended far beyond abortion. There are several books that survey the doctrinal positions of various religious groups on abortion, but this is the first book to provide not only an exposition of these beliefs but a detailed history of the internal denominational conversations and theological debates that shaped the official denominational positions about abortion in American Christianity from the pre-*Roe* era to the present. As this book shows, the positions on abortion that different Christian traditions adopted were historically contingent, but not accidental or capricious. In the end, they reflected a particular theological framework that began long before *Roe v. Wade* and continued long after it. And because these were *American* Christians who were debating the issue of abortion in a particular American context, their views on abortion closely reflected their larger vision for the nation, their understanding of their country's founding documents, and their own relationship to American politics. Although Christians throughout the world discussed the morality of abortion in the late twentieth century, the unique contours of the political debate over abortion in the United States and its inseparability from the landmark Supreme Court case *Roe v. Wade* meant that the discussion of abortion in the nation's churches would take on a uniquely American character that fused Christian theology with visions of the nation's identity.

This book therefore challenges two popular assumptions. One assumption is held by many religious people themselves who imagine that ideas about abortion within their own religious tradition have never changed, because they reflect timeless truths conveyed by sacred texts or the clear light of conscience and reason. This is clearly not the case. Every major Christian tradition in the United States—including Catholicism, liberal Protestantism, evangelical Protestantism, and Black Protestantism—has experienced significant internal debate and reevaluation of the abortion question during the past sixty years. Some religious denominations have gone so far as to directly reverse positions on abortion that they took a half century ago, but even those that have not have often reconsidered their framing of the abortion question or at least have had to address internal challenges to that position.

But if the assumption that religious positions on abortion are unchanging has been widespread in the nonacademic world, many academics have adopted another assumption about religion and abortion that is equally false: the position that theological views of abortion are capricious and subject to sudden reversals that have little connection to the historical theology of the particular religious group in question. Perhaps these religious groups' theological declarations on the subject are merely fig leaves that provide a thin covering for their real political interests. The oft-told historical myth that evangelicals didn't care about abortion (or perhaps were even pro-choice) before their religious movement was captured by the Religious Right in the late 1970s is a case in point. Those who tell this story want to convey the view that evangelical opposition to abortion is not grounded in scripture or historic evangelical theology, but was instead the creation of political Machiavellians.[3]

This book challenges such interpretations. Religious beliefs and historic theological traditions do shape views on abortion, and we have to take them seriously if we want to understand why Americans have such strong convictions on both sides of this issue. This book traces the historical narrative that led each of the religious groups in question to develop a particular position on abortion and demonstrates that that position was logically and coherently connected to the group's theological outlook. Our views on abortion are influenced by our larger views about human life, gender, sexuality, the purpose of law, and, for many people, God and humans' relationship to God. Theology is about the ordering and framing of those particular views. And for those on both sides of the abortion debate, abortion therefore was (and is) a deeply theological issue, an issue that connects to our deepest understandings of the meaning of human life, our place in the cosmos, and our relationship to the divine.

If this book is successful, readers will come away with a realization that those on the opposing side of the abortion debate have sincerely held, logically coherent, historically shaped reasons for their convictions. Furthermore, these convictions are often rooted in religious texts and theological principles that those on both sides of the abortion debate share. Even if the two sides disagree with each other sharply, they both "read the same Bible and pray to the same God," to use the words of Abraham Lincoln when he spoke of the division among Christians of his own day over slavery.

The first three chapters trace the Christian theological discussions of abortion before *Roe v. Wade* and discuss the views of the Christian traditions that had the greatest influence on the political debate over abortion in the 1970s: liberal Protestants, Catholics, and evangelical Protestants. Liberal Protestants (who have also been variously called "mainline Protestants" or "ecumenical Protestants") are members of established denominations that can trace their ecclesiastical and theological lineage to the early nineteenth century or before, but who have embraced twentieth-century liberal assumptions about the need to reinterpret the Bible in the light of contemporary science, human rights principles, democratic pluralism, and, above all, the principles of human equality and individual freedom.[4] American Catholics are members of the worldwide Roman Catholic Church. Evangelical Protestants are Protestants who can trace their theological heritage to an early twentieth-century fundamentalist movement that insisted on biblical inerrancy or infallibility and largely rejected higher criticism of the Bible, which means that they have continued to emphasize historic nineteenth-century American Protestant ideas about the importance of individual conversion, the role of the Holy Spirit in salvation and regeneration, and the need for a "personal" relationship with Jesus as Savior.[5]

Chapter 6 introduces a fourth group of Christians — Black Protestants — that in some ways straddled the divide between liberal Protestantism and evangelicalism while challenging the assumptions of whites in both traditions. As theological heirs of the form of Christianity that enslaved African Americans developed in the eighteenth and early nineteenth centuries, Black Protestants cared deeply about both biblical authority and social justice, but disagreed among themselves about how to apply those principles to the issue of abortion. Despite the deep differences between their theological traditions, evangelicals and conservative Catholics eventually arrived at a similar opposition to abortion, while most Black Protestants and white liberal Protestants, despite long-standing disagreements about the morality of abortion, eventually arrived at a similar support for abortion rights in the political sphere. This book argues that the Catholic–evangelical alliance was grounded in a similar concern about upholding a fixed standard of moral authority and a Christian framework for U.S. law, while the alliance between liberal Protestants and Black Protestants was based on a shared concern about upholding the values of religious liberty, equality, and pluralism in a democratic society.

In some ways, the boundaries between each of these traditions are porous, and the categorizations can feel a bit artificial at times. Most liberal Protestant denominations include members who are conservative evangelicals in their beliefs, and some of the nation's largest evangelical denominations have in turn included prominent members whose theological beliefs were influenced by liberal Protestantism. There are Catholics who think like liberal Protestants and others who have embraced a largely evangelical mindset. There are Black Protestants who are members of predominantly white denominations. And there are a few groups on the margins of American Christianity that do not fit into any of these categories and are mostly ignored in this study. Eastern Orthodox churches, along with conservative Anabaptists (such as Amish communities), have exercised very little sustained political influence in the United States, and they therefore receive no coverage in this book. The Church of Jesus Christ of Latter-Day Saints (Mormons), which has had a regional political influence in parts of the West, has had only a modest influence on national religious or political conversations about abortion, and is not covered in this study.[6]

Likewise, there are no chapters on non-Christian religious groups.[7] By focusing only on Christian churches, this study retains a cohesiveness that might be lost with a broader coverage, and it is able to examine in detail how different groups interpreted the same shared sacred text (namely, the Bible) and theological ideas that emerged in conversation with each other. Especially in the early 1970s, Americans widely understood the religious debate about abortion to be an exchange of views between Protestants and Catholics, and even today the vast majority who engage in religiously influenced discussions of abortion are interacting with arguments created within one of the major Christian traditions. By limiting this study to American Christians, I am framing the story in such a way that it has the maximum value for understanding the trajectory of the political conversation on this topic.

Yet even if the categorizations used in this book are sometimes approximate rather than absolute, and even if this framework leaves out a few Christian groups that may not comfortably fit into any of these categories, there is a lot to be gained by using this framework, because the religious categories used in this book allow us to make sense of a few major approaches to the abortion issue that transcended denominational lines but that closely followed particular theological contours that can roughly be categorized as "liberal Protestant," "evangelical," or "Catholic." By the end of the first three chapters of this book, I hope that readers will have a clear sense of the historical process by which members of a particular Christian tradition arrived at a particular understanding of abortion after a long period of internal debate and, most importantly, how that understanding relates to the religious group's larger view of God, humanity, politics, and society.

The last four chapters of this book explain how *Roe v. Wade* (1973), which was in many ways a liberal Protestant decision, galvanized a debate over abortion among mainline Protestants, evangelicals, Catholics, and Black Protestants that ultimately became a debate about much more than reproductive rights. In the end, the debate turned out to be a discussion of religious values, sources of moral authority, and the identity of the nation itself. By the end of this book, I hope that readers will gain a greater understanding of how and why these particular religiously influenced viewpoints have resulted in a polarizing political debate on abortion, and how we might engage with that debate in ways that respect the theological convictions of the various participants.

Our country's political and legal debate about abortion has always been inseparably linked to religious assumptions. The United States has never had — and quite likely, never will have — an abortion policy that is purely religiously neutral, with no influence from any religiously based assumptions. *Roe v. Wade* reflected liberal Protestant theological assumptions. Justice Harry Blackmun, who wrote the majority opinion, was a churchgoing liberal Methodist, and his decision closely echoed the principal assertions of liberal Protestant denominational resolutions on abortion and the editorial commentary on abortion policy in the *Christian Century*. As a liberal Protestant decision, *Roe* incurred opposition from people who did not share liberal Protestants' theological framework for thinking about abortion, the beginning of human life, and individual liberty. Their activism eventually succeeded in reversing *Roe v. Wade* in *Dobbs v. Jackson Women's Health Organization* (2022). But the Supreme Court's reversal of *Roe* in 2022 could not answer the question of what framework could replace the liberal Protestant assumptions that had guided abortion policy for half a century. The dismantling of the liberal Protestant framework for abortion policy left the United States with an ideological vacuum that each religious group involved in the abortion debate has tried (so far unsuccessfully) to fill.

This book is not primarily about politics, so it does not cover every significant abortion court case or every major abortion policy. But the religious views that this book analyzes have had profound political implications, since abortion is a deeply polarizing political subject in the United States. This book will therefore give readers a much deeper understanding of the philosophies that have shaped political debates over abortion. There are already numerous studies of the partisan political dimensions of these controversies (including a few that I have produced myself), but what is often missing in studies of the politics of abortion is a serious and comprehensive examination of the reasons why different groups adopted opposing viewpoints on this issue.[8] This book is a study of those reasons. It uses a study of the abortion debate within Christian churches to show that for large numbers of Americans those reasons are theological. And when it examines political controversies over abortion, it explores those political debates from the perspective of the competing theologies of the religious groups involved, which means that its coverage of abortion policy may look very different from typical treatments that use a political, legal, or social framework to understand this topic.

Because this book is a study of theologically influenced reasoning about abortion, it focuses heavily on denominational resolutions, papal encyclicals, and debates among clergy—the sort of thing that may seem boring or irrelevant for those who would prefer to read about the activities of activists or the opinions of the "average" person in the pew or others who never wore a clerical collar. But as public opinion surveys taken in multiple denominations have demonstrated, active churchgoers often adopt the views of their particular religious tradition on abortion. This means that the debates that occurred among the Protestant church leaders who participated in their denominations' general assemblies or among the Catholic clerics who were members of the United States Conference of Catholic Bishops really did matter for millions of Americans.[9] By paying attention to the language used in those debates, we can trace changes in theological approaches to abortion over time, and we can begin to construct a history of the different ways in which Christians have thought about abortion and the reasons why they have adopted those views. And by doing so, we will be better equipped to understand the convictions that lie behind the polarizing political debates about this issue.

Of course, a skeptic might argue that Christians do not adopt their views on abortion because they hold a particular theological conviction; instead, they adopt a theological view that reflects their preexisting views on abortion. After all, there is some political science scholarship that suggests that people's political party has more influence on their religious practices than their religious practices have on their choice of political party.[10] Yet regardless of whether this is true, it is still the case that our views on abortion are inseparably related to our larger convictions about theological matters. Whether our views on abortion shape our theology or our theological convictions determine our views on abortion, the end result is a larger worldview that has political and social implications extending far beyond the abortion debate. That larger worldview is usually both strongly cohesive and historically constructed, and it is therefore well worth studying because of the insight that it gives us into how we understand life and society.

This book is therefore a tool to understand how other people think about some of the most divisive and vitally important issues facing Americans today. At a time of deep political polarization, this book will give us the insights we need to reach across the partisan and religious divide and understand the views of people we think are wrong. In many cases, they read the same sacred texts, appeal to the same set of theological principles, and pray to a common God, but they interpret their theological tradition and its implications for abortion very differently. By the end of this book, you will understand why.

CHAPTER 1

LIBERAL PROTESTANTS BEFORE *ROE*

Abortion as a Personal Moral Decision

In 1957, a Florida woman facing a crisis pregnancy took the train to New York in search of an illegal abortion. For decades, New York City's illegal abortion industry, which was closely connected with organized crime syndicates, had performed perhaps 250,000 abortions or more per year, which meant that every year, thousands of women from up and down the Eastern Seaboard and across the Midwest traveled to New York for a pregnancy termination. Occasionally, the police broke up one of the criminal rings controlling the back-alley abortion business, but most of the time, they left it alone. Many women who lacked the connections to a sympathetic doctor near their home could therefore make their way to New York and take their chances among the unlicensed abortion providers offering a service that was against the law. This was the situation that the woman from Florida faced in 1957.

But this woman, like many others entering the city in search of an abortion, did not know where to find someone who was willing to transgress the law in order to perform the procedure, and especially where to find someone who was competent to perform it safely. After all, one would not expect those who offered an illegal service to advertise their business in the yellow pages. But fortunately for her, she had the next best thing: a church connection. A Protestant minister had given her the name of Howard Moody, the thirty-six-year-old pastor of New York City's Judson Memorial Baptist Church. Moody was sympathetic to the woman's plight and tried to help. In fact, he was so sympathetic that he decided that helping women to obtain safe abortions needed to become a permanent part of his ministry. Within ten years, he would be operating a national abortion referral service, with ministers and rabbis from across the United States participating in an effort to connect women to illegal abortion services in their cities.[1]

The idea that Protestant ministers would play a leading role in helping women obtain illegal abortions might seem strange to some people today, but it was not so surprising in the mid-twentieth century, when Protestantism was associated with progressive views on birth control and medical care. In the years leading up to *Roe v. Wade*, liberal Protestants were some of the nation's leading advocates of abortion legalization, and that included clergy and laity. Indeed, liberal Protestants played such a dominant role in framing the campaign for abortion legalization that one could even call *Roe v. Wade* itself a liberal Protestant decision.

NINETEENTH-CENTURY PROTESTANT SUPPORT FOR ABORTION RESTRICTIONS

Protestants were still the dominant religious group in the early 1970s, just as they had been throughout the entire history of the United States. And in the early 1970s, the most culturally influential and wealthiest Protestant denominations—those commonly known as "mainline," a group that included Episcopalians, Congregationalists, Presbyterians, Methodists, Lutherans, and a smattering of other groups, ranging from American Baptists to Disciples of Christ—were closely associated with the values of liberal democracy. They believed in science, progress, freedom of choice, and individual rights of conscience. Nearly every mainline Protestant denomination therefore endorsed abortion legalization before *Roe v. Wade*. But despite their general support for abortion's legality, mainline Protestants were ambivalent about its morality, and this ambivalence would shape *Roe v. Wade* and contribute to its ultimate instability.

Protestants had deeply rooted theological reasons for moral qualms about abortion. The two most famous Protestant Reformers of the sixteenth century—Martin Luther and John Calvin—had expressed objections to abortion, with Calvin clearly indicating that he viewed the fetus as a full human person. In his commentary on Exodus, he wrote, "The *foetus*, though enclosed in the womb of its mother, is already a human being (*homo*), and it is almost a monstrous crime to rob it of the life which it has not yet begun to enjoy. If it seems more horrible to kill a man in his own house than in a field, because a man's house is his place of most secure refuge, it ought surely to be deemed more atrocious to destroy a *foetus* in the womb before it has come to light."[2] Indeed, before the second half of the twentieth century, there was little discernible difference between Protestant and Catholic theological views on abortion, just as there was little difference between Protestant and Catholic official church teachings on contraception before the end of the 1920s. The doctrine of original sin, which received strong emphasis in both Luther's and Calvin's theology, naturally fit with the idea that a sinful human nature was transmitted at the moment of insemination and that the soul therefore originated at conception rather than being infused into a prenatal body at a later stage of fetal development. The Reformed Protestant emphasis on the sovereignty of God, God's foreknowledge and predestination of individuals, and the value of human life solely because of its relationship to God also seemed to undermine any arguments that humans had the right to take fetal life without God's explicit authorization or that they had the right to interrupt God's creative work in the womb. Late twentieth-century advocates of abortion rights would commonly emphasize the role of human choice in the process of procreation, but these ideas were alien to traditional Calvinist theology and Reformed ideas of God's sovereignty as creator. Even if the parents of an embryo or fetus did not value their prenatal child, that child could still have value because God valued it, later Reformed theologians, such as Karl Barth, would eventually argue.[3]

That did not mean that Protestants in the Reformation era and afterward talked about abortion very often. For most of the seventeenth, eighteenth, and early nineteenth centuries, references to abortion from Protestant ministers (or, indeed, from any American Protestants, including lay members who never authored a sermon) were extremely rare. After a pregnancy reached the "quickening" stage — the point at which a pregnant woman could perceive fetal movement, a moment that usually occurred late in the second trimester — abortion could be prosecuted as a capital offense under English common law, but before quickening, the common law tradition seemed to be more permissive. In practice, the abortion cases that went to trial in the American colonies of the eighteenth century seem to have been limited to unmarried women who had had sexual relations with a much older (often married) man and were therefore unable to marry the man who had impregnated them, which was the usual practice for young couples who didn't wait until the wedding night to conceive their first child.

Given the limited amount of historical evidence about colonists' opinions on abortion in the eighteenth century, historians of the subject have come to widely differing interpretations. The majority of historians, following the lead of James Mohr's landmark study of 1978, have concluded that because there were very few prosecutions of pre-quickening abortions in the colonial era and early republic, first-trimester abortions must have been widely tolerated, and that married (and unmarried) women commonly used abortifacients or procured the help of midwives to terminate unwanted pregnancies. But more recently, Marvin Olasky and Leah Savas published a detailed study of abortion cases in early America that concluded the opposite from the limited number of abortion cases. "Abortion in colonial times remained rare," Olasky and Savas claimed, because "God-fearing" people had "an internal sense that abortion was wrong."[4]

Given the silence of ministers on the subject, it may be impossible to know for certain what Protestants of the eighteenth century believed about abortion. But what appears most likely, in an era when the average married woman had seven children and when 90 percent of people lived on farms, is that most married women expected to have a large family and saw additional children as a blessing rather than a burden, and that any married women's attempts to limit their fertility through abortion or other means were therefore infrequent enough that they didn't attract commentary from the men who served as Protestant ministers. Nor do the women's writings that we have from the colonial era provide much record of abortion. Instead, we are reliant on sporadic court documents, which reveal both people's widespread familiarity with abortion in the colonies and their sense that it was something shameful, but not something that ministers felt the need to preach against directly. "Abortion was seen as blameworthy because it was an extreme action designed to hide a prior sin, sex outside of marriage," historian Cornelia Hughes Dayton concluded in her study of an abortion case in Connecticut from the 1740s. And because abortion was so closely associated with women who were perceived as "lewd or dissident," married women who resorted to abortion in this era probably felt the need to keep their pregnancy terminations a secret.[5] In Dayton's view, that had nothing to do with a belief that the fetus was a human being before quickening, a belief that Dayton did not think they had. Olasky and Savas disagree.

What we can say is that Protestant ministers of the time (such as Jonathan Edwards) strongly rebuked the sin of premarital sex, but they did not discuss abortion. But this silence probably did not convey approval. Because abortion was a largely covert practice that was closely associated in many Protestants' minds with sexual sin, it never received clerical approval in the eighteenth century. And in the nineteenth century, when abortion became more publicly discussed, some ministers began denouncing abortion in language that closely echoed the view that Calvin had expressed.

The issue of abortion attracted more attention from Protestants after the 1820s, because as young women began moving to rapidly expanding cities at the beginning of the industrial era, some of them wanted abortions, and there was a growing trade in abortifacients that could meet that demand. At the same time, some physicians (nearly all of whom were Protestant) began speaking out against abortion on biological and moral grounds. Appealing to new biological evidence about fetal life, they argued that "quickening" was not a medically meaningful stage of fetal development; the fetus was alive long before its movement could be detected, they said. And if that were the case, early-stage abortions should be illegal.

Historians such as James Mohr may be correct in thinking that nineteenth-century doctors and state legislators who favored abortion regulation were motivated at least in part by a desire to protect women from practices that were viewed as dangerous or unscrupulous while simultaneously protecting the professional authority of (male) physicians by regulating a procedure that (female) midwives often performed, but the physicians who led the campaign for abortion prohibitions—such as Boston physician Horatio Storer—believed firmly in the right to life of the fetus and made fetal life the center of their argument. State legislators found the argument persuasive. Beginning with Connecticut in the 1820s, states throughout the country moved to pass new abortion restrictions.[6]

The overwhelming majority of Protestants who wrote about abortion in the nineteenth century were medical doctors, but at the height of the campaign, in the late 1860s, a number of ministers also supported the campaign for fetal life. In 1867, the *Northwestern Christian Advocate*, a Methodist periodical based in Chicago, published an editorial that labeled abortion "infanticide" and "murder." Although the author of the unsigned editorial (who was presumably the paper's editor, the Methodist minister Thomas Mears Eddy) mentioned early church tradition against abortion, his greatest argument came from "medical science" and especially from Dr. Storer. Influenced by the latest scientific knowledge of fetal development, many state legislatures were quickly enacting restrictive abortion laws, the editorial encouragingly noted.

But, the *Northwestern Christian Advocate* also noted with disappointment, the Protestant churches were behind the times in this area. "Foeticide" was eschewed by the "Papal Church," but Protestantism was "blackly stained by this crime of child-murder." By the author's estimate, 15 percent of married women in Protestant churches had the "criminal hardihood to practice this black art"—by which he presumably meant that they had had abortions themselves or were skilled midwives who could perform abortions—and there was "an additional per cent who endorse and defend it." Whether or not the *Advocate*'s percentage estimates were correct, the editorial was no doubt accurate in saying that there were many lay Protestants who saw nothing wrong with abortion and many female church members who obtained abortions for themselves or performed them for other women. Like the physicians' arguments against abortion, the minister's editorial blended arguments in favor of the humanity of the fetus with a lengthy discussion of the health dangers of abortion and a dim view of midwifery. There was also a pro-natalist argument that appealed to widespread northern Protestant fears of Catholic immigration: If Catholics faithfully eschewed abortions while Protestant women obtained them, the Catholic population would grow in the United States and the Protestant population would shrink.[7] Above all, articles such as this one viewed abortion as an individual moral crime—an act of murder committed by selfish women, many of whom were married and chose to kill their unborn babies rather than take on the responsibilities of caring for an additional child. Earlier generations of New England women "never were spotted with the blood of innocents" and "never quenched life immortal for the sake of ease or fashion," the Pittsfield, Massachusetts, Congregationalist minister John Todd said, but the present generation of "degenerated" women in the pews refused to assume the "holiest position and duties" of motherhood and instead resorted to abortion.[8]

The Presbyterian Church (USA), which at the time was an active supporter of the temperance campaign and other Christian efforts to eradicate vice from the church and society, was so horrified by abortion that the denomination's General Assembly passed a resolution in 1869 declaring that "the destructing of parents of their offspring, before birth" was "a crime against God and against nature." "As the frequency of such murders can no longer be concealed," the Presbyterian General Assembly added, "we hereby warn those that are guilty of this crime that, except they repent, they cannot inherit eternal life."[9]

The Presbyterian denominational resolution and the antiabortion articles published in the late 1860s could not have been clearer—abortion was murder and the women who resorted to it would go to hell unless they repented. The seriousness of the charge might have led one to expect that these declarations would lead to a widespread ministerial campaign. Yet they did not. The overwhelming majority of Protestant clergy greeted the physicians' campaign against abortion with silence. And even the few Christian periodicals that had openly supported the campaign soon went on to other matters, probably because, in their view, the problem of abortion had been solved when state legislation made the midwives' practice of it illegal.

The Protestant ministerial discussion of abortion in the late 1860s, even if it was limited and short-lived, reflected the anxieties of some post–Civil War Protestants about vice on a number of fronts, from gambling to alcohol to pornography. Abortion, many Protestants of the time thought, was connected with other vices that perverted the sex act or prevented conception or childbirth. The most comprehensive federal antivice law of the era, the Comstock Act (1873), banned the possession or advertisement of instruments or medicines to perform abortion, but did so only in the context of a larger prohibition of obscene literature and contraceptive devices. By some measures, the Protestant campaign against abortion was one of the most spectacularly successful of these antivice campaigns—in this case, against the vice of the selfish taking of unborn human life by women who were unwilling to assume the duties of motherhood, as the Protestant antiabortion campaigners phrased it. By the end of the 1880s, every U.S. state and territory had a restrictive abortion law, which, in most cases, prohibited abortion except when it was necessary to save a woman's life, or, in the case of a handful of states, when it was necessary to protect the woman's health.[10] Although illegal abortion continued to be widely available in some places, many doctors vilified the practice. For much of the early twentieth century, physicians who wanted to deter women from abortions used illustrations of embryonic and fetal life to demonstrate that unborn human life developed along a continuum and that the popular idea that "quickening" marked a new stage of fetal life had no scientific basis.

But perhaps the rapid, overwhelming success of this campaign—which occurred with only the most limited pulpit mobilization for the cause—left Protestants without a tradition of antiabortion theological or philosophical reflection. Protestants of the late nineteenth and early twentieth centuries—and, indeed, most Americans in the Protestant-dominated culture of the era—seemed to believe that abortion was the taking of an unborn human life and was therefore rightfully illegal, but they did not say much about the precise point at which human personhood began or the reasons why they were sure that abortion was murder. Nor did anyone launch a campaign to reduce the number of illegal abortions. Sporadic police raids at the local level sometimes stopped individual abortion providers or broke up abortion rings that in the mid-twentieth century were often connected with criminal syndicates, but these police raids were not part of a nationally coordinated effort to stamp out abortion. Scattered comments against abortion can be found in the writings of some women's rights advocates of this era, but—in contrast to campaigns against prostitution or alcohol or in favor of women's voting rights or child labor laws—there was no systematic campaign against abortion in the early twentieth century. A few doctors gave traveling lectures on fetal development in order to deter women from having abortions, but the subject received hardly any attention in Protestant pulpits or periodicals.

Perhaps abortion received relatively little attention from Protestant pulpits because—as the few surviving late nineteenth-century ministerial writings against abortion suggest—Protestants at the time viewed abortion primarily as a private practice of middle-class married women rather than the resort of unmarried women or prostitutes. In practice, antiabortion laws were most likely to ensnare unmarried women, but the few ministers who expressed public concern about abortion instead viewed the practice as a way for married women to shirk their duty to have additional children. This pro-natalist view had limited traction among Protestants, because middle-class Protestants in industrialized cities of the late nineteenth century gave every indication of wanting to limit the sizes of their families, which did not bode well for any ministerial pro-natalist campaigns. If ministers had instead framed the antiabortion campaign as a way to save lower-class women from vice or rescue them from the sex trade—class-based frameworks that were key to the success of the era's moral campaigns against prostitution and alcohol—perhaps the campaign would have been more successful, but since they did not frame their campaign that way, it had limited appeal in churches. Instead, what did convince Protestants that abortion was wrong in most cases was the medical profession's successful campaign for antiabortion laws that framed abortion as an illegal and immoral activity that was nevertheless permissible when a professionally licensed physician deemed it necessary to save a woman's life. This framework for viewing abortion—that it was wrong, criminal, and dangerous in most circumstances, but acceptable when a professional physician used it to save a patient's life—continued to guide Protestants until the 1960s.

THEOLOGICAL CHANGES IN MAINLINE PROTESTANTISM IN THE EARLY TWENTIETH CENTURY

In the late nineteenth and early twentieth century a theological sea change occurred in Protestantism that would eventually lead decades later to a changed view of abortion. At the end of the nineteenth century, a large number of Protestant ministers began to see both sin and salvation primarily in societal rather than individual terms. For most of the nineteenth century, evangelical Protestants (a designation that characterized approximately 85 percent of the churchgoing Protestant population at the time) had viewed salvation as an entirely individualistic enterprise. The focus of revival preaching in the early nineteenth century was to save individual sinners from going to hell. And if salvation was individual, so was sin. Moral preaching for much of the nineteenth century focused primarily on individual vices; moral lessons in American Protestant-created schoolbooks, such as the *McGuffey's Readers*, did the same. Even when evangelical Protestants brought their moral campaigns into the political sphere, they still saw social legislation as a way to curb individual vice. The temperance movement of the early nineteenth century was a campaign to reform individual drunkards. The antislavery movement (which received significantly less support from white Protestants than the temperance campaign did) was a campaign against the immorality of the enslavers. But in the late nineteenth century, northern Protestant urban ministers, such as Walter Rauschenbusch and Washington Gladden, began to argue that both the kingdom of God and the gospel were primarily social in nature and that it was impossible to fully preach Christ's message without advocating for better working and living conditions for the working class or addressing the causes of poverty. When the Kansas City Congregationalist minister Charles Sheldon asked the question, "What would Jesus do?" in his best-selling novel *In His Steps*, the answer he gave was socially oriented: if Jesus were living in the 1890s, he would fight the saloon. In the hands of the Methodist activist Frances Willard and the other Protestant women who led the Women's Christian Temperance Union, a movement that had focused primarily on stopping individual drunkenness became focused instead on a much broader social platform. Ridding the country of liquor would be the key to alleviating poverty and improving family life and women's rights, Willard believed; for that reason, temperance advocacy should be accompanied with woman suffrage and other social reform causes. The Protestant college presidents of the early twentieth century echoed this emphasis on the social; in the sermons and college addresses they presented, they spoke of the lofty societal goals that a Christian education should equip college graduates to accomplish: the promotion of democracy, social and political reform, and world peace.[11]

Not all Protestants accepted this new emphasis on the Social Gospel, but most of the "modernists" (or mainline Protestants) who opposed the fundamentalists in the intradenominational fights of the early 1920s were sympathetic to it, and it shaped the priorities of some of the largest Protestant organizations of the time, including not only denominational agencies but also parachurch organizations, such as the Young Men's Christian Association (YMCA) and the Young Women's Christian Association (YWCA). The Federal Council of Churches, the nation's first major ecumenical interdenominational association, outlined the goals of the Social Gospel in "The Social Creed of the Churches," which it adopted as soon as it was founded in 1908. "We deem it the duty of all Christian people to concern themselves directly with certain practical industrial problems," the "Social Creed" said. "To us it seems that the Churches must stand: For equal rights and complete justice for all men in all stations of life." The Federal Council then listed a series of specific political stances it believed its constituent denomination had to take, including advocacy for a living wage, the end of child labor, and industrial regulations to protect worker safety.[12]

The new conception of morality as primarily social in nature prompted many Protestant ministers to become advocates of birth control. In the mid-to-late nineteenth century, when white middle-class Protestants thought of morality primarily in individual terms, it was easy for many of them to view birth control as a personal dereliction of duty on the part of women and closely akin to obscenity. That was the way that the few Protestant ministers who had spoken out against abortion in the 1860s had written about pregnancy termination, and it was the way that the supporters of the Comstock Act in the 1870s thought about contraceptives and birth control in general. Birth control was a vice, and it was associated either with sexual immorality among people who refused to accept the consequences for their fornication and adultery or with the selfishness of married women who refused to do their duty of bearing children. Such views had a long Christian history, because until the twentieth century, no Christian church endorsed birth control and one could find plenty of good Christian testimony against it, not only from Catholics but also from the Protestant Reformers Luther and Calvin.[13]

But beginning in the 1920s, the nation's liberal Protestant periodicals were filled with articles advocating birth control. Contraceptives and birth control information were still illegal in some states, but liberal Protestants—especially the most liberal denominations of New England, the Congregationalists, the Unitarians, and the Universalists—wanted to promote birth control as a positive social good. When the sociologist Melissa J. Wilde surveyed more than 10,000 articles on birth control from more than seventy denominational periodicals published between

1919 and 1965, she found that there was a very close correlation between a denomination's support for the Social Gospel and eugenics and its advocacy of birth control. In the 1920s, denominations that endorsed the Social Gospel and were concerned about the rapid population growth of Catholic immigrant groups in the nation's major cities were highly likely to endorse birth control, while periodicals from more theologically conservative denominations that did not endorse the Social Gospel (such as the Southern Baptist Convention or Missouri Synod Lutherans, for instance) did not.[14]

The periodicals that endorsed birth control argued that middle-class Protestants were already choosing to limit their family size; to reduce poverty, malnutrition, and the problems of child labor, the poor also needed to be introduced to the blessings of contraception. This was the argument of Harry Emerson Fosdick, a New York Baptist pastor who may have been the nation's most prominent liberal Protestant minister of the 1920s. "There is no hope for the solution of the population problem except in the scientific control of the birth rate," he said in a sermon at Park Avenue Baptist Church in Manhattan. "Starvation, unemployment and physical and moral decay" would result if the population growth rate was not kept in check.[15]

For the first time, Protestant ministers began to speak of "unwanted children" as a serious social problem and to view the prevention of their birth as the answer to the crisis. "Economic conditions [can] force upon unwanted children a premature life of labor, malnutrition, congested and unhealthy living conditions, and a pair of overburdened parents," the Episcopal church rector Richard Flagg Ayres wrote in *Living Church* magazine in 1930. "Chaining a man to a treadmill for the sake of unwanted children is a peculiar application of Christian principles!"[16]

As recently as 1908, the Anglican Church had condemned the use of contraceptives, but by the 1920s and 1930s, birth control was receiving support from a younger generation of Protestants. (Ayres, for instance, was only twenty-seven when he published his pro-birth-control article in *Living Church*). For young ministers who came of age in the era of the Federal Council of Churches' Social Gospel campaigns and were educated at colleges and seminaries that identified the kingdom of God with the alleviation of poverty, child labor, and other social ills, it was easy for them to be persuaded by Margaret Sanger's argument that birth control could reduce poverty and ill health, and if that was the case, it must be part of the mission of the kingdom of God. The old proscriptions against birth control had to be wrong.

Convinced that they had a positive duty to promote birth control, liberal Protestants moved quickly to change their stance on the issue. Between 1929 and 1934, eight Protestant denominations—starting with Quakers and Universalists but quickly expanding to include Unitarians, Methodists, Congregationalists, northern Presbyterians, and Episcopalians—passed liberalized resolutions on birth control.[17] Sanger, recognizing that Protestant clergy could be useful allies—especially in her effort to brand Catholic opposition to birth control as a sectarian viewpoint that did not represent all religion—wrote to Protestant ministers to recruit them for her cause. In the early 1940s, Planned Parenthood established a National Clergymen's Advisory Council; by 1946, it had 3,200 clergy supporters.[18] In the 1920s and 1930s, liberal Protestants who endorsed the birth control campaign saw this as a logical extension of the Social Gospel's emphasis on poverty relief and societal improvement, but by the 1940s and 1950s, their view of the issue may have been more individualistic. They began to describe birth control more routinely in terms of "responsible parenthood" for their middle-class parishioners—that is, as a moral decision that each couple needed to make for themselves (and which they had a duty to make "responsibly").[19]

This method of speaking about moral decision-making reflected a new liberal Protestant embrace of existentialist thinking in the early postwar era. Whereas Catholics cited natural law principles and the authority of the magisterium as a universal objective standard for moral reasoning and conservative evangelical Protestants emphasized biblical precepts, liberal Protestants eschewed such inflexible standards and instead argued that each person had a duty to arrive at their own moral conclusions based on a personal encounter with the "other," that is, through the "I–Thou" relationship, as the Jewish philosopher Martin Buber phrased it. Morality could not be dictated from above; it was discovered from within, through a thoughtful, reasoned reflection on principles of love. In the 1960s, the Episcopal theologian Joseph Fletcher took this mode of reasoning to its ultimate conclusion in his widely distributed ethics text *Situation Ethics*, which argued that there was only one absolute moral principle: the principle to love one's neighbor. Even the prohibition against murder, he argued, could legitimately be broken for the sake of love for one's neighbor.[20]

This new method of moral reasoning perhaps played a role in mainline Protestants' attraction to the utilitarian calculus that shaped the movement for abortion law liberalization in the mid-twentieth century. Protestant ministers did not start the movement for abortion law reform, but they were early converts to it, and they quickly began echoing its utilitarian arguments.

THE ARGUMENTS FOR ABORTION LAW LIBERALIZATION

The physicians who first argued for abortion law reform in the 1930s did so on the grounds that the current restrictive abortion laws were not working and were inhumane. They had not deterred women from seeking illegal abortions; even the most conservative estimates suggested that at least 200,000 women obtained illegal abortions every year in the United States. And perhaps 5,000 or more of these women died each year from abortion-related complications. Women's lives could be saved, the advocates of abortion law reform claimed, if abortion laws were liberalized. This remained the movement's primary argument in the 1950s and 1960s, even though by then the number of women who died from illegal abortions each year had fallen to only a few hundred, primarily because of the discovery of antibiotics, which greatly reduced the risk of dying from infections.[21]

The argument that restrictive abortion laws were inhumane also broadened to include the inhumanity of denying an abortion to a woman who had been raped or the inhumanity of forcing a woman to continue a pregnancy when the fetus she was carrying was deformed. In 1959, the American Law Institute proposed a model abortion law that allowed for abortions that occurred in cases when a woman's life or health was in danger or in cases of rape, incest, or suspected fetal deformity, but some liberal Protestant ministers and ethicists were already defending the morality of abortion on these grounds even before the legal profession spoke out. When a woman was raped by an insane person, "the most loving thing possible (the right thing)," Joseph Fletcher wrote in 1954, was for the woman to abort her pregnancy. Thus, when the American Law Institute proposed liberalizing abortion laws, the proposal accorded so closely with liberal Protestant ethical thinking at the time that the *Christian Century* endorsed it almost immediately on the grounds that it was the "humane" approach. "When a law offends the dignity of innocent human beings, destroys physical and psychic health and menaces life itself, that law is not civilized and humane but barbaric and cruel," the magazine's editors said in January 1961, when surveying existing antiabortion laws. At the very least, the *Christian Century* declared, abortion should be legal in cases of rape and incest, because "by what code of morality can we justify laws which compel such women to bear unwanted children forced upon them in criminal acts?" This continued to be the magazine's stance throughout the 1960s; the "humane" approach was to liberalize abortion laws in order to save women from the dangers of illegal abortions performed by "bungling quacks and filthy midwives" or the pain of carrying a rapist's baby to term. Abortion laws that did not allow for pregnancy termination in the cases outlined by the American Law Institute were "inhumane," the *Christian Century* stated in 1967.[22]

Yet although the *Christian Century* supported liberalizing state abortion laws, it was still opposed to removing all restrictions on abortion, which, the magazine said, "leaves to the unborn no rights at all." "New York's 84-year-old abortion laws [which allowed for abortion only in cases when pregnancy endangered a woman's life] need reforming, as do those of other states," the *Christian Century* said. But a repeal of all abortion prohibitions because of the claim that women had an absolute right to abortion might go too far, the liberal Protestant magazine suggested. "Few doctors and few responsible people outside the medical profession would argue that all restraints should be lifted or that pregnancies should be interrupted because of some married mother's whim or some unmarried mother's shame or fear," the *Christian Century* said in 1961. Protestant advocates of abortion law liberalization in the 1960s almost invariably envisioned a situation in which abortion access would be carefully controlled by the medical profession, with guidance from appropriate moral authorities. "The limits of legalized abortion should be drawn by the mutual agreement of the law, medicine and the church," the *Christian Century* stated.[23] Unlike contraception—which, by the 1960s, liberal Protestants endorsed as an unalloyed good that should be promoted internationally as part of government humanitarian aid—abortion raised troubling moral questions. In 1961, the National Council of Churches of Christ in the USA (an ecumenical organization that included most mainline Protestant denominations as members) adopted a resolution declaring that "Protestant Christians are agreed in condemning abortion or any method which destroys human life except when the health or life of the mother is at stake. The destruction of life already begun cannot be condoned as a method of family limitation."[24] Abortion, in other words, was acceptable only in very narrow cases of medical necessity, because the fetus was "human life."

Yet in spite of their strong moral reservations, the idea that the church, the law, and medical professionals could find a middle way in the tension between the historic Christian belief that the fetus had value as a creation of God and the twentieth-century belief that restrictive abortion laws harmed women pervaded liberal Protestant discussion of abortion. As early as the 1950s, when discussions of reforming abortion laws were just beginning—and when, as yet, no Protestant denomination had endorsed abortion law reform—a few Protestant ministers were appealing to the idea that when it came to "therapeutic abortions," Christians had to follow their consciences and avoid moral dogmatism. When one social science researcher asked the ministers of the leading mainline Protestant churches in Charlottesville, Virginia, to comment on the morality of therapeutic abortion in 1952, he encountered several who were already emphasizing the freedom of individuals to determine their own view of the matter after appropriate moral reasoning and consultation with medical and religious professionals. "The Presbyterian Church would certainly not take the absolutist position of the Roman Catholic Church with regard to therapeutic abortions," said the pastor of Charlottesville's Westminster Presbyterian Church in 1952. "The Presbyterian Church officially, having taken no stand on this subject, leaves its ministers and members a freedom to follow enlightened conscience with regard to the matter. Generally speaking, I would say that there would be very few of our ministers, officers or members who would take a stand against therapeutic abortion as such." The social science researcher received a similar statement from one of Charlottesville's Episcopal ministers: "The question of 'therapeutic' abortion is probably best decided among Episcopalians on the basis of the moral judgment of the individual, her family, the parish priest, and her physician."[25]

RIGHTS CONSCIOUSNESS AND SEXUAL LIBERALIZATION OF THE 1960S

As late as the mid-1960s, no Protestant denomination was willing to endorse the legalization of elective abortion, but by 1970, this was the official position of most mainline Protestant churches. Yet this sweeping change on abortion policy was only the tip of the iceberg when it came to theological and ethical changes in mainline Protestantism. During the same period, liberal Protestants mobilized against the Vietnam War and in favor of civil rights, with a few ministers going to jail for their protests. They became more vocal in their support of sex education. Some ministers began publicly supporting gay rights. A few denominations, such as the United Presbyterian Church, now the Presbyterian Church (USA), adopted new confessions or standards of faith that began emphasizing compassion and individual moral discernment rather than unchanging doctrines and moral precepts.

For decades, mainline Protestants had believed that Christianity as an institution was a necessary framework for American democracy, but when a younger generation of ministers and seminarians saw white churches oppose the civil rights movement and the nation's government authorize the bombing of Vietnamese villages in the name of democracy and a generic anticommunist civil religion, they lost confidence in either the government or the church to issue moral dictates. "Younger ministers," University of Chicago Divinity School professor Langdon Gilkey wrote in 1965, "are by no means sure of anything they learned in seminary—except perhaps on the subject of race relations."[26] That was certainly true for ministers-in-training at Gilkey's institution; a survey taken in 1966 showed that 95 percent of University of Chicago divinity students favored interracial marriage (which was still illegal in many states), but not a single respondent was willing to say that sex belonged only within a lifelong, monogamous marriage.[27] "Traditional Christian sexual norms . . . do not stand above history," the young Harvard Divinity School professor Harvey Cox wrote in 1965. "Like all human codes they stand in continuous need of revision so they will help rather than hinder God's maturation of man." The modern pluralistic secular environment showed that "all things are relative," Cox said.[28] In such an environment, it was not the place of either the church or the federal government to tell women whether they could have an abortion, because both institutions had lost their moral authority. What was clear, they thought, was that antiabortion statutes and rigid moral codes hurt women. And if that was the case, the only compassionate stance was to fight against restrictive abortion laws and help women violate them, just as some of those who opposed racial injustice protested against segregation statutes.

This was the philosophy behind the Clergy Consultation Service on Abortion, which the liberal Baptist minister Howard Moody—along with nineteen other Protestant ministers and one Jewish rabbi—founded in 1967 in order to counsel women facing crisis pregnancies and direct them to illegal abortion providers if they wished. Moody, like several other ministers involved in abortion counseling, was a strong supporter of the civil rights movement and an opponent of the Vietnam War, and his moral compass had been shaped by those movements. The task of a minister, he believed, was to advocate for the rights of the powerless and confront social injustice. Restrictive abortion laws were unjust, he thought, because they were inhumane for women, regardless of what one thought about the fetus. They disproportionately disadvantaged the poor and racial minorities, who were most likely to resort to dangerous methods of abortion when hospital abortions were illegal. "Belief in the sanctity of human life certainly demands helpfulness and sympathy to women in trouble and concern for living children," said the Clergy Consultation Service in its charter statement. "When a doctor performs such an operation [abortion] motivated by compassion and concern for the patient, and not simply for monetary gain, we do not regard him as a criminal, but as living by the highest standards of religion and of the Hippocratic oath." By 1969, at least 1,400 ministers were part of the Clergy Consultation Service on Abortion, and the organization was helping 10,000 women per year obtain abortions.[29]

Moody and his allies became alert to the abortion issue primarily because of changing sexual norms among the middle-class women who attended their congregations. In the 1960s, a majority of Americans still disapproved of premarital sex, according to public opinion polls, and pregnancy outside of wedlock was still considered shameful for the middle class. Yet half of brides in the 1950s were no longer virgins by their wedding night, and even more were opting for premarital sex by the late 1960s. In many places, birth control was still difficult for many unmarried women to access, both because of laws restricting the distribution of contraception to unmarried people and because of cultural taboos that discouraged doctors from prescribing birth control pills to women who were not married. Some middle-class white women who found themselves pregnant out of wedlock married the father of their child before giving birth, and others who remained single put their newborn children up for adoption with the hope that no one would find out their secret. But by the mid-1960s, a number of middle-class white women in college or graduate school were ready to reject all of these options. They saw nothing problematic with premarital sex, but they did not want to be pregnant before marriage. Rather than deal with an unwanted pregnancy by jumping into an undesired marriage or putting an unwanted child up for adoption, they instead sought out abortion services. To ministers such as Moody, this seemed reasonable, because they understood these women's frustration with a double standard that seemed to punish only women for the supposed sin of premarital sex. Though usually not directly rejecting the long-standing American Christian stricture against out-of-wedlock sex, the ministers in the Clergy Consultation Service were nevertheless ready to call out the hypocrisy in the uneven enforcement of this moral norm. They had compassion for the women who came to their pastoral office for help, and they thought the best answer to their dilemma was to empower them to access the medical services they needed to safely terminate their pregnancies if that was their choice.[30]

The ministers in the Clergy Consultation Service were more radical than many, since to join the group they not only had to be willing to support abortion access but also be willing to break the law, a practice that many of them were already familiar with because of their involvement with civil rights activism in the segregated South earlier in the decade. But their own denominations often proved receptive to their efforts to endorse much more liberal changes in abortion policy than most mainline Protestant clergy had envisioned only a few years earlier. In 1967, the American Baptist Convention (which changed its name to the American Baptist Churches USA in 1972) adopted a resolution urging the "churches of the American Baptist Convention" to "support legislation in their states to make abortion legal in cases of rape, incest, mental incompetence, or where there is danger to the health of the mother." Their stated rationale for this endorsement of therapeutic abortion laws was the same one that motivated both the *Christian Century* and the Clergy Consultation Service: the argument that the "widespread practice of illegal abortion" had produced "physical dangers and mental anguish" for too many women. Other mainline Protestant denominations passed similar resolutions, with some by the early 1970s calling for the legalization of all abortion, not merely the liberalization of abortion laws in cases of medical or therapeutic necessity. By the end of 1972, nearly every mainline Protestant denomination—including Baptist, Episcopal, Lutheran, Methodist, Presbyterian, and United Church of Christ—had officially endorsed the cause of abortion law reform, either by declaring the permissibility of abortion in cases of medical or therapeutic necessity or by calling for the repeal of all antiabortion laws.[31] These resolutions did not declare that abortion was necessarily right or that the decision to terminate a pregnancy should be taken lightly. Nevertheless, they suggested either that moral decision-making was the right of the individual Christian and that pregnant women had the responsibility to make this decision in light of their own consciences or that restrictive abortion laws harmed women and should be repealed on humanitarian grounds.

Liberal Protestants borrowed some of these arguments from secular and Jewish advocates of abortion rights, but their Christian theology of the "sanctity of life"—a phrase that liberal Protestant advocates of abortion law liberalization repeatedly invoked, along with the slight variation "sacredness of life"—prompted them to give greater weight to the value of the fetus as, at the very least, a potential life. Secular and Jewish advocates of abortion legalization often declared without qualification that they viewed embryos or first-trimester fetuses merely as a "mass of undifferentiated cells," and that they were not people because they lacked human association. They "had no consciousness, no life experience, no previous association with fellow humans," Alan F. Guttmacher, a doctor who had served as president of Planned Parenthood Federation of America, said in 1968. Such a view reflected to a certain extent the Jewish rabbinic tradition, which viewed the pregnant woman's life as more important than the fetus, but to an even greater extent, it reflected a modern humanist view that saw human personhood as intrinsically connected to rationality and the socialization process. Because, in the modern secular calculus, humans had no relationship to a transcendent God that could give value to human life, their value came from their relationships to each other; humans were valuable because other humans valued them. Guttmacher wrote, "To me, an early conception is not a human being created in God's image; it is a potential human being in man's image."[32]

But although some of the most liberal Protestants were attracted to some of these ideas, their theological belief that every human being was created in the image of God and that human life was "sacred"—combined with the Christian tradition's historic concerns about abortion—kept most of them from going as far as Guttmacher. Few of them were willing to say that abortion was a morally neutral operation. Instead, they said that abortion was a morally complex issue that every woman had a right to decide for herself; neither the church nor the state should make the decision for her. But although this view appealed to the majority of liberal Protestants (since it accorded well with liberal Protestant principles about moral decision-making), a significant minority of liberal Protestants insisted that it did not give enough weight to the possibility that the fetus really was a human life, and that if it was, it deserved legal protection.

OPPOSITION TO ABORTION AMONG A MINORITY OF LIBERAL PROTESTANTS

Even as many liberal Protestant clergy rushed to embrace the cause of abortion law reform in the name of compassion, a few argued that the principle of humanity required them to oppose abortion. Throughout the late 1960s and early 1970s, the *Christian Century* continued to receive letters from readers who believed that abortion was the taking of human life. Those readers were not necessarily theological or political conservatives; one, for instance, identified herself as a minister in the United Church of Christ, a liberal denomination that was an early leader in the call for abortion legalization.[33] Opponents of abortion argued that if the fetus was a human life, Christians had a duty to discourage murder and uphold the rights of the fetus, no matter how morally or socially progressive they might be. This was the stance of Paul Ramsey, a Methodist ethicist teaching at Princeton University. It was the view of Charles Carroll, a California Episcopal priest who had participated in civil rights marches with Martin Luther King Jr. and Cesar Chavez and who saw his opposition to abortion as a natural extension of those other campaigns. It was also the position of Karl Barth, the aging Swiss theologian who was revered as one of the most famous Protestant theologians in the world, especially by many American Presbyterians.[34]

Rather than seek to dismiss these views or minimize the moral tension involved in the abortion decision, liberal Protestants who favored the liberalization of abortion laws often highlighted the moral dilemma involved. Abortion was a "serious moral issue," *Christian Century* contributing editor and Methodist minister J. Claude Evans wrote in 1973. "Any decision for abortion is a sad decision, a choice between competing values of great complexity where no choice is perfect."[35] Abortion was "the agonizing decision," David R. Mace, another ordained Methodist minister (and college professor), stated in a book of that title in 1972.[36] Abortion decisions were painful, many liberal Protestant clergy conceded, not merely because abortion destroyed a *potential* human life but because it probably destroyed an *actual* life. "The dilemma before us is this," the University of California, Davis campus ministers John Moore and John Pamperin wrote in 1970: "How can we sanction the taking of life within a context that is life-affirming?"[37] Yet in the end, Moore and Pamperin did sanction the taking of unborn human life. So did several other writers in the same issue of *Christian Century*, including one of the ministers participating in the Clergy Consultation Service on Abortion who insisted that all of his actions were guided by the "ethic of the sacredness of life."[38]

Pro-choice liberal Protestant ministers believed they could maintain the tension between their adherence to the "sacredness of life" and their conclusion that abortions that terminated human life must sometimes be performed because of the distinction between human life and human personhood. Life, they admitted, might be present from the moment of conception, but that did not mean that personhood was. For mid-twentieth-century Protestants who believed in "personalism"—a theology that gave central emphasis to the personhood of God and the personhood of the individual human—this distinction was especially important. In the 1940s, the strong emphasis on personalism in Boston University's School of Theology had provided the theological framework for one of its PhD students, Martin Luther King Jr., to encourage the individual's resistance to the state in defense of human dignity. A quarter century later, the dean of BU's School of Theology employed the theological idea of personhood to find what he believed was a middle course between those who insisted that the fetus had no value and those who wanted to save the fetus at all costs, even if that cost included the mother's well-being. A person who identified life with personhood could not afford to be "callous to either the pregnant woman's *zoe* [a Greek word that the author used to mean a fuller life than mere biological existence] or to the well-being of society."[39] Fetal life had value, he argued, but not necessarily the full value of personhood. To treat fetal life as equivalent to the life of a woman was to diminish the personhood of the woman, and that was fundamentally wrong. A woman's well-being might not be strictly part of her physical biological life, but it was part of her personhood or fullness of life, and it was therefore unethical to use the arm of the law (or perhaps even the moral authority of the pulpit) to force a woman to sacrifice the qualities that were intrinsic to her fullness of life and dignity for the sake of a fetus. But neither was it right for a woman to terminate her pregnancy casually or thoughtlessly.

None of the liberal Protestant denominational resolutions in favor of legalizing abortion in the late 1960s or early 1970s directly stated that the fetus was not a person, and several directly highlighted the value of fetal life. The closest that any denomination came to declaring that human personhood did not begin at conception may have been when the United Methodist Church's Board of Christian Social Concerns adopted a resolution in 1969: "Since personhood is more than physical being, we affirm that the fetus is not a person, but rather tissue with potentiality in most cases for becoming a person."[40] But this was the statement of a denominational agency—not a general assembly with authority to speak for the entire denomination—and its use of the phrase "tissue" to describe the fetus received immediate pushback from at least one of the denomination's prominent theologians. The Methodist board had attempted to ground this declaration on fetal nonpersonhood in the Christian ethic of love: "Personhood develops as one is loved, responds to love, and in that relationship comes to fulness as a child of God." But Princeton University Christian ethics professor Paul Ramsey was aghast. Ramsey was a Methodist who said that he might not necessarily object to the liberalization of abortion laws, but to call the fetus merely "tissue" was outside the pale of what either Christian theology or medical science would allow, he thought. "This must be the first time in the history of religion (certainly, of Christianity) that some of its leading spokesmen have endorsed the 'tissue' interpretation of unborn human life," he wrote.[41] The word "tissue" did not appear in the resolution on abortion that the General Conference of the United Methodist Church (UMC) adopted in 1972. Nor did any suggestion that the fetus was not a valuable life. Instead, in contrast to the stance that one of its denominational agencies had taken in 1969, the UMC proclaimed the grave moral considerations involved in any termination of fetal life, even as it declared that abortion might be a necessity in some cases. "We reject the simplistic answers to the problem of abortion, which on the one hand regard all abortions as murders, or on the other hand, regard abortions as medical procedures without moral significance," the UMC stated in its declaration on "Responsible Parenthood." "We believe that a profound regard for unborn human life must be weighed alongside an equally profound regard for fully formed personhood, particularly when the physical, mental and emotional health of the pregnant woman and her family show reason to be seriously threatened by the new life just forming." the resolution said. "To support the sacred dimensions of personhood, all possible efforts should be made to insure that the infant enters the world with a healthy body, and is born into an environment conducive to realization of his/her full potential."[42] But when that was not possible, abortion might be a legitimate choice, the UMC suggested. This was a pro-choice resolution, but it was a far cry from saying that the fetus was merely "tissue." In contrast to some secular pro-choice activists who at times used terms such as "tissue" or "cellular mass" to describe the embryo or fetus, most of the Protestant denominational resolutions on abortion from the late 1960s and early 1970s declared their respect for unborn fetal life. "Since the fetus is the organic beginning of human life, the termination of its development is always a serious matter," the Lutheran Church in America (now part of the Evangelical Lutheran Church in America) said in 1970. "Nevertheless, a qualitative distinction must be made between its claims and the rights of a responsible person made in God's image who is in living relationships with God and other human beings."[43] God has "shown his concern for the quality and value of human life," the United Presbyterian Church said in 1972, but restrictive abortion laws "do not insure the right of all children to be born as wanted children" and were therefore out of harmony with God's concern for the "quality . . . of human life."[44]

In an attempt to balance their concern about fetal life with their desire to reduce the harm of restrictive abortion laws and protect the liberty of conscience for women and their doctors, many liberal Protestant ministers in the mid-to-late 1960s supported therapeutic abortion laws (that is, laws that allowed for abortion only in specific cases, such as rape, incest, suspected fetal deformity, or dangers to a woman's health) as a middle path between "abortion on demand" and abortion prohibitions. Such laws, after all, recognized that abortion was a morally serious matter that was legitimate only when the good it accomplished outweighed the harm, an argument that closely accorded with the prevailing liberal Protestant view on the issue. The Episcopal Church, like the American Baptist Convention, adopted a resolution in 1967 that advocated the legalization of abortion in a few narrowly defined circumstances: "Where it has been clearly established that the physical health of the mother is threatened seriously, or where there is substantial reason to believe that the child would be born badly deformed in mind or body, or where pregnancy has resulted from forcible rape or incest."[45]

But liberal Protestants soon abandoned their support for this middle pathway at about the same time that the general public did—that is, at the beginning of the 1970s, less than five years after the first therapeutic abortion laws were enacted. These laws did not accomplish their promoters' goal of reducing the number of illegal abortions, because the number of abortions permitted by these laws was low, and the process that women had to go through to prove that they needed an abortion (especially in cases of rape) was humiliating, at least in some states. And, as a resolution of the Episcopal Church Women pointed out in October 1970, therapeutic abortion laws also discriminated against the poor, who had less ability than wealthier women to jump through the bureaucratic hoops needed to secure a hospital board's permission for an abortion.[46]

Without necessarily changing their theology of abortion, liberal Protestant ministers pivoted to advocating for the repeal of nearly all prohibitions on the procedure, at least during the first or second trimesters, not because they thought that all abortions were morally justified but because they believed that women alone should make that choice. To say otherwise was to violate their personhood. When the *Christian Century* informally surveyed its female staff members in early 1970, fewer than half said that they would ever be willing to have an abortion themselves, but they were unanimous in saying that the procedure should be legal.[47] For liberal Protestants in the early 1970s, there was a clear distinction between the morality of abortion and its legality. As a moral issue, abortion was ambiguous, but as a matter of law, the issue was clear: neither the church nor the government could make women's moral decisions for them, which meant that they had to have the legal freedom to determine this matter in their own consciences, after consulting with their doctors and perhaps their religious advisors.

"I've always said what personal issue is more important and significant than the issue of bringing a life into the world?" said Michael D. Smith, the Presbyterian campus minister at the University of Arizona in the early 1970s, who was also a member of the Clergy Consultation Service on Abortion. "And that, of all places, is where a woman has the right to decide for herself. . . . It's a religious issue because women are created in the image of God . . . with among other things, moral agency. That means they have the power to make moral decisions. That is how God creates each one of us . . . We have the capacity, as well as the right, to make moral decisions. . . . In the case of the woman who is pregnant, nothing is more personal than that. It affects her more than anyone else, so that issue of God creating us with moral agency comes down to a bottom line in relation to women having the right to decide for themselves."[48]

Behind all of this was a suspicion of moral dogma and authority. In the 1950s, mainline Protestants had championed the idea of personal moral reasoning (and had criticized both Catholics and fundamentalists for their reliance on moral dogma), but with the assumption that those who engaged in the rational task of moral reflection would reach the correct conclusions. Their views about sex and other controversial matters were still generally conservative, and they believed that rational inquiry would support these conclusions. By the late 1960s, they were even more suspicious of ardent champions of personal moral reasoning than they had been in the 1950s, but they no longer assumed that moral reflection would arrive at a universal set of norms. The civil rights movement and the Vietnam War shook their faith in the moral establishment. They were sure that the civil rights movement was right and that the U.S. military effort in Vietnam (with its use of napalm against civilians) was wrong. These were bedrock convictions for a young generation of liberal ministers. And if the white church establishment was wrong about those matters, perhaps it was also wrong about matters of sex. Perhaps, in the end, one could never be morally certain about the matters about which the church was once so certain. In a 1973 editorial opposing legal restrictions on pornography, the *Christian Century* remarked that it was impossible to know whether pornography was really immoral — but what it said about pornography could just as easily have applied to its view of premarital sex, homosexuality, or abortion. "The assumption that we already know what is 'good' and what is 'bad' in such areas stands in direct contrast to the liberal notion that openness to the future is essential, for God's word to the world continues to approach us from the future," said the *Christian Century*. "Since everything of human construction — form or idea — is continually in need of re-formation, we must constantly guard against the heresy of worshiping our own creation."[49] For Protestants who were now more open than ever to moral change and resistant to fixed moral dogma, the idea that it was now up to each individual pregnant woman — not the state or the church — to determine whether abortion was right or wrong made perfect sense.

Perhaps it was no surprise, then, that the most vocal critics of the U.S. government's actions in Vietnam were sometimes equally ardent critics of the state's efforts to impose its own moral understanding of abortion to constrain women's choices. In 1971, the United Church of Christ (UCC) passed resolutions opposing the Vietnam War, supporting the Berrigan brothers' acts of civil disobedience to protest the war, and calling for "the right of women to choose abortion unfettered by the state."[50] The UCC was hardly alone in this matter; most of the nation's mainline Protestant denominations—including Baptist, Lutheran, Methodist, and Presbyterian—passed resolutions in support of legal abortion sometime between 1968 and 1971. Several of these resolutions specifically highlighted freedom of conscience as the primary justification for supporting abortion legalization. But at the same time, many of them also highlighted the need to safeguard the "sanctity of life" as a reason to be concerned about fetal life.

The American Baptist Convention's abortion resolution of June 1968 was typical in attempting to preserve this delicate balancing act. The previous year, the denomination had endorsed modest abortion law reform efforts to allow for abortion for specific medical reasons, but by 1968, the denomination was ready to go beyond this, since there was a growing perception among some ministers in the denomination—especially those, such as Howard Moody, who were involved in the Clergy Consultation Service—that these laws did not go far enough to help the large numbers of women who wanted to terminate their pregnancies and were willing to go to almost any length to do it. The American Baptist Convention therefore endorsed a trimester division for abortion law reform. During the first twelve weeks of pregnancy, abortion should be legally available for any reason, but after the twelfth week, it should be available only for the therapeutic reasons listed in the American Law Institute's abortion law reform proposal. "Because Christ calls us to affirm the freedom of persons and the sanctity of life, we recognize that abortion should be a matter of responsible personal decision," the American Baptists said.[51] These potentially conflicting twin concerns of "freedom" and "sanctity of life" would be resolved in typical liberal Protestant (and especially liberal Baptist) fashion in the form of "responsible" personal decision-making, the resolution suggested. The pregnant woman would have the freedom to make her own moral decision in this area, but she should do so in a morally "responsible" manner. And, once her pregnancy reached the second trimester, she could no longer make this decision alone, but only in consultation with her physician for approved medical reasons. This framework closely presaged the approach that the Supreme Court would adopt four and a half years later in *Roe v. Wade*.

The United Methodist Church's official statement on abortion in 1972 went further than the American Baptist Convention's resolution in calling for the "removal of abortion from the criminal code," which, in practice, would mean decriminalizing or legalizing all abortions, even those performed in the second trimester and beyond. But at the same time, the statement was even more direct in expressing grave moral reservations about abortion. "Our belief in the sanctity of unborn human life makes us reluctant to approve abortion," the UMC declared in its opening line on the subject. "But we are equally bound to respect the sacredness of the life and wellbeing of the mother, for whom devastating damage may result from an unacceptable pregnancy. In continuity with past Christian teaching, we recognize tragic conflicts of life with life that may justify abortion." After endorsing the legalization of abortion, the UMC then concluded with an exhortation that abortion not be considered a casual or morally unproblematic decision: "A decision concerning abortion should be made only after thorough and thoughtful consideration by the parties involved, with medical and pastoral counsel."[52]

Despite this new emphasis on women's moral decision-making responsibility in the abortion question, most of the mainline Protestants who spoke out on behalf of women's right to control their own reproductive cycle were men. Abortion, in the minds of the earliest advocates of abortion law liberalization, was a legal, medical, and moral issue, and men had a near monopoly on the leadership in each of those spheres. In 1970, 92 percent of medical doctors in the United States were men, as were approximately 95 percent of lawyers. The ministerial profession was even more heavily male dominated. Although both the United Methodist Church and the United Presbyterian Church had been ordaining women since the 1950s, only 1 percent of Presbyterian ministers in the United States were women in 1973.[53] And some mainline denominations, such as the Episcopal Church, had not yet allowed any women to serve as pastors. Thus, in the 1960s, the nation's main organizations that advocated abortion law liberalization—such as the Association for the Study of Abortion and the Abortion Law Reform Association—were led mostly by male professionals: doctors, lawyers, and the occasional Protestant clergyman, such as the Episcopal priest Lester Kinsolving. But this began to change at the end of the 1960s. The National Organization for Women endorsed abortion rights in 1967. Two years later, in 1969, the second-wave feminist icon Betty Friedan wrote an article entitled "Abortion: A Woman's Right," and became one of the cofounders of NARAL, which at the time stood for the National Association for the Repeal of Abortion Laws.[54] In response, women in the pro-life movement began taking on greater leadership roles and founding their own organizations, such as Women Concerned for the Unborn Child, which the Pittsburgh Catholic pro-life activist Mary Winter organized in the spring of 1970.[55] The male ministers whose voices had dominated the conversation about abortion in liberal Protestant circles were caught off guard.

In the summer of 1970, after the *Christian Century* published several articles on abortion, some readers wondered why the magazine had not asked a woman to write any of the pieces. This omission was "passive rather than active discrimination," the magazine's editor responded. "To our knowledge, we have never received an article from a woman on the subject of abortion. However, the door remains open."[56]

Women began rushing through the door more quickly than the editors may have expected. The feminist movement was making rapid political and cultural headway in 1970, and it was quickly recasting the abortion issue as a women's rights issue. After all, 1970 was the year in which the Boston Women's Health Collective published *Our Bodies, Ourselves*, which marked a revolt against the male medical establishment and an encouragement for women to take personal control of their own health care, including abortion. It was the year that Bella Abzug, a strong advocate of women's rights and abortion law repeal, was elected to the U.S. House of Representatives from New York. It was the year that tens of thousands of women participated in the Women's Strike for Equality that Betty Friedan organized to demand three main goals: free childcare centers, equality in the workforce, and "free abortion on demand."[57]

Most liberal Protestant women did not go as far as their more radical secular feminist counterparts in adopting the revolutionary language of women's liberation or in arguing for "free abortion on demand," but they did begin using the language of women's moral decision-making power to argue that women needed to be given the choice to make their own personal moral decisions about pregnancy termination. "Our Christian concern for the human rights of all persons, whether as individuals or as groups, compels us to support the right of women to make the final decision about termination of an unwanted pregnancy in which a woman has strong reason for not bearing a child," the ecumenical organization Church Women United said in March 1970. "A woman does not make a decision for abortion easily or lightly and every encouragement and support should be offered to avoid this extreme solution. But this recourse must be open to her and she must be free to make the final decision with the help of her family, doctor, and spiritual advisor for she is the one who is required to go through the pregnancy and childbirth and will be expected by society to be primarily responsible for any child that is born."[58]

It was a subtle shift rather than a revolutionary one. The members of Church Women United were not arguing, as Friedan had in 1969, that the "right of woman to control her reproductive process must be established as a basic and valuable human civil right" because it was "essential to equality for women."[59] They were instead arguing that if the right to abortion was fundamentally the God-given right to be a moral decision-maker in the presence of one's Creator, that right did not belong only — or even primarily — to a woman's doctor, let alone to her church or her minister. Each pregnant woman should be accorded the respect as a human person to make that moral choice for herself. Given the moral ambiguities of abortion and the tragic circumstances surrounding the choice, it was imperative for Christians to offer the social help that would free women from the situations that led them to seek abortions, but it was equally imperative for Christians to recognize that if women did find themselves in those situations, their right to make the final moral determination about abortion for themselves should be honored. To do otherwise would be to deny women the right to be full human persons, since for liberal Protestants, the right to freely make moral choices was an essential characteristic—perhaps even the most important characteristic—of human personhood.[60] Other women's denominational organizations passed resolutions expressing the same principle. Instead of grounding the cause of abortion rights in the principle of women's equality (as Friedan had), they instead grounded it in the principle of freedom of conscience for both men and women. "The Church stands for the exercise of freedom of conscience by all and is required to fight for the right of everyone to exercise that conscience," Women of the Episcopal Church said in 1973. For that reason, women should have the freedom to "exercise their conscience in the matter of abortion."[61]

By grounding abortion rights in conscience rights for women, liberal Protestant women may have promoted gender equality in moral decision-making and advanced a strong argument for the repeal of restrictive abortion laws, but they did little to remove the moral stigma associated with abortion. Indeed, as Church Women United's abortion resolution suggested, many liberal Protestants who supported abortion legalization still believed that there were real ethical dilemmas associated with abortion. Only by arguing that the fetus was definitely not a person or that women had the absolute right to control their own bodies could liberal Protestants free the abortion decision from its moral ambiguities and suggest that abortion was a positive thing, as some pro-choice secular feminists argued. But only a few liberal Protestants were willing to make this argument. One who did was Rachel Conrad Wahlberg, a Texas Lutheran married to a United Lutheran Church minister. In 1972, she wrote in the *Christian Century* that "even though the fetus has the characteristics of a human being, it cannot be a separate human being until it is outside the mother's body."[62] Although Wahlberg was hardly the first liberal Protestant to reject the idea of fetal personhood (the United Methodist Church's Board of Christian Social Concerns had already done so in 1969, after all), she did break new ground in basing this declaration on the idea of bodily autonomy and women's rights. Any being that was still in utero and fully dependent on the mother's body for survival could not be a full human person, no matter how many other "characteristics of a human being" it had, Wahlberg suggested. And women should have an absolute right to abortion because they should have full freedom to control their own bodies. "There is a cannibalistic aspect here," Wahlberg declared in 1971, when writing about the relationship between the pregnant woman and the fetus she was carrying. "The fetus actually feeds on the mother's body. . . . Is it any wonder that a woman wants to have the right to decide whether to be used in this fashion? Helpless, the fetus feeds on the mother. Helplessly, she is fed on. Because of this interaction, she feels that the fetus *is* her own body." This was very closely parallel to the argument of secular feminists of the time who grounded the right to an abortion in the right of women's bodily autonomy, among other things. It seemed congruent with the secular philosopher Judith Jarvis Thomson's 1971 article, "A Defense of Abortion," which argued that even if the fetus was a human person, abortion could still be ethically justifiable, since no one had the right to live parasitically in another person's body without that person's consent.[63] This was an argument for bodily autonomy and women's liberation grounded in the moral principle of free choice, but despite its popularity in the secular sphere, only a few liberal Protestants were willing to make it. The appeal to freedom of conscience sounded far more Christian to many liberal Protestants than the insistence that women had the right to abortion because they deserved the freedom to control their own bodies or that the fetus was not a person because it was living in utero. Indeed, the fact that the fetus was fully dependent on its mother seemed to some liberal Christians like a reason to sympathize with it and protect it, since a core aspect of the Christian message was helping the weak and championing the rights of the marginalized, they believed.

Wahlberg's articles resulted in pushback from both women and men. Glenda Adams Hess, a New York biology teacher, responded to Wahlberg with a two-page article outlining the biological case for fetal personhood. She took issue not only with Wahlberg but also with Joseph Fletcher's view that personhood was identified only with "freedom," "self-determination," and "rationality," qualities that, she noted, newborn infants also lacked.[64] Hess's firm defense of fetal personhood was more common among

Catholics than among Protestants, but the *Christian Century*'s willingness to publish it indicated the editor's belief that it was within the range of views that the magazine's liberal Protestant constituency might share or be interested in reading. The claim that human personhood could not be defined by rationality or self-awareness sounded deeply egalitarian, and it resonated with a minority of liberal Protestants who became convinced that the campaign for abortion legalization was part of a larger culture of death and dehumanization that had led to the Vietnam War.

This argument was not quite strong enough to overcome most liberal Protestants' belief that antiabortion laws were inhumane and hurt women, but it did strike a chord, and it may have played a role in ensuring that liberal Protestants continued to treat abortion as far more morally ambiguous than contraceptives. But their history of sparring with Catholic bishops over legal access to contraception in New England from the 1940s through the early 1960s influenced their response to the Catholic Church's declarations on abortion and prompted many of those who were somewhat ambivalent about abortion's morality to take a firm stance in favor of legalizing it on the grounds of religious and personal freedom. Abortion legalization would "show respect for the pluralism of our society," the *Christian Century* said in January 1973, shortly before *Roe v. Wade* was decided on the 22nd. "Antiabortionist individuals and churches would be free to teach their faith views," the magazine said, but "without leaning on the state to do its dirty work of enforcement."[65]

Howard Moody also made this a central part of his argument for the repeal of antiabortion laws, which he said represented a sectarian religious view that had no place in the legal code of a pluralistic society. "No church or religious body has any right to expect the state to enforce its particular rules or moral tenets," he wrote in January 1973. Although Catholics opposed to abortion claimed that what they were asking the state to enforce was not Catholic dogma but instead a universal moral principle based on reason, Moody did not buy the argument. Most Americans who were not Catholic did not view abortion as murder in the way that the Catholic Church did. Therefore, he argued, this moral view was a sectarian religious view that had no place in public law. "To base laws on the theological and moral beliefs of any particular group is to create a dangerous paradigm for a pluralistic society," Moody wrote. Only laws that stemmed from a broadly shared consensus that transcended religious divisions would be enforceable and enduring in a religiously diverse society. In his view, abortion prohibitions did not meet that test.[66]

But how could a legal policy on abortion honor the values of personal conscience and religious pluralism while also recognizing the moral dilemmas involved and the fact that many people considered the fetus either an actual human being or at least a potential one? Methodist minister J. Claude Evans, who served on the *Christian Century*'s editorial board and was also a member of the Clergy Consultation Service on Abortion, suggested that abortion should be fully legal for the first eighteen weeks of pregnancy and illegal thereafter. This would give legal imprimatur to people's freedom of conscience to make their own decisions on abortion during the early stages of pregnancy, while honoring the value of fetal life in the later stages.

Evans's recommendations were printed in the January 31, 1973, issue of the *Christian Century* under the headline "Defusing the Abortion Debate," but by the time they reached subscribers' mailboxes, the abortion policy recommendations of another devout Methodist—Supreme Court Justice Harry Blackmun—had made Evans's proposal a moot point. The majority opinion that Blackmun authored in *Roe v. Wade* closely resembled Evans's suggestions in that it mandated the full legalization of abortion in the early weeks of pregnancy while also allowing for restrictions on abortion in the later stages. But perhaps its most important resemblance was its assumption that legalizing abortion (at least within limits) would honor religious pluralism and, in Evans's words, "defuse" the abortion debate. In essence, both Evans and Blackmun expected that Americans would accept the liberal Protestant view on the subject if it were enshrined in the law, since doing so would allow freedom of conscience on the issue while retaining some vestiges of the traditional Christian respect for fetal life.

ROE V. WADE

Justice Blackmun, a Nixon nominee and lifelong Republican, was also probably the most devout churchgoer on the bench. He was a Methodist and was in church every Sunday when he was in Washington, DC. He even preached on a few occasions, delivering sermons that invariably centered on a socially oriented theme with a strong endorsement of democracy.[67] He saw the preservation of democracy and constitutional liberty as a fundamental part of his Christian faith. When it came to abortion rights, his thinking closely accorded with the prevailing trends among liberal Protestants, and it was this thinking that he enshrined in *Roe v. Wade*.

The right to an abortion, Blackmun and other justices on the Court believed, had to be grounded not only in the right to privacy of the pregnant woman but also in a substantiation of the claim that the fetus had no constitutionally protected rights. Opponents of abortion argued that the fetus's life was constitutionally protected. To support that claim, Americans United for Life submitted an amicus curiae brief (written by University of Notre Dame law professor Charles Rice) that relied heavily on a combination of biological evidence and tort case law to prove that the embryo or fetus had a unique genetic composition from the moment of conception and that for decades courts had treated the fetus as a person in prenatal injury cases. In his majority opinion, Blackmun dismissed these arguments not with scientific evidence but with the argument that the evidence was irrelevant as long as philosophers, scientists, and theologians disagreed on the point at which human life began. Like other liberal Protestants of the time (such as Howard Moody), Blackmun appealed to a plurality of religious and philosophical opinions on the issue as justification for adopting a liberal opinion that would honor the views of the more permissive members of that plurality, an approach that was in keeping with the twentieth-century liberal Protestant value of pluralism. "We need not resolve the difficult question of when life begins," the Court said in *Roe*. "When those trained in the respective disciplines of medicine, philosophy, and theology are unable to arrive at any consensus, the judiciary, at this point in the development of man's knowledge, is not in a position to speculate as to the answer." Like other liberal Protestants, Blackmun decided that the presence of a range of views on the question meant that the question of abortion's morality—like faith or religion in general—would have to remain in the private sphere; it could not be a matter of government regulation. This was what liberal Protestants had been saying for several years leading up to *Roe*. Blackmun noted regarding Protestant opinion, "Organized groups [of Protestants] that have taken a formal position on the abortion issue have generally regarded abortion as a matter for the conscience of the individual and her family."[68] This is exactly what *Roe v. Wade* did for all Americans, extending the liberty of conscience on this issue to everyone, just as liberal Protestants wanted.

In keeping with prevailing opinion among liberal Protestants, Blackmun grounded the right to an abortion in the right to privacy, a right that the opinion characterized primarily as the right to an "abortion decision," not the right for a woman to have full control of her own body, as many abortion rights supporters wanted. The right to control one's own body was not absolute, *Roe v. Wade* said. Neither, for that matter, he conceded, was the right to an "abortion decision." In a close parallel with the United Methodist Church's declaration that "a decision concerning abortion should be made only after thorough and thoughtful consideration by the parties involved, with medical and pastoral counsel," Blackmun's opinion in *Roe v. Wade* spoke of multiple interests that needed to be considered along with the woman's decision. "The right of privacy, however based, is broad enough to cover the abortion decision," he wrote, but "the right, nonetheless, is not absolute, and is subject to some limitations; and that, at some point, the state interests as to protection of health, medical standards, and prenatal life, become dominant."[69] This was secular legal language of rights rather than moral obligations, but it was also closely reflective of the spirit of liberal Protestant ecclesiastical views at the time. Sarah Weddington, the lead plaintiff attorney in *Roe v. Wade*, had urged the Court to go further and give women an absolute right to an abortion (which is what abortion rights organizations of the time were demanding), but Blackmun explicitly rejected this approach and opted instead for a trimester framework that was more comfortable for liberal

Protestants. Women would have an absolute, unimpeded right to elective abortion in the first trimester, but in the second trimester, the government could regulate abortion on health grounds. After the fetus reached the point of viability (which was at approximately the end of the second trimester), the state could prohibit abortion altogether as long as it retained exceptions for abortions that were performed to protect the life or health of the pregnant woman.

Some liberal Protestants of the time noted the close parallels between this framework and the resolutions their own denominations had already passed in the years leading up to *Roe*. "The statement adopted by the Eighth General Synod [of the United Church of Christ] in June 1971 was virtually identical with the Supreme Court ruling," UCC members Mary Ellen Haines and Helen Webber observed in the spring of 1973.[70]

Blackmun presented *Roe*'s trimester framework as a matter of science and common sense, but it echoed both the *Christian Century*'s proposal of an eighteen-week cutoff for abortion legalization and the American Baptist Convention's abortion resolution of 1968 (which had endorsed the legalization of elective abortions in the first trimester but only abortion for medical or therapeutic reasons in the second trimester and beyond). A month before the Court issued its decision in *Roe*, Blackmun sent a memo to his colleagues on the bench suggesting that he favored limiting the legalization of abortion to the first trimester and allowing states to regulate abortion at the end of the twelfth week. William O. Douglas agreed. But Lewis Powell and Thurgood Marshall favored allowing unrestricted abortions up to the point of viability, arguing that if access to abortion was cut off at the end of the twelfth week that might not give some women enough time to make their abortion decision. Blackmun conceded that any cutoff point was a bit artificial. "I have concluded that the end of the first trimester is critical," he told his colleagues. "This is arbitrary, but perhaps any other selected point, such as quickening or viability, is equally arbitrary." But Blackmun insisted that he did not want to repeal all abortion restrictions altogether; there was a point during pregnancy where he believed that a state's interest in protecting fetal life justified legal intervention. He was willing to compromise on anything between the twelfth and twenty-eighth week of pregnancy, but he could not imagine mandating the repeal of abortion restrictions beyond the point of viability, "when independent life is presumably possible." In the end, he adopted a trimester framework that was no one's first choice but was instead was a compromise measure that he hoped would appeal to all justices and "avoid excessive fractionation of the Court."[71] There would be some (albeit very limited) regulation of abortion allowed in the second trimester, but most women who wanted an abortion in the second trimester would presumably still be able to get one, and the Court would still preserve the differentiation between the first and second trimesters, as Blackmun had originally wanted.

In presenting his opinion to the public, Blackmun characterized it as a moderate decision that did not remove all restrictions on abortion. "It should be stressed that the Court does not today hold that the Constitution compels abortion on demand," Blackmun declared. "It does not today pronounce that a pregnant woman has an absolute right to an abortion. It does, for the first trimester of pregnancy, cast the abortion decision and the responsibility for it upon the attending physician. Thereafter, the decisions [including *Doe v. Bolton*] permit the state, if it chooses, to impose reasonable regulations for the protection of maternal and fetal health. And, after viability, they give the state full right to proscribe all abortions except those that may be necessary, in appropriate medical judgment, for the preservation of the life or health of the mother."[72]

Because Blackmun—like other liberal Protestants of the time, including the editors of the *Christian Century*—believed that the legal solution to the abortion issue that liberal Protestants generally favored represented a broadly shared consensus that most people would accept as imminently reasonable, he was taken aback by the level of protest that *Roe v. Wade* engendered. He was immediately deluged with letters comparing the decision to *Dred Scott v. Sandford* (1857) and legalized abortion to the policies of Hitler and the Nazi government. "The mail has been voluminous and much of it critical and some of it abusive," he complained to a friend on January 31, 1973. "I suspect, however, that the furor will die down before too long. At least I hope so."[73]

But the furor did not die down. By enshrining the values of liberal Protestantism into constitutional law, Blackmun inadvertently set in motion a process that would polarize both national politics and Christianity in the United States.

Immediately after the ruling, the most fervent advocates of abortion law repeal, such as NARAL, threw their support behind a short-lived effort by Representative Bella Abzug (D-NY) to repeal all abortion restrictions in the nation.[74] But NARAL leaders quickly realized that repeal efforts would never pass at the national level, and they then—like nearly all pro-choice advocates—abandoned that attempt and rallied around the effort to protect *Roe v. Wade*.[75] It might have been a liberal Protestant decision that did not fully line up with the demands of pro-choice feminists who wanted full repeal of all abortion restrictions, but with a campaign to reverse *Roe* through a pro-life constitutional amendment already well under way by April 1973, NARAL leaders and their allies in Planned Parenthood forgot about whatever reservations they might have once had about *Roe* and began a campaign to protect the decision. "Could the Supreme Court 'Abortion' Decisions Be Lost? Yes!" a Planned Parenthood brochure issued in April 1973 stated in a bold headline designed to alarm potential allies and mobilize them for action.[76] From that point on, *Roe* became the symbol of abortion rights, even if its rationale was not quite what some abortion rights activists had wanted.[77]

As *Roe* quickly gained the support of even the most fervent advocates of abortion rights, it became an icon of feminism and secularism, even though it had been produced by an all-male, largely Protestant Court and authored by a devout Methodist who was also a pro-business Republican. And as *Roe* took on this added ideological symbolism, opposition to it increased, not only from Catholics but also from many Protestants who may not have been interested in the pro-life cause before. Blackmun soon discovered that the values of liberal Protestantism he drew on when writing the opinion were not nearly as widespread as he had assumed.

CHAPTER 2

CATHOLICS BEFORE *ROE*

A Theology of Unborn Life

"Monday January 22, 1973 was the darkest day in the history of the United States, our beloved Country," a Michigan woman named Grace Burns declared in a letter she sent to Justice Harry Blackmun a week after he delivered the majority opinion in *Roe v. Wade* on behalf of the Supreme Court. Didn't Blackmun know that the biological evidence clearly indicated that each person had a unique genetic composition from the moment of conception, and that therefore human life began at conception and was worthy of legal protection from that moment? She feared for the future if society accepted "abortion and other similar evils of lack of love of life." All of these "evils," she believed, were a product of a "contraceptive society." But she had chosen a different path for herself and was determined to stand against these societal horrors. She was a "God-fearing woman, a wife, a mother of twelve children," she said. "I love my Country."[1]

Burns's letter was one of thousands that Blackmun received from conservative Catholics in opposition to his opinion in *Roe*, and it was noteworthy not because it was unique but because it was typical. Burns, who was in her late forties at the time she wrote Blackmun, had come of age at a time when the Catholic Church preached strongly against both contraception and abortion, and she had evidently taken those values to heart. In many ways, her life was typical of other women of the World War II generation. She had married a Michigan State graduate and high school teacher who had served in the navy during the war, and together they had settled into small-town Michigan life that revolved around their parish and around the activities that many other middle-class members of their generation also enjoyed: gardening, road trips, and raising a large family. But for devout Catholics such as Grace Burns and her husband, being Catholic also came with a set of values and practices that shaped their understanding of what it meant to be an American.[2] Tellingly, Burns never identified herself as Catholic in her letter to Blackmun nor did she appeal directly to Catholic doctrine. Instead, she argued that her views of abortion were based on science and on her love for her country and love for human life. She was aghast to discover that the Supreme Court evidently did not share her views, which she thought were based on obvious truths.

The other letters that Blackmun received from Catholics opposed to abortion were similar. Occasionally, they left hints that clearly indicated that the writers were Catholic, either through a reference to an unusually large number of children (which, in the case of Burns, far exceeded the number of children that any middle-class white Protestant family of the early 1970s was likely to have), a negative reference to contraception (which most Protestants and other non-Catholics of the 1970s accepted as legitimate), or a reference to the "Fifth Commandment" against killing (which most Protestants, unlike Catholics, numbered as the sixth commandment). But otherwise, unless they were priests or nuns who signed their names using a title that clearly indicated their Catholic vocation, most Catholics who wrote Blackmun didn't say anything about their church affiliation. They didn't quote papal encyclicals. They didn't mention Catholic natural law theory. Whereas some of the conservative evangelical Protestants who wrote to Blackmun quoted scripture, Catholic letter writers tried instead to position themselves as nonsectarian advocates of a commonsense position that all Americans of a broadly based, ecumenical Judeo-Christian heritage could support. In their view, they opposed abortion not because they were Catholics, but because they were Americans who loved God and human life.[3] Yet as they belatedly realized, many other Americans did not support their views. This created a dilemma for them. In his *Roe v. Wade* opinion, Blackmun had suggested that their pro-life principles were sectarian dogma that had no place in public law. Yet this consignment of Catholic moral thinking to the sectarian world of the private sphere—which had seemed imminently reasonable to the liberal Protestant Blackmun—was unimaginable to millions of devout Catholics, such as Grace Burns. Everything in their background had led them to believe that what Blackmun viewed as sectarian beliefs were in fact universal moral truths that should have been obvious to any rational person.

THE DEVELOPMENT OF A CATHOLIC MORAL PERSPECTIVE ON ABORTION

Unlike Protestants' views of abortion, the view of abortion that the Catholic Church in the United States held in the mid-twentieth century had developed almost entirely outside of the country. In opposing abortion, twentieth-century Catholics believed that they were drawing on a centuries-old tradition that dated back to the earliest days of the church. And for Catholics, that tradition was inseparably tied to the value of fetal life. Liberal Protestants might appeal to other moral claims when discussing abortion, but for many Catholics the discussion of abortion's morality centered above all else on the value of unborn life, and on this issue, they thought, the tradition was clear.

From the first century onward, followers of Jesus had emphasized the need for Christians to care for the weak and marginalized, just as he had taught. The early church provided for widows, the sick, and orphans, and made these principles key tenets of the faith. Some of the earliest Christian writers highlighted respect for the lives of newborn infants and unborn fetuses as one application of the Christian principle of concern for all human beings. Although the New Testament never directly mentions abortion, the procedure was condemned in several of the earliest Christian writings, including the *Didache* and the Epistle of Barnabas (both of which were written only a few decades or less after the New Testament canonical writings were penned). In the *Didache*, an anonymously produced set of rules for a second-century Christian community, the stipulation against abortion occurs in a list of sins included in the commandment "You shall not murder." One 1903 translation of the *Didache* rendered the Greek phrase as "Thou shalt not destroy a child by abortion, neither shalt thou slay him that is born." Other translations use slightly different wording but convey a similar idea: "You shall not murder a child by abortion nor kill that which is born"; "You shall not murder a child, whether it be born or unborn"; "Do not murder a child by abortion or kill a newborn infant."[4] Two things are clear from the passage: the Christian community that produced the *Didache* considered abortion to be a form of murder, and it equated abortion with infanticide.

Numerous other ancient Christian writings included strong affirmations of the value of fetal life even from the moment of conception. Two of the clearest come from the late second-century Christian apologist Athenagoras of Athens and the North African Christian Tertullian, who wrote in about 200 CE. Athenagoras's reference to abortion came in a work of apologetics in which he refuted the pagan charge that Christians were secret murderers or cannibals. The idea was absurd, Athenagoras said, because Christians abhorred all forms of murder, including abortion. "And when we say that those women who use drugs to bring on abortion commit murder, and will have to give an account to God for the abortion, on what principle should we commit murder?" he asked. "For it does not belong to the same person to regard the very foetus in the womb as a created being, and therefore an object of God's care, and when it has passed into life, to kill it; and not to expose an infant, because those who expose them are chargeable with child-murder, and on the other hand, when it has been reared to destroy it." In other words, if Christians were universally known as strong opponents of both abortion and infanticide (as Athenagoras expected his pagan critics to admit), it would be unthinkable for them to murder people or cannibalize them in secret, as some pagans who had heard distorted accounts of Christ's body and blood being consumed in the Eucharist may have assumed.[5] Tertullian argued in his *Treatise on the Soul* that even in its earliest embryonic form, unborn human life had a soul and was fully human: "Now we allow that life begins with conception, because we contend that the soul also begins from conception; life taking its commencement at the same moment and place that the soul does."[6] Abortion was therefore murder, he argued in his *Apology*. In a section designed to demonstrate to pagan readers that Christians were thoroughly nonviolent, he noted that Christians opposed even feticide, which many pagans of the time accepted as legitimate: "In our case, murder being once for all forbidden, we may not destroy even the foetus in the womb, while as yet the human being derives blood from other parts of the body for its sustenance. To hinder a birth is merely a speedier man-killing; nor does it matter whether you take away a life that is born, or destroy one that is coming to the birth. That is a man which is going to be one; you have the fruit already in its seed."[7]

The Council of Ancyra (314) prescribed a penalty of ten years penance for any woman who had an abortion or those "who are employed in making drugs for abortion." The council viewed this as a merciful approach, because "a former decree excluded them until the hour of death, and to this some have assented." But this council, "being desirous to use somewhat greater lenity," offered women who had abortions a path back to the sacraments and full acceptance in the church after they completed only ten years of penance. Basil, a fourth-century bishop of Caesarea, clarified that this penalty applied to all abortions, "whether the embryo were perfectly formed, or not."[8]

The penalty of ten years of penance for abortion left no doubt that abortion was a grave offense, but it was still less than the twenty years of penance that Basil imposed for murder, and identical to the penance that Basil imposed for involuntary homicide. Basil did not explain why both he and the Council of Ancyra treated abortion similarly to involuntary homicide rather than murder, but Theodore Balsamon, a twelfth-century patriarch of Antioch, who wrote a commentary on Basil's letters, speculated that it was because women who had abortions did so because of shame or fear, which was different from murders committed out of anger or malice.[9]

For Basil and the Council of Ancyra, then, all abortion was killing, but the motivation behind it led them to treat those involved in it somewhat more mercifully than murderers. Yet shortly after Basil's death, Christian theologians began debating an issue that would call into question the assumption that even when performed at the earliest stages of pregnancy, abortion ended a human life. That question was ensoulment. When did a soul enter the embryo or fetus?

A few theologians of late antiquity, such as Maximus the Confessor (ca. 580–662), agreed with Tertullian that ensoulment began at conception, which meant that every embryo or fetus was just as much a person as a newborn baby or a full-grown adult. In making this argument, Maximus relied on the Christian doctrine of the Incarnation. Christians had long believed that the Son of God entered the world at his conception, at the Annunciation, and that Jesus's soul and body had been fused together and present in Mary's womb from the moment that the Holy Spirit had "overshadowed" her, described in the first chapter of the Gospel of Luke. But other theologians, such as the fifth-century bishop Theodoret of Cyrus (or Cyrrhus), argued that in the penalties for homicide and manslaughter given in Exodus 21, the Mosaic law distinguished between a formed and unformed fetus, and that in Genesis 2, God did not infuse Adam with a soul until his body was created. This argument was based on a Greek mistranslation of the Hebrew text of Exodus 21. Jewish rabbinic tradition, in contrast to medieval Western Christianity, followed the Hebrew text closely and did not imitate medieval Christians in differentiating between "formed" and "unformed" fetuses, but since most Christians of late antiquity had more facility with Greek than Hebrew, they accepted the idea that Exodus 21 differentiated between earlier and later stages of fetal development. Human souls did not exist without human bodies, the theologians argued, and if the embryo or fetus at the earliest stage of pregnancy was "unformed," it could not have a soul. Augustine equivocated on this point; some of his condemnations of abortion were so strong that they seemed to suggest that from the moment of conception, the fetus had a soul, but he also suggested the difficulties of imagining an unformed fetus that had died in the earliest weeks of pregnancy participating in the general resurrection. He had no doubt that abortion was a grave evil, and he thought that the doctrine of original sin suggested that both ensoulment and inherited sin began at conception, but like other theologians of his time, he also found the idea of the ensoulment of an unformed mass that lacked human shape difficult to fathom.[10]

After the twelfth century, the rediscovery of Aristotle seemed to settle the question for most theologians, including Thomas Aquinas, the church's most influential theological writer since Augustine. Since Aristotle said that animation of the fetus occurred at forty days for males and eighty days for females, this became the generally accepted view among theologians. It was never universally held; there were still at least a few theologians who continued to argue for ensoulment at the point of conception. And even those who strongly held to the position of delayed ensoulment, such as Aquinas, made an exception for the ensoulment of the Son of God at the Annunciation. Jesus's soul, Aquinas held, had been fused with his body from the moment of his conception; in contrast to the usual course of human development outlined by Aristotle, there had been no delayed animation for the Son of God.[11]

Yet though Aquinas's Aristotelian view of delayed ensoulment was the predominant view among Catholic theologians for several centuries in the late medieval and early modern eras, it was at odds with earliest church teaching on the issue, and it was also difficult to harmonize with other aspects of Catholic theology. The doctrine of the transmission of original sin seemed to require that the transmission of a human soul, made in God's image but marred with the guilt of Adam's sin, occur at the moment of conception. Without the doctrine of original sin, one could easily imagine a divinely created human soul being implanted in a human body at a later moment of pregnancy, as some theologians taught, but with Western Christianity after Augustine firmly committed to the doctrine of original sin, the notion of later ensoulment created almost insuperable theological difficulties. So did the doctrine of the Incarnation and the Christian theology surrounding Jesus's ensoulment at the moment of his conception. But the widespread Christian understanding that identified ensoulment with a body—not with a free-floating spirit or an unformed blob—made it hard for theologians to accept the idea that the implantation of a rational soul could occur before the fetal body was fully formed. Accordingly, following Aristotle, they imagined the transmission of a series of souls: first a vegetative soul that was transmitted at the moment of conception, then an animal soul that developed later, and finally a rational soul that entered the fetal body forty days after conception in the case of males or eighty days in the case of females. But by the seventeenth century, some theologians had begun to argue that this scheme seemed needlessly complex, and they favored the idea of a single soul that began at conception. In the modern era, embryological studies that showed that humanlike features and the general outlines of a conventional human shape formed in the fetus long before people in Aquinas's day had assumed made it much easier for the church to identify rational ensoulment with the moment of conception, as at least a few theologians had argued all along.[12]

But during the centuries when a distinction between the "formed" and "unformed" fetus prevailed in the church, this distinction affected only the penalties assigned to various types of abortion, not the question of whether abortion was a sin. Even when many Catholic theologians believed in delayed ensoulment, the church never suggested that the notion of delayed ensoulment was official doctrine or anything more than an educated guess. Nor did it ever suggest that abortion at any stage of pregnancy was acceptable. Indeed, all theologians who commented on the issue agreed that abortion was a sin, and canon law treated it as such. For centuries after the Council of Ancyra, church authorities generally assigned the same penalties to all abortions, regardless of the stage of gestation in which they occurred, and even when Pope Gregory XIV adjusted canon law in 1591 to differentiate between abortions before and after "quickening," the church still considered abortion even in the earliest stages of pregnancy to be a sin, even if it could not be equated with homicide. This was not surprising in view of a uniform tradition that considered contraception and sterilization grave evils. All of these were attacks on God's right to create human life through the sex act, and they violated the natural law. The church considered sterilization such an egregious evil that some medieval canon law codes treated deliberate sterilization as homicide, a categorization that the church later dropped (even though it still considered sterilization a grave sin). Thus, even as the church equivocated on the question of when a fetus became a full human person with a rational soul, its high regard for God's creation of human life, as expressed in its strong condemnation of contraception and sterilization, kept it from accepting any form of abortion. And in 1869 the Catholic Church officially returned to a position that all abortions were equally evil when Pope Pius IX issued a revised penal code for abortion that specified that anyone who performed an abortion, procured an abortion, or even attempted an abortion would be excommunicated, regardless of the stage of development of the fetus. These penalties were then included in the code of canon law published in 1917 and have remained in force ever since.[13]

In issuing this penal code, Pius IX essentially returned church penal law on abortion to the spirit of the Council of Ancyra's declaration and moved the church away from the notion of delayed animation that had held widespread theological influence for much of the medieval and early modern eras. Although he never officially defined the moment of human ensoulment, Catholic theologians and ethicists after that point generally identified ensoulment with conception, and this became the popular understanding for many Catholics. From then on, whenever popes or bishops wrote about abortion, they treated it as a grave evil that destroyed a human person, regardless of the stage at which it was performed. And since this doctrine accorded well with early church teaching on the issue and with the findings of modern science, many Catholics considered it unassailable. Unlike, say, the doctrine of the Immaculate Conception (which Pius IX declared in an encyclical in 1854), the church's teaching on abortion was not based primarily on a papal declaration nor was it controversial among Protestants, at least at first. The ecclesiastical penalties for abortion were defined by a papal declaration and by canon law, but the moral teaching itself—the idea that all abortion was wrong, because it was the unjustified taking of human life—was based on embryological science and universally accepted moral principles, Catholics believed. Those moral principles were part of the natural law, which, in its Thomistic formulation, was the foundation for nearly all Catholic moral reasoning in the early twentieth century. And though not all people might recognize it, the natural law was "engraven on the human mind for every intelligent and honest person to read," said Fr. Francis Connell, a theology professor at Catholic University of America, in 1946.[14] Aquinas himself might have misunderstood embryological development and ensoulment, but that was only because of scientific ignorance, not because of a defect in moral reasoning or the natural law. Now that embryological and genetic science was clear, there was no excuse for poor moral reasoning on abortion. For Catholics of the mid-twentieth century, there was only one relevant question when it came to determining the morality of abortion: Was the fetus a human life? Science and natural law provided compelling reasons that it was, they thought, which meant that the question should have been settled for any reasonable person, whether Catholic or not.

AMERICAN CATHOLIC DEFENSES OF UNBORN HUMAN LIFE

The development of Catholic doctrine on abortion occurred almost entirely outside of the United States. When Catholic immigrants arrived in the United States in large numbers in the nineteenth century, they brought this doctrine with them, but for several decades, it was not a source of division with Protestants, because there was little difference between the perspective of the Catholic Church and the American Protestant establishment on the issue. The first major wave of Irish and German Catholic immigration to the United States, which occurred between 1830 and the mid-1850s, came at a time when state legislatures were beginning to enact abortion restrictions in response to a campaign from doctors who argued that medical evidence of fetal development suggested that even in its earliest stages, fetuses were human lives that deserved legal protection. This was the same medical evidence that convinced European Catholic theologians that distinctions between the formed and unformed fetus needed to be abandoned, so when Protestant-dominated state legislatures passed restrictions on abortion that also rejected these distinctions, it paralleled what the Catholic Church was doing in Europe, or what the British government had done at the beginning of the nineteenth century. Disputes between Protestants and Catholics in antebellum America could be vituperative, and there was little comity between the two groups, but on abortion and contraception, there was no cause for argument. By the time significant numbers of Catholics entered the medical and legal professions, Protestants had already enacted abortion restrictions across the nation that Catholic clerics happened to agree with. And on birth control, the Protestant-inspired Comstock Act (1873) made it illegal to send contraceptive information through the mail.

If Protestants of the late nineteenth century saw any difference between their own views and those of Catholics on the issue of abortion, it was only on the matter of the one exception that nearly all state laws against abortion allowed for: abortions that were necessary to save a pregnant woman's life. Although such abortions would become extremely rare by the mid-twentieth century, they were much more common in the late nineteenth century, when caesarian sections were nearly impossible to perform safely. Although few Protestant theologians or ministers had ever commented on the matter directly, the legal permission for abortion in such emergency cases, combined with the general practice of physicians in performing such abortions when needed, led people to assume that Protestantism allowed for abortions in cases when it was necessary to save a woman's life. But Catholic theologians, after debating the matter for centuries, did not arrive at this conclusion. The fetus was not an aggressor, the church said, and therefore the canon law against abortion applied even when a pregnancy endangered a woman's life. On this point, some Protestants attacked Catholic Church doctrine as inhumane. In practice, Catholic theological views on abortion in these exceptional cases were not so inflexible; some theologians did allow for pregnancy termination if the direct killing of the fetus was not intended.[15]

It was not until the 1920s, though, that significant differences between Protestant and Catholic views of unborn life emerged as a dividing point between the two Christian traditions. At the time, the conflict centered on birth control rather than abortion, but the fault lines that developed in the debates over contraception were very closely parallel to the divisions on abortion a few decades later. These divisions centered not only on sex, marriage, and human life, but also on questions about the purpose of the family and the value of people who were poor or marginalized. The Catholic Church in the United States was an immigrant church, composed primarily of the working class and the poor. From the first decade of the twentieth century, some Catholic priests, such as Fr. John A. Ryan, advocated for a living wage. In 1919, the National Catholic Welfare Conference (the national organization of Catholic bishops) endorsed a living wage and several other programs to improve the lives of the poor.[16]

Liberal Protestants also wanted to improve the lives of the poor, but unlike the Catholic Church, they believed that decreasing birth rates among the poor and recent immigrant groups could reduce poverty. In 1929, the Universalist Church became the first Christian denomination to endorse the use of birth control. Because the Universalists were a very small group—and because they were so theologically liberal that their influence on mainstream Protestant thought was limited—the Universalists' action probably could have been ignored if it had not been closely followed by similar resolutions from more influential Protestant denominations. In 1930, the Lambeth Conference, a global conference of the bishops of the Anglican Communion, adopted a resolution allowing married couples to use contraceptives, a reversal of the position that the conference had previously adopted. Several Protestant denominations followed in the 1930s with their own endorsements of birth control. In response to this mainline Protestant shift on birth control, Catholics responded with a reaffirmation of the church's traditional doctrine on the issue. Birth control campaigns would lead to a "cheapening of human life," the Jesuit magazine *America* warned in 1924.[17] Discouraging the poor from having more children was no way to respect their dignity or value their lives, they believed. And despite the Lambeth Conference's stated opposition to abortion—and the claim of some contraceptive advocates that birth control devices would prevent abortions—Jesuits such as the medical ethicist Fr. Ignatius Cox and some of the editors of *America* magazine claimed that birth control would actually increase the abortion rate, because it "created the mentality which abhors births," thus encouraging people to terminate their pregnancies by abortion when the contraceptive devices on which they relied failed.[18]

The connection between contraception and abortion was implicit in the first major papal encyclical on birth control, *Casti Connubii*, which Pius XI issued in December 1930 as a response to the Lambeth Conference's endorsement of contraception and to new social developments that favored the liberalization of laws restricting divorce and birth control devices. In the midst of the pope's defense of binding, lifelong, Christian marital covenants that were undertaken for the purpose of procreation, he also devoted several paragraphs to abortion, since he viewed divorce, birth control, and abortion as similar attacks on marriage and human life. Laws that allowed abortion in cases of perceived medical necessity were wrong, the pope said in the encyclical: "However much we may pity the mother whose health and even life is gravely imperiled in the performance of the duty allotted to her by nature, nevertheless what could ever be a sufficient reason for excusing in any way the direct murder of the innocent? . . . Those who hold the reins of government should not forget that it is the duty of public authority by appropriate laws and sanctions to defend the lives of the innocent, and this all the more so since those whose lives are endangered and assailed cannot defend themselves. Among whom we must mention in the first place infants hidden in the mother's womb. And if the public magistrates not only do not defend them, but by their laws and ordinances betray them to death at the hands of doctors or of others, let them remember that God is the Judge and Avenger of innocent blood which cried from earth to Heaven."[19]

Although small Catholic minorities in a few countries in the 1930s and 1940s (including Sweden and Japan) faced the imminent legalization of abortion as a real political issue, no state legislature in the United States during this period considered legalizing abortion, which meant that American Catholic bishops in the country focused most of their effort in this period not on campaigning against abortion but on lobbying against proposals to legalize contraception. In Massachusetts, Archbishop Richard Cushing (a future cardinal) led a successful campaign to defeat a referendum in 1948 that would have legalized the sale of birth control devices in the state. In the weeks leading up to the election, the Catholic Church put up billboards in Boston: "Birth Control Is *Still* against God's Law! Vote NO on Question No. 4 on the Ballot." Catholic priests delivered homilies explaining why birth control should remain illegal. One Sunday homilist declared that legislation against contraception was appropriate because "the prohibition of Birth Control is not a law peculiar to the church any more than are the laws against murder, theft, perjury or treason. . . . The Catholic Church does not initiate these laws. They are rooted in our very natures and are written by God in the very heart of every man, woman and child."[20] In essence, Catholic clergy of the 1940s generally believed that civil law should echo the universally accessible natural moral law. Sectarian doctrine should not be enshrined in the law; the law should protect religious freedom. But legislation against obscenity and birth control should be encouraged, because those behaviors damaged social well-being by encouraging a disrespect for human life and sexuality, and because the moral arguments against them were based on principles that were not explicitly Catholic. And if that were true of contraception, it was even more true of abortion.

Although Catholic magazines did not devote as much attention to abortion as they did to the much more imminent threat of birth control in the 1930s and 1940s, they periodically published antiabortion articles that noted the horrors of legalized abortion in the Soviet Union and lamented the lack of interest in more rigorously enforcing antiabortion laws in the United States. The prevalence of large criminal abortion syndicates in New York City was evidence of the public's unwillingness to treat illegal abortion providers as a serious social menace. Most of all, though, Catholic magazines warned that the contemporary birth control campaign, which had the support of many prominent Protestant ministers, would eventually lead to the acceptance of both abortion and euthanasia, since it stemmed from a devaluation of human life, they thought.[21]

How often a Catholic family of the 1940s heard such warnings might have depended partly on the breadth of their Catholic periodical reading, but even families that did not read religious magazines regularly might have encountered several reminders of the value of fetal life in the course of their religious activities. That would have been most obvious in the realm of contraception. At a time when many of the nation's most prominent Protestant denominations were endorsing birth control and when numerous middle-class Protestant and Jewish couples practiced contraception, the Catholic Church's insistence that birth control was a violation of the natural law and a "grave sin" set Catholics apart from their non-Catholic neighbors. Couples who followed the church's teaching in this area—as two-thirds of Catholic couples of childbearing age did in the mid-1950s—received constant reminders of their church's countercultural insistence on the value of children and prenatal life. Families received regular reiterations of this teaching from their priest's homilies, their diocesan paper, and their catechism lessons. "The end to which marriage is primarily directed is that children be brought into the world and properly reared for happiness in this life and in the next," the third edition of the *Baltimore Catechism* (1949) declared. "Hence, when a married couple make use of their right to sexual union but perform the act in such a way that the conception of children is positively frustrated, they are guilty of a grave sin."[22] Even apart from the issue of whether human life began at conception, Catholics who followed the church's teaching on sex and contraception would have acquired a high view of childbearing.

But in addition to valuing the birth of children, Catholics of this era also had a theology that identified ensoulment and the beginning of human personhood with the moment of conception. In Catholic hospitals, medical personnel received a daily reminder of that theology from the "Ethical and Religious Directives," which the nation's leading Jesuit medical ethicist, Fr. Gerald Kelly, had asked every Catholic hospital to display, beginning in 1948: "Every unborn child must be considered a human person, with all the rights of a human person, from the moment of conception."[23] For most lay Catholics outside of the medical profession, this theology was reinforced most frequently in remembrances of Jesus's miraculous conception and the immaculate conception of the Virgin Mary. Every year, devout Catholics observed the Feast of the Immaculate Conception on December 8, which reminded them that the Virgin Mary's sinlessness began at the moment of her conception. They regularly prayed, "Mary, conceived without sin, pray for us who have recourse to thee."[24]

A theology that identified the beginning of original sin in a person's life at the moment of that person's conception—and, conversely, the beginning of the Virgin Mary's state of sinlessness with her own conception—was of necessity a theology that thought of conception (not birth) as the point of ensoulment and the beginning of personhood, since the guilt of sin or the holiness of sinless grace belongs only to persons, not to impersonal clusters of cells. The conceptus might look like a microscopic brainless mass that had no resemblance yet to the shape of a human body, but devout Catholics knew that it already had an eternal soul that was in relationship with its creator and that would never die. For Catholics who studied the third edition of the *Baltimore Catechism* (as all American Catholics of the 1950s were supposed to do), the catechism's description of the qualities that the Virgin Mary had when she was still a zygote would have provided strong confirmation of the value of embryonic life: "*In the first instant of her conception* the Blessed Virgin Mary possessed the fullness of sanctifying grace, the infused virtues, and the gifts of the Holy Ghost. She was, however, subject to pain and suffering, as was her Divine Son" (emphasis added).[25] In other words, from the moment she was conceived, the Virgin Mary was, for Catholics, a person with all of the divine grace and qualities of her later development. Catholics who believed and regularly thought about this and celebrated it periodically would probably have thought it obvious that a person's life, soul, and personhood began at conception. They didn't think of a zygote as just a microscopic clump of cells; they thought of it as a miniature person, with an eternal soul whose divine gifts and lasting qualities of personality were already stamped upon it.

This was the backdrop against which Catholics received regular reminders of the church's prohibitions on abortion. Even in the 1950s, when proposals to liberalize abortion laws were receiving only occasional attention in the secular press (and even less attention in Protestant churches), Catholic periodicals were quick to line up rebuttals against them. When the secular general-interest periodical *Woman's Home Companion* published an article in 1955 that advocated abortion law liberalization on the grounds that antiabortion laws did not work, the Archdiocese of Dubuque, Iowa, encouraged Catholic women to write letters of protest to the magazine, an exhortation that diocesan papers in other parts of the country also echoed. Catholic diocesan papers also regularly published articles arguing against therapeutic abortion, publicizing the legalization of abortion in the communist countries of Eastern Europe, and highlighting Catholic resistance against these policies. In a 1958 series on "The Commandments for Adults," for instance, the *Catholic Transcript* (the journal of the Archdiocese of Hartford, Connecticut) included an entire article on "therapeutic abortion" as an application of the commandment "Thou shalt not kill." Abortion "constitutes a direct lethal attack upon an innocent human being, and is therefore immoral," the article stated. But this was not a uniquely Catholic teaching, the *Catholic Transcript* insisted; it rested on scientific evidence and assumptions about the value of human life that were widely shared.[26] The Catholic stance on abortion was simply "the traditional moral teaching of our Western culture," the *Catholic Standard and Times* stated in 1955. The Catholic Church may have upheld that standard more consistently than Protestants did, but it was not a uniquely Catholic sectarian stance.[27]

Yet Catholic ethicists also took pride in the fact that the Catholic Church was more consistent and more vocal than most Protestants and other non-Catholics in its uncompromising defense of human life. Although the Catholic Church allowed for just war and killing in self-defense, it was firmly opposed to taking any *innocent* life, even when many people argued that such killing would be justified on utilitarian grounds. In the 1930s, Jesuits in the United States spoke out against euthanasia. During World War II, the Jesuit ethicist John Ford denounced the bombing of civilians, because "to take the life of an innocent person is always intrinsically wrong, that is, forbidden absolutely by the natural law." After the United States dropped atomic bombs on Hiroshima and Nagasaki, Ford condemned the action as "the greatest and most extensive single atrocity of this period." He declared in 1950 that "the Catholic Church will always defend the sanctity of life against all comers."[28]

THE CATHOLIC CHURCH'S REACTION TO EARLY ABORTION LIBERALIZATION PROPOSALS

When conversations about abortion law reform began in a few state legislatures in the early 1960s, the Catholic press's reaction was swift and firm: Because the fetus was a human being from the moment of conception, any loosening of abortion restrictions was unconscionable. This was true even in the case of the most modest liberalization proposals. In 1961, Catholic bishops in New Hampshire denounced the state legislature's narrowly focused effort to make abortions legal before the twentieth week of pregnancy in the rare cases when abortion was necessary to save a pregnant woman's life, because even this limited measure was a step too far toward a denial of humanity to the fetus. That put them at odds with Protestant denominations in the state.[29] No Protestant denomination at the time approved of elective abortion, but most Protestants believed that abortion was justified in cases of medical necessity, which included, at the very least, cases in which pregnancy threatened a woman's life. But the Catholic Church viewed Protestants' willingness to allow for abortion in such cases as a sign of moral relativism. In the view of some Catholic writers of the time, Protestants who had accepted a violation of natural law in the case of birth control lacked the philosophical framework to defend the value of fetal life or, for that matter, any moral absolutes that were no longer culturally popular. "The absence of principles and laws in Protestant morality makes one wonder about the future," the Catholic journalist Robert Hoyt wrote in December 1959. If they wouldn't stop at birth control or abortion legalization, would they "gradually find it possible to regard acts of homosexuality as morally neutral?" he asked. "For that matter, what action of any kind—no matter how shockingly evil or perverse it may appear to the Protestant conscience today—can be definitely and permanently outlawed as un-Christian, unnatural, inhuman?"[30]

For Catholics of the early 1960s, the struggle against abortion law liberalization was a fight against moral relativism and a defense of the unchanging principles of the natural law, which they believed were accessible to every human being's conscience, but which Protestants, for whatever reason, seemed to have partially ignored. But it was also a fight against the potential totalitarian horrors of an amoral state. This was evident in the "diary" of a fetus that the Jesuit magazine *America* published in June 1962. In a half-page article that would be reprinted countless times over the next decade in a wide variety of Catholic and pro-life periodicals, an unborn baby girl recounts every moment of her life over the course of twelve weeks, from conception through the development of a heartbeat and the growth of "tiny fingers" and hair, until finally the article abruptly ends with the line, "December 28: Today my mother killed me." The article was issued under the byline of the Polish cardinal Stefan Wyszynski, with the explanation that he had used the piece "as a pastoral aid in his battle against pressure from the Red Polish government for relaxation of the Church's stand on abortion."[31] Legalized abortion was something that communist governments were trying to force on their populations, American Catholics knew, but the church was faithfully resisting the effort. They were faithfully defending the idea that human beings were fully persons at the moment of conception. The diary of a fetus declared, speaking in the voice of a newly formed zygote, "I am as small as the seed of an apple, but it is I already. And I am to be a girl. I shall have blond hair and azure eyes. Just about everything is settled though, even the fact that I shall love flowers."[32] Advocates of abortion legalization routinely invoked the importance of choice, contingency, and socialization in the formation of a human being, so they never would have conceded that from the moment of conception "everything is settled." But pro-life Catholics instead emphasized the idea of God's plan for human beings from the moment of conception, and they saw the unique genetic composition of each zygote or embryo as the blueprint of that divine plan. Each zygote or embryo was therefore neither an accident nor merely a "potential" human being that could become a full person through the human socialization process, as some abortion rights advocates argued in the 1960s. Instead, each zygote or embryo was a divine gift of incalculable worth, because it was a full human being with a determined gender, personality, character traits, and a God-ordained life plan.

Two months after *America* magazine published this article, Sherri Chessen Finkbine's nationally publicized abortion brought the debate over abortion law to the United States. Finkbine was a nationally known star of the popular children's television program *Romper Room*, and she was a happily married mother of four children. In 1962, she became pregnant for a fifth time, but during her first trimester, she learned that a thalidomide-based medication she had been taking was known to cause birth defects. Rather than risk giving birth to a deformed infant, she sought an abortion, only to discover that Arizona law did not permit her to have an abortion unless her pregnancy endangered her life (which it did not). Most other states had similar laws at the time.

When Finkbine traveled to Sweden, with her husband, for an abortion, newspapers across the United States covered the event. Her action galvanized a nascent campaign to liberalize abortion laws so that people could legally terminate their pregnancies in cases of suspected fetal deformity. Many conservative Protestant churches were silent about Finkbine's case, but because American Catholic clergy had already been talking about abortion and fetal personhood, they were ready with a counterargument against her line of thinking. Finkbine's "efforts represent a violation of God's law and of right reason," *America* magazine's editors declared. "From the fertilization of the ovum, through the successive stages of fetal development and up to the last moment of adult life, there is a direct and unbroken continuity. It is, therefore, just as immoral to kill the human embryo as it would be to kill the child after birth, or to end the life of a comatose and helpless invalid." Expressing sympathy for the challenges that a couple might face in caring for an infant with severe disabilities, they nevertheless declared, "To agree that a human life may be sacrificed on the altar of emotional tranquillity, or that a child may not be born because, in the judgment of others, its life may be complicated by physical deformity, is as unreasonable and unfair to the child as it is immoral."[33]

Public opinion polls showed that Catholics were substantially more likely than Protestants or other Americans to object to Finkbine's abortion decision. A Gallup poll taken in late August 1962, immediately after Finkbine's abortion, showed that 49 percent of Catholics said that Finkbine did the "wrong thing" in terminating her pregnancy in order to avoid giving birth to a deformed child; only 33 percent said that she did the "right thing." Among Protestants, by contrast, 56 percent said that her abortion was the "right thing"; only 27 percent thought her decision was the "wrong thing."[34] This survey, which was the first Gallup poll ever taken on American views on abortion, indicated a stark religious divide on the question, with Catholics far more opposed to abortion than Protestants were. Nevertheless, the poll also indicated that Catholic opinion on the question was not monolithic; 33 percent of Catholics, after all, insisted that Finkbine had done the "right thing," even though the Catholic press at the time said that she had not. Subsequent studies have shown that in the late 1950s, approximately one-third of married Catholic women of childbearing age were using forbidden forms of contraception, so the fact that one-third of Catholics also defied church teachings by supporting therapeutic abortion in at least a few exceptional cases is perhaps not surprising. On both birth control and therapeutic abortion, the church's teachings, though still widely honored, were not accepted by all Catholics.

VATICAN II'S EFFECT ON THE ABORTION DEBATE

Only a few weeks after the international debate over Finkbine's abortion, bishops from across the world gathered in Rome for what was arguably the most significant event in the Catholic Church in five hundred years: the Vatican II ecumenical council (1962–65). The last ecumenical council, Vatican I, had been interrupted in 1870 by the Franco-Prussian War and was remembered largely for its declaration on papal infallibility. But aside from that doctrinal statement, it left the Tridentine structure of the church largely intact. Vatican II, by contrast, involved three years of debates among the largest and most global assembly of bishops in the church's history and resulted in hundreds of pages of conciliar documents that collectively introduced more changes in church liturgy and political theology than had ever occurred since the Council of Trent in the sixteenth century. When Pope John XXIII unexpectedly convened the council, saying that it was time to "open the windows and let in the fresh air," no one knew quite what to expect. Some conservative bishops hoped the council would definitively reaffirm traditional teaching on questions about which there was some debate. As the council progressed and it became apparent that it would do far more than merely reaffirm existing doctrinal understandings, other more progressive bishops hoped that the council would be open to a liberalization of church teaching on birth control.

Neither group got exactly what it hoped for. There were surprises for almost everyone, both in what the council said and what it chose not to address. The church that emerged from Vatican II looked in some ways profoundly different from the way it had appeared at the beginning of the 1960s. Masses could now be said not only in Latin but also in the vernacular, and indeed, most were. Personal Bible reading was now encouraged. Protestants were now "separated brethren" (not heretics), and Catholics were encouraged to cooperate with them and with other non-Catholics through genuinely ecumenical dialogue. And the Catholic Church was now defined as the "people of God"—both the clergy and the laity, not merely the hierarchy. All of this would have a profound effect on the Catholic Church's response to abortion. But exactly what the council's declarations meant for abortion policy was subject to competing interpretations.[35]

One of the most significant developments of Vatican II was its strong affirmation of religious freedom, which was based in part on the work of the American Catholic theologian John Courtney Murray. "The human person has a right to religious freedom," the council declared. "This freedom means that all men are to be immune from coercion on the part of individuals or of social groups and of any human power, in such wise that no one is to be forced to act in a manner contrary to his own beliefs, whether privately or publicly, whether alone or in association with others, within due limits."[36] Did this therefore mean that coercive abortion laws were inappropriate in a pluralistic society in which some people's consciences led them to seek abortions?

This was the way that a few of the most progressive Catholics interpreted it. By the end of the 1960s, Fr. Robert Drinan, a Jesuit academic and Boston College Law School dean who ran for Congress (and won), was arguing that because of Vatican II, it was inappropriate for Catholics to use the law to force their views of abortion on others.

Similarly, some of the most progressive Catholics interpreted Vatican II's definition of the church as the "people of God" to mean that the hierarchy did not have the authority to impose an interpretation of Catholic doctrine that did not accord with the laity's own consciences, especially if that hierarchy was all-male and therefore did not fully represent the "people of God." This was the view that some Catholics took on birth control in the 1960s, and in the 1970s, some Catholics, such as the founders of Catholics for a Free Choice (later, Catholics for Choice), would apply this argument to abortion also. If the bishops could define doctrine, so could the laity—if not for the whole church, at least for themselves. For decades, both the global Catholic Church and the predominantly Irish-led Catholic Church in the United States had been hierarchically organized, with a clergy that expected the laity to respond in obedience even to teachings that they personally disagreed with, such as contraception. In the years leading up to Vatican II, the movement of an increasing number of Catholics into the educated, suburban middle-class had begun to strain the traditional immigrant networks that had sustained the laity's willingness to acquiesce to the rigid strictures of a Catholic enclave. Now it appeared to some Catholics that the church might finally be ready to modernize by accepting the democratic argument that the laity could make their own decisions about official church teachings by letting their own personal consciences rather than the church magisterium become their ultimate moral authority.[37] In essence, they could begin to act more like liberal Protestants and less like traditional Catholics.

But this was not the intention of most of the bishops who drafted and ratified the conciliar documents of Vatican II, and it was not the way that American bishops interpreted the council's declarations. Instead, George Weigel argues that Vatican II's political theology was an attempt to move Catholic politics beyond merely protecting Catholic interests or codifying the Catholic understanding of the natural law and instead to promote a "Christocentric humanism" that centered on human dignity, human needs, and the "Lordship of Christ" over all creation.[38] The principle of human dignity was the foundation for Vatican II's "Declaration on Religious Freedom" (*Dignitatis Humanae*), so the council's advocacy of noncoercion in civil regulation of religion and morality could not extend to matters touching on human dignity and human life.

Immediately after Vatican II, several bishops backed away from their political campaigns against contraception, since they believed that these were no longer appropriate. Cardinal Cushing, who had led the campaign in Massachusetts against legalizing contraception, decided not to lobby against a birth control legalization proposal in the state in 1965, since he now believed that contraception, at least if it were made available only to married couples (as the proposal stipulated), was a matter of "private morality" that did not need to be the focus of public law. This was also the view of John Courtney Murray, a participant in Vatican II. It was not "the function of civil law to prescribe everything that is morally right and to forbid everything that is morally wrong," Murray said.[39]

But abortion was a matter of human life. If any practice justified legal coercion, surely the killing of innocent people did. Vatican II said in *Gaudium et Spes*, "God, the Lord of life, has conferred on men the surpassing ministry of safeguarding life in a manner which is worthy of man. Therefore from the moment of its conception life must be guarded with the greatest care while abortion and infanticide are unspeakable crimes."[40] Such a statement was hardly surprising, given the Catholic Church's long opposition to abortion. Indeed, this was largely just a reiteration of what Pius XI and Pius XII had said about abortion during the decades leading up to the council. But what Vatican II did was to frame the context for Catholic campaigns against abortion as a matter of advancing a Christocentric humanism focused on human dignity and the protection of human life in all contexts. Campaigns against abortion were only one component of a broader campaign for human freedom, life, and dignity. *Gaudium et Spes* also stated, "Whatever is opposed to life itself, such as any type of murder, genocide, abortion, euthanasia or wilful self-destruction, whatever violates the integrity of the human person, such as mutilation, torments inflicted on body or mind, attempts to coerce the will itself; whatever insults human dignity, such as subhuman living conditions, arbitrary imprisonment, deportation, slavery, prostitution, the selling of women and children; as well as disgraceful working conditions, where men are treated as mere tools for profit, rather than as free and responsible persons; all these things and others of their like are infamies indeed. They poison human society."[41]

Many bishops in the United States had already been thinking of the right to life for the unborn as part of a broader campaign of human rights advocacy, so they were receptive to the framing of the issue that Vatican II reiterated. In 1947, the National Catholic Welfare Conference had issued a model declaration of human rights that began with an affirmation of the "right to life and bodily integrity from the moment of conception," but then enumerated several other rights that accorded well with the New Deal liberalism of American Catholic bishops: the right to a "living wage," collective bargaining, education, and "assistance from society."[42] In grafting the right to life for the unborn onto this larger set of rights and social obligations, the bishops were building on a tradition of Catholic social welfare teaching that began in earnest with Leo XIII's encyclical *Rerum Novarum* in 1891 and that continued through Pius XI's *Quadragesimo Anno* (1931) and beyond. Under the influence of these encyclicals, American bishops had long campaigned for a living wage—that is, a "wage sufficient to support [a worker] and his family," as Pius XI defined it. They had spoken of the need for the state to promote human dignity and social well-being and to steer a middle course between laissez-faire capitalism and socialism. In 1963, in the midst of Vatican II, John XXIII expanded on these ideas in his encyclical *Pacem in Terris*, parts of which closely echoed the language that American bishops had employed in their declaration of human rights from 1947.

"Man has the right to live," the pope declared. "He has the right to bodily integrity and to the means necessary for the proper development of life, particularly food, clothing, shelter, medical care, rest, and, finally, the necessary social services. In consequence, he has the right to be looked after in the event of ill health; disability stemming from his work; widowhood; old age; enforced unemployment; or whenever through no fault of his own he is deprived of the means of livelihood."[43]

Some of these rights accorded far more closely with the Democratic Party's New Deal liberalism than with the libertarian-leaning conservatism of right-wing Republicans, such as Barry Goldwater. But Catholic theology was much less supportive of individual autonomy than either secular liberals or liberal Protestants generally were. Although John XXIII and Vatican II affirmed individual freedom of conscience when it came to religious liberty, they grounded this declaration in the principle of human dignity, not individual autonomy. And they also believed that the nuclear family—not the state or the individual—was the "the natural, primary cell of human society," said John XXIII.[44] Government policy therefore must have the goal of strengthening the family and supporting parental rights, not replacing the family.

Although John XXIII and Vatican II recognized the religiously pluralistic nature of modern states, they did not support the idea of a secular society, if "secular" is defined as the absence of religious values in the public square. Instead, John XXIII argued, "We must think of human society as being primarily a spiritual reality. By its means enlightened men can share their knowledge of the truth, can claim their rights and fulfill their duties, receive encouragement in their aspirations for the goods of the spirit, share their enjoyment of all the wholesome pleasures of the world, and strive continually to pass on to others all that is best in themselves and to make their own the spiritual riches of others. It is these spiritual values which exert a guiding influence on culture, economics, social institutions, political movements and forms, laws, and all the other components which go to make up the external community of men and its continual development."[45] Vatican II expanded on this framework to promote a broadly based Christian vision for a modern society that would not be theocratic or a restoration of a now-defunct Christendom, but would instead be a just and equitable society, with notions of justice stemming from the foundational natural law principles of human dignity, social obligations, and the right to life from conception to natural death.

THE CATHOLIC CHURCH'S PRO-LIFE ACTIVISM IN THE LATE 1960S

Immediately after Vatican II, Catholic clergy and theologians in the United States brought the principles of human dignity and the right to life into the political sphere in response to legislative proposals to pass more permissive abortion laws. When Fr. James McHugh, director of the church's Family Life Bureau, surveyed a few leading theologians teaching at Catholic universities in 1966, all of them agreed that "from the moment of conception, the human person exists, and any assault on its life is gravely evil," and all of them therefore agreed that the church should oppose proposals to liberalize state abortion laws. Direct ecclesiastical involvement in politics was appropriate on this issue, they said, on the grounds that they were defending the innocent.[46]

This was the view of most Catholic lawyers and ethicists who wrote on abortion in the mid-1960s. The principle of religious pluralism meant that many church teachings—including moral teachings, such as those on contraception—could not necessarily be translated directly into civil law, as Catholics now recognized in the wake of Vatican II and the aftermath of the Supreme Court's decision to strike down some state anticontraceptive laws in *Griswold v. Connecticut* (1965). By 1965, even bishops who had recently given support to campaigns to restrict access to contraception through legislation, such as Cardinal Richard Cushing, archbishop of Boston, were turning away from those campaigns and affirming the value of church–state separation on such matters.[47] But abortion was an exceptional case, they believed, because it involved human life. "To allow the state to permit the killing of innocent human beings through abortion 'strikes at the common good so gravely that it endangers the fabric of society and so should be suppressed by law,'" the *Catholic Lawyer* said in 1964, quoting Norman St. John-Stevas, a member of the UK Parliament. If Catholics did not oppose proposals to liberalize state abortion laws, they would be complicit in moral evil, the *Catholic Lawyer* said.[48] *America* magazine took a similar stance in 1965: "If a person is convinced that abortion is an attack on human life, he has as much right and duty to say so as he has to denounce racial discrimination as an offense against human dignity."[49] The magazine explained in another article published two years later, "When persons of any persuasion protest that they would never impose their standards on persons of other faiths what they usually mean is that they do not consider the observance of their religious standards essential for the welfare of the community. If they thought such observance was essential, how could they possibly vote in conscience against it? All of which helps explain why many Catholics could vote for reforming the divorce law in New York but not for 'liberalizing' the State's abortion laws. Broadening the divorce law didn't kill anybody. . . . But abortion laws would kill people."[50]

In response to those who claimed that laws against abortion did not work and were inhumane, Catholics argued that the law had a didactic value that went beyond its mere utilitarian function. "Where fundamental human values are at stake, law must be judged by other criteria than its mere effectiveness in preventing crime," *America* magazine stated in 1965. "Here, above all, law is the voice of society's conscience. If that voice wavers or falls silent, on the plea that it is better to legalize and thus to control actions that we cannot prevent, the conscience of multitudes will be corrupted. Human life is too sacred for society to encourage disrespect for it in the womb in order to have abortions legally performed in hospitals under ideal antiseptic conditions."[51] The primary question for pro-life Catholics was thus not whether the law "worked" (though they hoped that it did) but whether the law reflected the values that they believed were the foundation for a just and humane society.

These were foundational American principles, rooted in both the Declaration of Independence's assertion of a "right to life" and in the Constitution's promise that no one could be deprived of life without "due process." Accordingly, church authorities who were arguing against abortion commonly cited these secular founding documents instead of scripture or church teachings, and connected them to the natural law, since they viewed their political campaign against abortion as a campaign not only to enforce a moral precept but as a defense of the country's most important founding principle. "Those who would weaken laws which protect human life are posing a threat both to society itself and to the fundamental moral principles on which it is based," the bishops said. "The right to life and the necessity of protecting it were deemed essential in the Declaration of Independence following the Judeo-Christian heritage of the dignity of man. . . . In preserving respect for the principle of the sanctity of life man sustains the basis of society in liberty and equality."[52]

When their opponents charged them with opposing abortion only because of their Catholic faith, many pro-life Catholics took offense, because in their view, the arguments against abortion were based on universal moral and legal principles that should be important to everyone, regardless of their religious belief. "Sometimes we tend to lose sight of what is at stake," the Catholic New York lawyer and pro-life activist Robert Byrn wrote in 1965. "At such times it is necessary to remind ourselves that, theological considerations aside, an induced abortion is the deliberate destruction of an innocent human life and that the liberalization movement is based upon an ethic both alien to our jurisprudence and at odds with the general trend of the law."[53]

As they saw politicians, the media, and voters ignore their warnings and liberalize state abortion laws over their opposition, some pro-life Catholics feared that the country they loved would soon abandon all moral restraint and jettison all respect for human life. "If the present campaign for abortion continues to mount and make progress, the final resultant can be nothing less than a depreciation of the sanctity and value of human life," Msgr. Paul Harrington of Massachusetts wrote to a fellow Catholic pro-life activist in Hawaii in 1966. "Once abortion is acceptable and made respectable in a culture, then, logically, consistently and necessarily, infanticide and euthanasia must follow. When this eventuates, I fear that the value of human life between peoples will diminish and that it would seem inconsistent with our pattern and culture to be able to oppose personal assaults or homicide. If, when and as, this happens whatever culture and refinement our civilization may have had will be lost and the law of the jungle will prevail. I certainly hope that this does not occur, but the seeds are now being planted."[54] Such warnings were common in pro-life publications, but this note of despair was part of Harrington's private correspondence, which suggests that such warnings were not merely issued for rhetorical or political effect but were instead a deeply held belief for many pro-life Catholics of the time.

Pro-life Catholics in the mid-1960s saw their opponents as utilitarian relativists who would allow fetal life to be destroyed simply because it was a barrier to someone else's happiness. Only an absolute insistence on the inviolable right of all people to live would protect the lives of those whose existence was inconvenient for someone else. This conviction was why numerous Catholic pro-life activists (not just Harrington) expected that infanticide, euthanasia, or other horrors would quickly follow the legalization of abortion. "As soon as one allows direct suppression of innocent human life in any form, he has priced human life," the Jesuit theologian Richard McCormick wrote in 1965. "That is, he has subordinated it to some temporal value: economic advantage, physical well being, the good life, protection of reputation or whatever it may be. Once he has done this, there is nothing *in principle* that prevents his destroying human life at other stages and in other circumstances: the aged, the infirm, the socially or economically burdensome, the crippled, the suffering. It is only a matter of waiting until the going price has been reached."[55]

McCormick was one of many priests of the mid-to-late 1960s who held liberal views in both politics and theology. Like numerous other liberal Catholics at the time, he questioned the church's prohibition on artificial contraception. When Paul VI reaffirmed the Catholic Church's opposition to artificial contraception in the encyclical *Humanae Vitae* (1968), it set off a firestorm in the church, since many Catholics had expected the pope to loosen restrictions on contraception rather than reiterate them with his endorsement. Although theological conservatives in the church welcomed the pope's pronouncement, dozens of more liberal theologians and priests publicly dissented, and a majority of Catholics of childbearing age simply disregarded the instructions. One study conducted shortly after *Humanae Vitae* found that 43 percent of American priests "rejected its teaching" on birth control, with 79 percent of priests under the age of thirty-five saying that they approved of contraception.[56] But although there was such widespread disregard in the church to official church teaching on birth control that many bishops—with the exceptions of a few conservatives, such as Cardinal Patrick O'Boyle, archbishop of Washington, DC—were willing to tacitly tolerate defections from official Catholic doctrine on this point, there was much greater unanimity among the clergy on the issue of abortion. McCormick's defense of the church's pro-life teaching suggested why. A generation earlier, the church had argued vehemently that both contraception and abortion were attacks on human life, and *Humanae Vitae* had reiterated that connection, but McCormick's writings suggested a new framing for abortion legislation that connected the issue to concern for the marginalized and the disabled without reference to the now-controversial natural law principles on contraception. Fr. Marvin O'Connell, a history professor at the University of St. Thomas and an advocate for the right to life, wrote in 1970, "The two matters [contraception and abortion] are very different, and Catholics who might disagree violently over the morality of preventing conception surely can be of one mind about the sacredness of life once conceived."[57]

In the 1930s and 1940s, when they were engaged in arguments with Protestants who accepted artificial birth control but not abortion, Catholics had insisted on the connection between contraception and abortion, saying that one would lead to the other. Those predictions seemed to come true in the late 1960s, when secular abortion rights advocates, such as Larry Lader, began arguing that abortion should be the "accepted back-up" for contraceptive failure.[58] But rather than take credit for predicting this chain of events, most Catholic bishops tried to say as little as possible about the connection between contraception and abortion. They knew that in an era when an overwhelming majority of non-Catholics, along with at least half of all Catholic couples of childbearing age, were using contraceptives, they had nothing to gain and much to lose by pressing this argument.

A few theologically conservative Catholics—including lay pro-life activists, such as Randy Engel, and clergy, such as Fr. Paul Marx—continued to echo papal encyclicals, such as *Casti Connubii* and *Humanae Vitae*, in linking abortion to what Georgetown University philosophy professor Germain Grisez called a "contraceptive mentality." In their view, Americans were beginning to accept abortion only because they had already accepted the principle that unwanted pregnancies should be prevented, and if they could not do that before conception, they would do it after conception.[59] But most American Catholic clergy disagreed. Several of the most prominent right-to-life advocates in the church—including James McHugh, Richard McCormick, and John Noonan—had given strong hints that they would have liked to see the church liberalize its stance on contraception; they now saw birth control and abortion as very distinct issues. And even some bishops who might have supported the church's conservative stance on contraception recognized that if they were to win the fight on abortion, they would need a very different framing of the issue. "I hope we can do better on it than we did on birth control," said Bishop Paul F. Tanner, the National Catholic Welfare Conference director, in a letter to a fellow bishop in 1966, when he was contemplating how the church could mount an effective campaign against abortion.[60]

Unlike the earlier Catholic campaign against contraception, which had relied heavily on natural law arguments about the purpose of sex—and the suggestion that if contraception were legalized, sexual immorality would be encouraged—the documents of Vatican II offered an alternative framing of the abortion issue that the clergy believed would have much broader appeal: the framework of human dignity and concern for all people, including the marginalized. The head of the church's Family Life Bureau, Fr. James T. McHugh, promoted this framing of the issue in the communications that he sent out as the coordinator of the church's pro-life campaign and as the creator of the National Right to Life Committee in 1968. As a young, moderately politically liberal priest who was a strong supporter of Vatican II, McHugh drew on widely shared human rights concerns in his campaign to frame the abortion issue in the context of the "Christian value on human life."

In January 1969, McHugh sent a sermon outline to bishops throughout the nation so that priests in every diocese could preach a uniform defense of the pro-life position to those who attended Sunday Mass. The sermon outline began with the principle that humans were created in the image of God. Every human being had a "heavenly destiny." As creatures bearing the image of God, humans had rights and responsibilities, just as Vatican II had declared. They were not merely individuals, but individuals in community, connected first of all to God through Christ, but also in relationship with other humans. The "bond" of that communal unity was "love." "Order in community requires law," the sermon outline said. "Individual ethical convictions are inadequate." Foremost among the rights that the law had a duty to protect was the right to life and "bodily integrity." That right was threatened by abortion, euthanasia, infanticide, and "killing—war." The last example, which reflected McHugh's left-of-center political convictions, might have played particularly well among parishioners who had become concerned about the war in Vietnam.

McHugh's sermon outline included a wide range of citations from Vatican II documents and from John XXIII's *Pacem in Terris*, a reflection of the fact that he saw the church's right-to-life campaign as deeply grounded in the social teaching of the church from the 1960s and its "Christo-centric humanism." The sermon outline noted that the value of human life was connected to humans' status as divine image-bearers and to their "eternal destiny." If humans were created to live forever with God, their lives had incalculable value, and the state and society therefore had a "responsibility to safeguard human life at every stage of its existence."[61]

When preaching a sermon in church, a Catholic priest was free to ground the right to life in the principle of humans' "eternal destiny," but when speaking in a secular space, pro-life Catholics commonly grounded their arguments in science and in the language of the U.S. Constitution. The Fifth and Fourteenth Amendments' prohibition on depriving anyone of "life, liberty, or property" without "due process" protected the unborn if they could show that the fetus was a human being, they thought, which they believed science and natural reason could show.[62] But even if they thought that one could make the case for a right to life on completely secular grounds, the Christocentric humanist framework outlined by Vatican II and papal encyclicals such as *Pacem in Terris* gave them an additional theological impetus for their campaign. Their fight against abortion was a foundational step toward the creation of a just society that would protect the life, freedom, and dignity of every person as an image-bearer of God who was created for eternity and for a life in community with God and others.

Because this was a political and social vision grounded in the principle of human rights, it was impossible to separate it from the world of politics; opposition to abortion could not therefore be merely a private conviction or an internal church teaching. "The function of the law is to protect and support the rights of every person," the National Conference of Catholic Bishops (NCCB) declared in November 1970. "Proposed liberalization of the present abortion laws ignores the most basic of these rights, the right to life itself. . . . The law must establish every possible protection for the child before and after birth." The NCCB cited one of the declarations of Vatican II for this political mandate. But in keeping with the liberal social vision of the Catholic Church in this era, the bishops envisioned antiabortion laws as positive, rights-based affirmations, not punitive laws that punished individuals who obtained or provided abortions. They thought the solution to the problem of abortion would come from an ethic of social responsibility that would include "compassion and justice for the expectant mother," expressed in the form of "medical and other insistence." "The evil of abortion is not exclusively the responsibility of one person," the bishops stated. "Government and all voluntary agencies" needed to do their part to offer assistance to pregnant women.[63]

This framework was inspiring not only for Catholics on the political right but also for many on the political left. In the 1960s and early 1970s, many even of the most theologically conservative Catholic clergy and theologians were liberals when it came to African American civil rights and the Vietnam War. Cardinal Patrick O'Boyle, who threatened disciplinary measures against priests in his diocese who publicly dissented from *Humanae Vitae*, delivered an invocation at the March on Washington in 1963 and was a strong supporter of the rights of African Americans.

He saw the legalization of abortion in Washington, DC, as a form of "genocide" against the city's majority-Black population.[64] Germain Grisez, who was a strong defender of the church's teaching on contraception even when many bishops were downplaying it, opposed not only abortion but also capital punishment, nuclear deterrence, and the Vietnam War, which he said "poses many problems from an ethical point of view."[65] And if this was true of some of the church's theological conservatives, it was even more true of some of the more progressive bishops. Cardinal John Dearden, archbishop of Detroit, who was famous for supporting labor causes and civil rights campaigns in the city, explicitly connected the antiabortion campaign to opposition to the Vietnam War in 1972. "We cannot be selective in our love for life," Dearden said in September 1972. "The very same reasons call on us to protect it wherever and however it is threatened, whether through the suffocation of poverty or in villages ravaged by napalm or unborn life in a mother's womb."[66]

This liberal framing of the issue made the pro-life cause appealing to some politicians on the left, especially if they were Catholic. In the early 1970s, the best known liberal Democratic U.S. senator, Ted Kennedy, took a position on abortion that closely paralleled Dearden's. "Wanted or unwanted, I believe that human life, even at its earliest stages, has certain rights which must be recognized — the right to be born, the right to love, the right to grow old," Kennedy said in 1971. "When history looks back to this era it should recognize this generation as one which cared about human beings enough to halt the practice of war, to provide a decent living for every family, and to fulfill its responsibility to its children from the very moment of conception."[67]

To be sure, not every pro-life Catholic was a social or political liberal or an opponent of the Vietnam War. Some in the movement, such as Notre Dame law professor Charles E. Rice and National Right to Life Committee administrator and lawyer Juan Ryan, were political conservatives who strongly supported the military. Ryan was a Republican and a member of the National Rifle Association (NRA); Rice was a veteran of the U.S. Marines.[68] But in the late 1960s and early 1970s, the bishops who took the lead in framing the abortion issue were often sympathetic to the liberal wing of the Democratic Party. Dearden, for instance, served as president of the NCCB from 1966 to 1971; he thus took a leading role in framing the bishops' official responses to social issues at the time, including both abortion and the war. At a time when the vast majority of Catholic voters were still Democrats and when the priesthood was attracting an unusually high number of social justice-minded liberals, the political orientation of both the American Catholic Church and of the pro-life movement was still reflective both of New Deal liberalism and the social teaching of papal encyclicals, such as *Quadragesimo Anno* and *Pacem in Terris*. And even if not all Catholics agreed with the entire social framework that McHugh encouraged priests to present in their homilies on abortion, what united both liberals and conservatives in the pro-life cause was a belief that abortion killed unborn people, and that if it were legalized nationwide, it would open the door to a rash of other horrors, including possibly the legalization of suicide, euthanasia, or compulsory abortion in the name of population control.[69] These were things that both political liberals and conservatives among Catholics agreed would be disastrous. Regardless of their partisan ideology, their position on contraception, or their attitude toward the changes in the church that Vatican II had introduced, pro-life Catholics across the political spectrum agreed that protection for the right to life from the moment of conception was an essential foundation for a just society and for the other values they held.

CATHOLIC POPULAR OPINION ON ABORTION

Compared to the contentious issue of contraception, there was relatively little internal dissent in the Catholic Church about the issue of abortion in the late 1960s and early 1970s. No bishops expressed any objections to the church's teaching on abortion, which was a marked contrast with their private (and sometimes not-so-private) grumblings about the church's opposition to contraception. And in the early 1970s, some of the very few priests who publicly dissented from the church's teaching on abortion faced church discipline—as did Fr. Joseph O'Rourke of New York, who defied the decision of a parish priest in Marlborough, Massachusetts, to refuse the sacrament of baptism for the infant son of an unrepentant abortion rights supporter. O'Rourke was expelled from the Jesuit Order for his action.[70] Critics of the church hierarchy's stance on the issue attributed the church's apparent homogeneity on the abortion issue to the bishops' strong-arm tactics to quell dissent, but more than the bishops' actions seemed to be at play. John Deedy, the managing editor of *Commonweal* magazine, noted in early 1973 that although "there has been some Catholic dissent to certain tactics of the bishops in their anti–abortion fight . . . on the whole there appears to be a wide and in some quarters deeply felt Catholic sharing of the bishops' concern for the integrity of fetal life."[71] Public opinion polls seemed to bear this out, at least to some extent. Only 36 percent of Catholics favored the legalization of abortion for any reason during the first three months of pregnancy, according to a Gallup poll conducted in December 1972.[72] Approximately two-thirds of Catholics were thus opposed to the scale of abortion legalization permitted by *Roe v. Wade*.

Politicians in heavily Catholic states were well aware of this, and they were therefore hesitant to support the legalization of abortion. According to a NARAL estimate, only about 10 or 11 percent of the members of the members of the Massachusetts legislature were pro-choice in 1973. And in Rhode Island, the nation's most heavily Catholic state, popular opposition to abortion was so strong that the state did not comply with *Roe v. Wade* and repeal its prohibition on abortion until 1975.[73]

But if most Catholics in the 1960s and early 1970s were opposed to the full-scale legalization of elective abortion—and if most had strong moral reservations about abortion that reflected the church's teaching on the value of fetal life—large numbers of Catholics were nevertheless unwilling to take the absolutist stand on the issue the bishops did. In response to the 1966 Gallup poll question, "Do you think abortion operations should or should not be legal when the child may be deformed?" 46 percent of Catholics said that abortions in such cases should be legal; only 43 percent said that such abortions should be illegal. And in cases in which pregnancy endangered a woman's health, Catholics were even more willing to permit abortion; 70 percent said they favored legalizing abortion in cases when a woman's health was in danger. This was only slightly less than the 79 percent of Protestants who favored legalizing abortion in such cases.[74]

Still, though, Gallup polls throughout the 1960s consistently showed that Catholics were less supportive of abortion than Protestants, even if the gap between the two religious groups was narrowing. And polls also consistently indicated during this decade that the vast majority of Catholics opposed the legalization of elective abortion. The majority were willing to legalize abortion for narrowly defined medical reasons, but only 16 percent of Catholics in January 1966 said that abortion should be a legal option "when a family does not have enough money to support another child," compared to 78 percent who said that abortion should not be legal in such cases. Three years later, in November 1969, 58 percent of Catholics said that they would oppose a law that "would permit a woman to go to the doctor to end a pregnancy at any time during the first three months"; only 31 percent of Catholics said that they would support such a law. In 1973, immediately after *Roe v. Wade*, Catholic support for the legalization of elective abortion during the first trimester of pregnancy increased to 36 percent, but that was as high as it got for a while. In March 1974, only 32 percent of Catholics said that they approved of the Supreme Court's decision in *Roe v. Wade*, and 61 percent opposed it. Opposition to the decision may have been even higher among Catholic women. A poll taken only of women in 1973 showed that only 27 percent of Catholic women approved of the Court's decision in *Roe*; 69 percent disapproved. By contrast, 46 percent of Protestant women approved of the Court's decision; only 44 percent disapproved.[75]

Based on all of these polls, it seems fair to say that approximately two-thirds of Catholics generally opposed elective abortion and more or less accepted the church's views on the issue, even if a substantial number of them were also willing to allow for abortion in a few areas where the church was not, especially in cases where pregnancy endangered a woman's health. At a time when church attendance rates and levels of religious devotion were higher among women in the Catholic Church than they were among men, it is perhaps not surprising that public opinion polls also seemed to indicate that opposition to abortion was slightly higher among Catholic women than among Catholic men. And opposition to abortion was far higher among Catholic women than among Protestant women. They might have been willing to legalize abortion for exceptional situations, such as when pregnancy endangered a woman's life or health. But most did not want it to be easy to obtain for just any reason. The unborn child was too valuable.

CATHOLIC ENGAGEMENT WITH CRITICISM OF THE PRO-LIFE POSITION

If the truth of the church's general teaching on abortion seemed obvious to most Catholics (even if some of them might have quibbled about its particular applications in extraordinary situations), it was not so obvious to many of those outside the church. Catholics who argued for the legislation of their views on the basis of science and universally accessible natural law had to deal with the uncomfortable fact that most Americans outside the church did not take their position. Supporters of abortion rights were wrong to assert that *only* Catholics opposed abortion or that the right-to-life movement was *merely* a Catholic cause; substantial numbers of Black Protestants and theologically conservative white Protestants (and even a few Jews and liberal Protestants) also supported legal restrictions on abortion in the early 1970s. Nevertheless, Catholic arguments against abortion had their greatest appeal to Catholics, and when one moved outside the church, those arguments did not have quite the same resonance.

This was true even of what many pro-life Catholics considered a watertight argument: the argument that because the zygote had a unique genetic composition from the moment of conception, and because the fetus, even during the early weeks of the first trimester, was not a formless blob of cells but was instead a body with a beating heart and a growing brain, the fetus was a person and abortion was a form of killing. But even though science could reveal *what* was happening during fetal development, it could not explain its meaning or its implications for abortion policy. Pro-life Catholics may have been a bit taken aback when the author of one of the science books they used to demonstrate the unique genetic composition of the zygote—*Life before Birth*, published in 1964 by the Princeton anthropology professor Ashley Montagu—stated that he did not agree with the political and philosophical implications that pro-life advocates drew from the scientific facts that his book presented. "From the moment of conception the organism thus brought into being possesses all the potentialities for humanity in its genes, and for that reason must be considered human," Montagu conceded. He then added, "But in point of fact the embryo, fetus, and newborn of the species does not really become functionally human until it has been humanized in the human socialization process. Humanity is an achievement, not an endowment. The potentialities constitute the endowment, their fulfillment requires a humanizing environment."[76] Montagu's phrasing, which suggested that even the newborn "does not really become functionally human" until it underwent the "human socialization process," seemed to confirm pro-life Catholics' warning that the same arguments used to justify legalized abortion would eventually lead to the acceptance of infanticide, even though this was presumably not Montagu's intention. But it also demonstrated that science alone could not solve the abortion debate, despite pro-life Catholics' argument that their pro-life views stemmed from clear scientific facts. Scientific facts were not self-interpreting, as Montagu's statements indicated; they depended on a larger philosophical context for their meaning.

Some Catholic pro-life activists recognized this. Robert Byrn, a Fordham University law professor who was one of the most prominent activists in the pro-life movement in the early 1970s, explained that Montagu's scientific findings about the zygote and embryo were clearly "based on fact," but "his relegation of the unborn and the newborn to the 'potentiality of humanity' is based, not on the facts of life, but on several personal value judgments." Montagu and other pro-choice activists, he thought, believed that "the right to live depends, not on the existence of life, but on the social quality of the life."[77] This was probably a correct assessment. Many of the arguments in favor of the liberalization of abortion laws in the late 1960s and early 1970s focused on the negative quality of life that would result if abortion were restricted. Women would die or experience severe injuries if they sought out dangerous illegal abortions. Unwanted children would be born into the world who would experience abuse or a life of poverty and crime. The world would become overpopulated. And women would be denied gender equality and bodily autonomy.

In defending their position, pro-life Catholics suggested that some of these predictions of negative consequences if abortion requests were denied were exaggerated. The problems commonly blamed on overpopulation were actually problems of "distribution," not population growth, Fr. James McHugh said, and the solution to those problems was not to limit births but rather to provide better housing, transportation, education, and employment opportunities outside of major cities.[78] Abortion, pro-life Catholics argued, would not solve these problems. Nor would it solve the problem of child abuse, which they said was more likely to occur to "wanted" children who ended up disappointing the parents than to "unwanted" children who might have been considered candidates for abortion. Catholics believed there were technological, legal, and social solutions to some of the problems that their critics said that legalized abortion would ameliorate, but they also acknowledged that abortion prohibitions might require suffering and self-sacrifice on the part of people who would have to care for disabled children and others who might be a difficult emotional and financial burden. Some called for greater government assistance to help families caring for disabled children. But in keeping with Catholic theology, Catholics also spoke of the redemptive value of suffering, including the suffering of those who cared for the "unwanted" and the needy and the suffering of women who endured severe health setbacks in order to carry a pregnancy to term.

The church had long taught the value of self-denial and redemptive suffering in imitation of Christ, and it reiterated this teaching in Vatican II: "By suffering for us He [Jesus] not only provided us with an example for our imitation, He blazed a trail, and if we follow it, life and death are made holy and take on a new meaning," said *Gaudium et Spes* (1965). In 1969, Fr. James McHugh applied this call to suffer to the specific task of choosing life for the unborn: "Without denying the sacrifices that are sometimes required to safeguard human life, we find 'that man's basic responsibility is to eliminate the bases of evil, ignorance, and injustice rather than to provide for an easier termination of developing human life.'"[79]

Such calls to self-sacrifice might have been difficult to accept under any circumstances, but they were especially challenging when they came from an all-male hierarchy and were directed at women who accepted the premises of second-wave feminism. In the first few years of the abortion debate, during the early 1960s, the church's all-male hierarchy had not necessarily been a public relations problem in the abortion debate, because the most prominent proponents of abortion law liberalization were also men; abortion had not yet become a feminist issue. But after the late 1960s, when the National Organization for Women and other second-wave feminist organizations began championing abortion rights as a signature cause, the debate about abortion became a debate about women's rights, and in this debate, the Catholic Church appeared to be at a serious disadvantage. It was hard to convince people that the defense of the unborn was a liberal human rights cause when it seemed to be diametrically at odds with the freedom and equality of women. To convince people that this was not the case, the Catholic Church and the pro-life campaign would have to promote a different version of feminism, a version that was based not on bodily autonomy or even on gender equality but on biological difference.

ABORTION AND THE FORMATION OF A CONSERVATIVE CATHOLIC FEMINISM OF BIOLOGICAL DIFFERENCE

In 1971, Clare Boothe Luce, a Catholic convert who was also an accomplished writer and former member of the U.S. House of Representatives and U.S. ambassador to Italy, told an audience that she agreed with the church's teaching on abortion, but the church had failed to "convince *women*" of abortion's horrors. The abortion question would ultimately be decided in "the political arena of a pluralistic society, and by an electorate that is now 50 percent female," she noted, so unless the church persuaded non-Catholic women to oppose abortion, the church would lose the political battle. The Jesuit editors of *America* magazine agreed. For years, they had run editorials on abortion from an all-male cast of theologians, but now, in the era of second-wave feminism, they decided that "the Church's presentation of its position must be more modern, more feminine, more self-consistent." They did not think that the teaching itself needed to be changed, but it needed to be presented in a way that honored women's perspectives to a greater degree.[80] Although some of the bishops had previously sidelined women's voices in the abortion debate during the 1960s, they changed their tune at the beginning of the 1970s and began giving pro-life women speaking opportunities in an effort to counteract feminist criticism. In New Jersey, several parishes that had never before allowed a woman to preach invited lay married Catholic women in 1970 to present sermons against abortion from the pulpit during Mass.[81]

Public opinion polls at the time indicated that Catholic women were more likely than Catholic men to oppose abortion, so recruiting women as spokespersons for the pro-life cause was not difficult. Catholic women such as Elizabeth Goodwin in California, Alice Hartle in Minnesota, Mary Winter in Pennsylvania, and Ellen McCormack in New York had already taken the lead in organizing pro-life groups in their states and mobilizing women in the campaign. From the moment that state legislatures began considering abortion liberalization bills, Catholic women had written numerous letters to their state senators and representatives to urge them to vote against the legalization of abortion.[82] In doing so, they articulated not only a commitment to unborn human life but also a vision of gender difference that contrasted with the views of second-wave feminists, such as Betty Friedan. Pro-choice feminists like Friedan argued that women's equality depended on their right to have abortions in order to avoid unwanted pregnancies, but pro-life Catholic feminists argued that instead, women's equality depended on society's willingness to protect and support pregnancies and to affirm the important role that women had in giving birth.

"Full feminine humanity includes distinctly feminine functions," Sidney Callahan, a self-identified pro-life feminist wrote in the *National Catholic Reporter* in 1972. "Women need not identify with male sexuality, male aggression, and wombless male lifestyles in order to win social equality." "In my feminist view, every abortion represents an abandonment of women and children."[83] Such a view accorded well with Catholic social teaching that argued that the government had a responsibility to support families, and other Catholic pro-life feminists also championed it.

Like Callahan, many of the Catholic women who opposed abortion embraced a version of "difference" feminism that advocated rights for women within a framework that emphasized biological differences between the sexes. Women's ability to bear children was especially important to them. In their view, abortion was an attack not only on human life but also on women and their childbearing role. Pro-choice advocates commonly emphasized women's bodily autonomy and personal choice—an approach that often depicted fetal rights claims and women's rights as competing concerns—but pro-life women saw an inseparable relationship between fetal rights and women's rights, because they saw the connection between mother and child as the closest of all human relationships. "There is no relationship so intimate as that between a woman and her unborn child," Mary Winter, founder of Women Concerned for the Unborn Child, told the Pennsylvania legislature in 1972. After introducing herself as a "mother of seven children, the youngest as yet unborn," she argued that mothers had special insight into the abortion question—but not because they alone had a right to decide what happened to their own bodies (as pro-choice advocates argued) but because they had an instinctive and intimate knowledge of fetal life that no one other than a mother had ever experienced. "Science has been increasingly confirming over the last 100 years what we women have known instinctively since Eve," Winter said. "Since human life begins at conception, motherhood begins at conception also and women instinctively know this, whether or not we like to admit it."[84]

For Catholic women who had long prayed to the Virgin Mary as the ideal mother and who had reflected on her role in carrying the unborn baby Jesus for the nine months between the Annunciation and the Nativity, the idea that motherhood began at conception did seem instinctive. So did the idea that the motherly connection with their children, beginning even before the children were born, was the ultimate expression of femininity, and that an attack on that connection was by implication also an attack on women. Abortion was "the ultimate exploitation of women," Winter said. "The anti-life mentality is so foreign to the feminine mentality which, I believe, is biologically, instinctively geared toward the protection and nurturing of the young and the helpless."[85]

Whereas pro-choice feminists saw legal, safe abortion as a way for women to protect themselves against the consequences of unwanted pregnancy, especially in the cases of rape or short-term sexual relationships, Catholic pro-life feminists saw abortion as a way for other people—such as the woman's family, the woman's sexual partner, and society at large—to exploit women and then abandon them. "In the vast majority of cases it is not the woman who rejects her unborn child, but it is the pregnant woman who is rejected by a society that looks upon the unwed mother as an outcast or that sees the woman with more than two children as a threat," Winter said. "Women are literally deserted by the society at large in their role as mother. . . . When she is offered abortion as the only answer, she then submits to a degrading procedure that is mentally and physically hazardous—but society is satisfied, her family breathes a sigh of relief, the baby's father has been spared responsibility and the physician smiles as he rings up another sale."[86]

Instead of an alleviation from personal responsibility, Catholic women who were active in the pro-life movement called for a more compassionate society, just as Vatican II had. Winter herself advocated an expanded social safety net—"progressive humanitarian solutions" for the "distressed pregnant woman," as she phrased it. "She should be able to be confident that if some problems rise that are beyond her capacity she can trust her community, like a larger family surrounding and supporting her, to provide the assistance she needs," Winter said. This was very much in keeping with the spirit of traditional Catholic social teaching and practice. It was also a rejection of the philosophy of personal autonomy and a call for everyone to sacrifice their own personal interests in order to support human life, including the lives of the most vulnerable. To pro-choice feminists who said that abortion rights were necessary for women's liberation,

Winter had one question: "What are we being liberated from? From caring about the smallest and weakest and most disadvantaged members of society?"[87]

Above all, pro-life women's view on abortion stemmed from their firm conviction that the fetus was a baby and that laws against abortion were a way to protect them from murder. They often minced no words in their description of what they thought abortion really entailed for the fetus. "People have been fooled into thinking that the unborn are not human and . . . this misconception has led people to close their eyes to both the fact of the killing that occurs in abortion and the cruel method by which this killing is accomplished," Mary Ann Knight said on a local Southern California radio program in 1970. "Aborted babies die by being cut into pieces, suffocated or pickled alive. . . . Abortion permits no survivors. Society has the obligation to help the pregnant woman who has a problem but it cannot allow her to kill her unborn child any more than it could allow her to kill those children already born."[88]

The letters that pro-life Catholic women sent to their state legislators expressed a similar conviction. Blending invocations of God's sovereignty over human life, the Judeo-Christian prohibition on murder, and an appeal to constitutional principles and to natural law, they inveighed against abortion legalization proposals with the full conviction that the fetus was a human person with the right to life. "Every Catholic I know is opposed to this Bill," Eileen King told California state senator Anthony Beilenson, author of an abortion liberalization bill, in 1967. "Since when do we have the right to take a life? To kill an unborn child is just as wrong as killing a child or a full-grown person. . . . As a Catholic and as a person, I am offended by this Bill." Abortion liberalization "would pave the way for abortion for almost any reason, leading to a slaughter of the innocents," Rosa Belonzie wrote. "The Therapeutic Abortion Act seriously offends the Christian position, because it means killing a child who has both a natural and a constitutional right to life." "As a citizen, wife, and mother of four children I am much against legalizing the Therapeutic Abortion Bill," Mary Miani stated. "This bill is not only against my principals [sic], but against the natural laws of humanity." "God alone is the author of life,"

Mary Dowd told Beilenson. "We the people of the state of California do not want murder legalized. . . . May God grant you the courage to protect the babies."[89]

The letter writers often argued that there were more humane solutions to the problems that abortion liberalization bills would allegedly address. Instead of "taking of thousands of innocent unborn children's lives each year," Mary Kay Rennard said, "I believe there are other alternatives to be taken if a woman or young girl becomes pregnant outside of marriage. We have adoption agencies, social services, & medical care." Just as Catholic male clerics did, some of these women predicted that euthanasia and other horrors would follow the legalization of abortion. They wanted to promote the value of life, not destroy it. "As a mother, I believe each new life is to be nurtured," said Maria Wagner.[90]

Many Catholic women held these views even when it came to very difficult pregnancies. When Eunice Kennedy Shriver, a disability rights advocate who was the younger sister of President John F. Kennedy, was invited to square off against abortion rights advocate Alan F. Guttmacher in a forum on abortion in *McCall's* magazine in April 1968, she began her article with one of the most difficult questions that pro-life advocates had to confront: "Should a woman be forced to bear within her body the product of a rape?" The question was difficult, Shriver conceded. But she then proceeded to discuss what abortion did to a woman and to the society that legalized it, and she said that the solution was not to legalize abortion but instead to help the pregnant woman in crisis. "Instead of becoming the Hard Society, we could become a just and compassionate one," Shriver wrote. "Instead of destroying life, we could destroy the conditions that make life intolerable. In this society, every child, regardless of his capacities or the circumstances of his birth, would be welcomed, loved, and cared for—and abortion would cease to preoccupy us, because abortion would not be necessary."[91]

Like many other pro-life Catholics, Shriver presented an argument for fetal personhood from genetics. Every embryo and fetus had a unique DNA that differed from the DNA of the mother. Every embryo and fetus, if allowed to grow and continue living without interruption, would be born and develop into a toddler, a teenager, and then an adult, using the same genetic material that it had at the moment of conception. "Arguments favoring abortion generally proceed on the assumption that life outside the womb is somehow essentially distinct from life inside the womb," Shriver wrote. But genetics undercut these arguments by showing the continuity between life in its earliest stages in the womb and life after birth.

Shriver's use of a scientific argument to prove her case was hardly surprising; pro-life Catholics almost invariably used this argument in secular spaces, since it was designed to be acceptable to all people, regardless of their faith tradition. But Guttmacher brushed away the argument, seeing no particular value in an "undifferentiated mass of cells" even if they did have a unique genetic composition. Perhaps recognizing that the full effect of her argument depended not merely on science but on a theistic presupposition, Shriver followed up her scientific argument with a statement of her religious reasons for believing that human life had value from the moment of conception. "I believe that God is our creator, that He made us to his own image and likeness, that He is the steward of our life, and that He has not granted us power over other innocent lives," Shriver said. "For everything we know of God tells us that he values the life of every human being and commands us to respect and safeguard it at every stage, in every condition and circumstance. Having sure knowledge of the uniqueness and potential of the life within a mother's womb, I cannot grasp how we can righteously claim authority to destroy it."[92]

That was the Catholic argument in a nutshell—science, reason, and theology demonstrated the continuity between the embryo and the adult human, and an understanding of God as the creator and sustainer of every human life was the basis for the moral imperative to fulfill the mission of God by protecting life and creating the social conditions that would support the vulnerable. The alternative, Shriver said, was the "Hard Society."

At the time Shriver wrote, abortion was still illegal in most states, and likeminded politically liberal Catholics still thought they had a chance of creating a society that valued human life from conception to natural death. But *Roe v. Wade* struck a decisive blow at the foundation of this vision. In the days immediately following the decision, pro-life Catholics wrote to Justice Harry Blackmun not only to excoriate the Court ruling but also to lament the loss of their Christocentric humanist vision for society and their fear for a future in which the right to life was no longer legally honored. They felt like they had lost their country. "When the Supreme Court defaults in protecting the innocent, to whom do we turn?" Robert O'Malley of El Paso, Texas, asked Blackmun. "Is America to become a land of little hitlers playing God and deciding who is to live or die?" Nancy Fillion of Minneapolis said the Court ruling left her "sorrowful and despairing." "Why do we work so hard to end the killing in Viet Nam and practically on the same day begin a war on countless unborn children in America?" she asked. "It used to be that civil law was a good index to use to form one's conscience," Maureen Tauer wrote, using the Catholic language of conscience formation. "But your recent actions have erased that principle." "We say one nation under God. Are we?" a "Mrs. Paul Niemhalt" asked. "When the 5th Commandment of God says 'Thou shalt not kill,' and we tell any woman she is free to have her own baby murdered? . . . I am sure most of our Doctors when taking an oath to preserve life, didn't expect to be forced into mass murder of innocent babies." "The insane court decision to liberalize abortion is an attack upon the family and thus will weaken this country," a couple from Everett, Massachusetts, told Blackmun. The decision was a "catastrophe for America," Cardinal Patrick O'Boyle, archbishop of Washington, DC, declared.[93]

Many Catholics — including O'Boyle and the nation's other bishops — decided that they had to fight back. In this fight they were joined by a group they had considered unlikely allies: evangelical Protestants. Most evangelicals did not necessarily share the larger social vision that had shaped Catholic thinking on abortion, but they had their own reasons for opposing *Roe*, and eventually their political theology would reshape the pro-life movement.

CHAPTER 3

EVANGELICALS BEFORE *ROE*

A Moderate Conservatism on Abortion

In the summer of 1971, *Christianity Today* issued a firm denunciation of abortion. The magazine had waffled on the subject for the previous four years, suggesting that the procedure was morally problematic and generally objectionable, but also publishing articles by evangelicals who argued that it was legitimate in at least some circumstances. *Christianity Today's* editors had cautiously accepted the early abortion liberalization laws of the late 1960s, which had permitted abortion only for a narrow range of medically related reasons. But when New York and three other states legalized elective abortion through most of the second trimester, the editors decided they had had enough. Abortion was evil because it was "murder," they said.

L. Nelson Bell—the father-in-law of the magazine's founder, Billy Graham, and one of the magazine's editors—wrote one of the pieces denouncing abortion. This was especially fitting, since Bell was a physician who had served as a medical missionary to China in his younger years and who therefore was uniquely qualified to weigh in on this medical procedure. Bell pulled no punches in his diatribe against abortion. "Abortion on demand," he said, was "the wanton destruction of life." But then he mentioned what to a later generation of evangelicals might have seemed a shocking fact. He himself, as a physician, had performed a few abortions that he believed were medically necessary. And he did not indicate that he was sorry for doing so.[1]

Bell's position as both an unrepentant performer of a few medically necessary abortions and an opponent of abortion who considered the procedure to be the "destruction of life" typified the evangelical stance toward abortion at the beginning of the 1970s. Unlike Catholics, evangelicals lacked a clear theological position on when human personhood began or a clear sense that abortion was always sinful. Unlike liberal Protestants, they also lacked a clear reason for supporting abortion rights, since, with only a few exceptions, evangelicals were not attracted to the population-control movement, second-wave feminism, rights consciousness, or relativistic views of morality that had led many on the Protestant left to champion the idea that the abortion choice should be left to individual women. For years, they approached the issue with caution, taking a generally conservative stance, but one that still left enough flexibility to countenance a few abortions in exceptional circumstances or continue fellowshipping with those whose views on abortion were somewhat more permissive. But white evangelicals eventually found the theological and political framework to make sense of the abortion debate, and when they did so, they became the nation's strongest opponents of abortion, a stance from which they did not waver even as other religious groups dropped out of the antiabortion coalition.

EVANGELICALS' EARLY VIEWS OF CONTRACEPTION AND ABORTION

For evangelicals, discussions of abortion were never far removed from discussions of the Bible, either debates about what the Bible said about abortion specifically or larger conversations about biblical authority. That was not surprising, because modern evangelicalism in the United States could trace its roots to an early twentieth-century coalition of conservative Protestants who wanted to champion the authority of the Bible against liberal Protestant critiques of the doctrine of biblical inerrancy. For most of the nineteenth century, the majority of Protestant churches placed a primacy on the authority and historicity of the Bible and emphasized a personal relationship with God through faith in Jesus and belief in Christ's substitutionary atoning death. But in the early twentieth century, some Protestant ministers and theology professors began to see the Bible as a product of historical evolution, which meant that it was still a source of divine wisdom, but not inerrant in every detail. They also began to see sin in structural rather than merely individual terms, which meant that the call of the gospel was not primarily aimed at individual conversion but at social transformation. And though not necessarily giving up belief in the divinity of Christ, they began to give more emphasis to Jesus's inspiring moral example than to either his divine identity or his work of atonement on the cross. Theologically conservative Protestants who were known first as fundamentalists resisted all of these trends. They continued to champion the hallmarks of nineteenth-century Protestantism: the authority and historical accuracy of scripture, the necessity of individual conversion, the literal reality of all the biblical miracles, and the doctrine that Jesus's death on the cross literally paid the penalty for sin and that this pardon for sin was available for anyone who placed their faith in Jesus. In the 1940s, some of these fundamentalists began calling themselves "evangelicals" because of their desire to highlight the traditional gospel message (that is, the "evangelical" message) of the Christian faith.[2]

Compared to other Christians, evangelicals took a more individualistic view of sin, salvation, and morality. Sin was individual rather than structural, salvation was obtained through an individual act of faith rather than mediated through the church or sacrament, and morality was primarily about individual holy living rather than social transformation. The Bible—which they thought individuals could read and interpret for themselves, with minimal input from church or clergy—was their primary guide to individual ethics. Such individualism was in part rooted in the Reformation doctrine of *sola fide* ("faith alone") and *sola scriptura* ("scripture alone"), but evangelicals took this individualism to new heights. In the mid-twentieth century, this theological emphasis was especially prevalent among Southern Baptists (and among some Methodists and Presbyterians in the South) and among northern conservative Protestants who opposed the theological liberalism of the North's major Protestant denominations.

Fundamentalists (or evangelicals) differed with liberal Protestants on many things in the early twentieth century, but initially abortion did not seem to be one of them. Abortion was illegal everywhere in the United States, and no minister at the time suggested that it should be legalized. No denomination had yet taken an official stand in favor of birth control, let alone abortion. None countenanced premarital sex. But in an early sign of political divisions that would become more evident later, fundamentalists often went well beyond modernists in their opposition to flapper culture and their anxiety about potential cultural threats to the family and to traditional gender roles. They preached sermons warning that the nation's survival depended on the maintenance of a divinely mandated family structure. The Chicago-based fundamentalist magazine *Moody Monthly* said in 1928 that "America will go as her homes go. If her homes are Christian, she and the world are safe. But if her homes are godless, Ichabod is already written on her flag."[3]

A similar anxiety about family life and motherhood had prompted a few Protestant ministers to preach against abortion in the late 1860s, and in the 1920s and 1930s fundamentalists returned to this theme, especially as liberal Protestants of the era began embracing the cause of "planned parenthood" as a natural outgrowth of the Social Gospel. Fundamentalists believed that birth control was wrong not because it violated natural law (as Catholics believed) but because it was a way for women to avoid the God-given responsibility of motherhood. There "is no greater sin on earth to-day" than the refusal of a married woman to have children, John Roach Straton, pastor of New York City's fundamentalistic Calvary Baptist Church, said in 1920, because "the home life of the people is at last the hope of the Republic."[4] But if birth control was an evasion of the God-given duty of parenthood, abortion was worse because it was "murder," as Bob Jones Sr. termed it in 1930. To many fundamentalists, it was unthinkable. "Abortion," the Texas Baptist evangelist and *Sword of the Lord* editor John R. Rice said in 1945, was "the willful murder of the little one where conception has already taken place and life has already begun" and was "a crime prohibited by law and condemned by all decent people."[5]

Rice's statement suggests that many fundamentalists assumed as a matter of course that the fetus was a human being and that abortion deserved to be treated as a "crime." This view was hardly surprising, because the antiabortion laws—which few people other than a very limited number of doctors were then challenging—reflected this assumption. Even liberal Protestant publications at the time echoed this view. One mainline Protestant book published in 1957—Evelyn Millis Duvall's *Facts of Life and Love for Teen-agers*, written by a marriage counselor affiliated with the National Council of Churches' Joint Department of Family Life and published by the Young Men's Christian Association—declared that induced abortion was "a criminal offense in most states, unless it is done by a doctor to save the life of the mother. Even then it is considered a sin by some church groups. Since the purposive killing of the unborn baby not only destroys its life but also may endanger the health of the mother, any abortion is a serious affair."[6] The differences between conservative evangelical Protestants and liberal Protestants on abortion became evident only in the 1960s, when many liberal Protestants embraced the cause of abortion law reform. But by then, some conservative Protestants were also ready to reconsider their traditional views on reproductive issues. Most did not want to go as far as liberal Protestants who supported abortion rights, but at the same time, they wanted to avoid the condemnatory attitudes toward birth control that had characterized their fundamentalist predecessors' sermons on the issue a generation earlier.

In the 1920s, no Protestant denomination officially supported birth control, and the movement was still associated with feminism and with the political left, including with radicals such as Margaret Sanger and a few liberal Protestant ministers who supported her. It was therefore easy for fundamentalists such as John Roach Straton to oppose it. But by the 1950s, birth control had become thoroughly domesticated as a part of middle-class Protestant married life. Married women were using it not as a way to avoid childbearing altogether (as Straton had feared) but as a way to space pregnancies and end their childbearing after giving birth to three or four children. In an era of the largest baby boom in decades, it was difficult to argue that birth control was a threat to motherhood, family, or the republic. Some mainstream evangelicals therefore began suggesting that married couples could use contraception as long as they did not seek to avoid parenthood altogether, which they believed would violate God's creation mandate in Genesis 1 to "be fruitful and multiply." "I don't think there's anything wrong with birth control per se," said Harold J. Ockenga, a Boston pastor who had served as the first president of the National Association of Evangelicals (NAE). Other evangelicals were more cautious, with NAE president Herbert Mekeel opposing birth control categorically as late as 1959.[7] But by the mid-1960s, Mekeel's conservative position had been largely swept aside.

Evangelical magazines in the early 1960s began promoting the idea that God intended marital sex for far more than procreation, an idea that liberal Protestants had embraced in the 1920s but that conservative evangelicals had not. Conservative evangelicals had never said that the only purpose for sex was having children, but they had once placed so much emphasis on the duty of married women to embrace the role of motherhood that any discussion that married couples could engage in sex without the intention of conceiving a child had been largely muted. But by the early 1960s, they were singing a somewhat different tune. By then, millions of married couples with children were using contraception to time their childbearing more precisely and find greater enjoyment in both parenthood and marital intimacy. The widespread popularity of the birth control pill in the 1960s made this even easier and in turn prompted evangelical magazines to revisit the issue of birth control. This time, they came out more strongly in favor of contraception than they ever had before. *Eternity* magazine, which had published an article against birth control as late as 1961, reversed course in 1966 and endorsed married Christian couples' use of the birth control pill on the grounds that sex was about far more than conceiving a child. "More of us have found our way back to the Bible concept that sex is a fact of God's creation, a means of expressing love between husband and wife as well as the means of procreation," *Eternity* writer Irene Soekren said. "Those who believe that sex in marriage is significant in its own right, not requiring procreation to justify it, can accept birth control."[8] This became the near-universal line among evangelicals: God gave sex to married couples as a gift that strengthened a marriage and was intrinsically good in itself, even when not used for procreation. Married couples had a divine mandate to have children if possible, and sex must remain only in marriage, but not all marital sex needed to be open to the possibility of conception, because the sacred gift of marital sex had spiritual purposes that went far beyond the conception of new life, as important as that was. "Perhaps the primary purpose for which God has given every normal man and woman the sex drive is to have a miraculous means of expressing the depth of spiritual love by physical means," one Presbyterian minister wrote in *Christian Life* in 1964.[9]

One of the many evangelical leaders of the era who accepted contraception was Billy Graham. He and his wife had five children, and he strongly affirmed the value of children and parenting, but he saw nothing wrong with married couples using contraceptives to decide when to have children. "There is nothing in the Bible which would forbid birth control," he said in 1959. At the same time, though, neither Graham nor other evangelicals favored the international birth control campaigns that many liberal Protestants supported.[10] Birth control should not be illegal (as American Catholic bishops still insisted), nor should it be funded by the U.S. government as part of an international aid package. But married couples who wanted it should have the freedom to use it within limits, provided that they were not trying to avoid the duty of childbearing altogether.

Like other evangelicals, Graham preached that sex belonged only in marriage. His view of gender roles was traditionally conservative, but by the standards of the 1950s, this hardly set him apart from mainstream culture. Yet there was a distinctly evangelical flavor to his belief that if illicit sexual behavior and a feminist challenge to traditional gender roles succeeded in undermining the family, the nation itself would collapse, since the two-parent nuclear family was the divinely ordained foundation for society. "The home is the citadel of American life," Graham said in 1956. "If the home is lost, all is lost."[11] This was exactly what fundamentalists had said in the 1920s, but by the 1950s, Graham had succeeded in packaging what had once been an anti-birth-control message with a limited endorsement of contraception within marriage.

Most of the evangelical discussions of birth control in the late 1950s and early 1960s did not mention abortion. This was hardly surprising. In the mid-1960s, few married middle-class women used abortion as a form of birth control; the procedure, which was still mostly illegal throughout the United States, was much more likely to be a resort of unmarried women who were panicked about their pregnancy or, in a few instances, the reluctant refuge of women whose pregnancies were not progressing normally. It was also rarely discussed in the news. In 1961, the word "abortion" appeared in only one of the thousands of articles the *New York Times* published that year, and in this case, it was only a small article on page 18 about the arrest of a New York provider of illegal abortions on charges of homicide after a twenty-three-year-old unmarried magazine writer died in his office following a botched abortion. By contrast, the phrase "birth control" appeared in forty-six articles published in the *New York Times* in 1961. "Pornography" appeared in twenty-nine articles, and "homosexuality" in eleven. And "communism"—the focus of much of Graham's preaching during the early years of the Cold War—appeared in 464.[12] Some Catholics and a few abortion law reform advocates may have been talking about abortion at the beginning of the 1960s, but the mainstream news media had not yet tuned into the conversation, and neither had most evangelicals. *Christianity Today* did not begin publishing articles on abortion until 1967.

Theologically conservative Lutherans were one of the few groups of evangelical Protestants systematically discussing abortion in the late 1950s and developing antiabortion arguments that emphasized the high value of fetal life. In 1959, Alfred Martin Rehwinkel, a professor of Christian ethics and church history at the Lutheran Church—Missouri Synod's

Concordia Seminary in St. Louis, included a discussion of abortion in a book that he published on birth control. His views on contraception were the same as those of many evangelicals from other denominational traditions who were writing about birth control at the same time. The use of birth control in marriage was legitimate, he said, as long as it was not used by "the immoral or social parasites who for selfish reasons refuse to assume the responsibility of parenthood." An endorsement of birth control "does not even encourage small families unless circumstances demand them." Instead, it "encourages married couples to have children when safe and otherwise desirable," while giving them a way to prevent pregnancies at times when they might be "dangerous and for various legitimate reasons undesirable."[13] This was a standard view among evangelicals across the denominational spectrum who were beginning to embrace the idea that Christian married couples could legitimately use contraception to space childbirths. But unlike most other evangelical writings on birth control in the late 1950s, Rehwinkel's book also included a one-page discussion of abortion, which he categorically opposed. "There is a fundamental difference between abortion and the use of contraceptives," he wrote. Contraception did not destroy human life, but abortion "always means destruction of a new life that has come into existence by the union of the male sperm and the female ovum." Rehwinkel was willing to allow for the possibility of abortion "only in the most extreme emergencies to save the life of the mother," but said that when someone resorted to abortion "merely to terminate an undesired and undesirable pregnancy," it was a "willful destruction of human life" that "must be placed in the category of murder."[14] Rehwinkel's purpose in mentioning abortion was not so much to convince his readers that abortion was evil—a point he seemed to think they already acknowledged, since, he noted, abortion for reasons other than saving a woman's life was already generally illegal—but rather to convince theologically conservative Christians who were reluctant to accept birth control that contraception and abortion were very different entities. He was not responding to the fledgling abortion law reform movement (a movement that he likely didn't even know existed) but rather to

Catholic arguments of the time that saw a connection between the prevention of unborn human life through contraception and the destruction of unborn life through abortion. The two acts were very different, Rehwinkel argued. Eventually, in the late twentieth century, Rehwinkel's answer to this potential Catholic objection would become evangelical orthodoxy. But at the time he wrote, few evangelicals were even aware of the question.

If evangelicals had paid attention to the very limited public conversation about abortion at the beginning of the 1960s, they would have seen nothing in news stories of botched illegal abortions performed on unmarried young women that would have led them to champion the cause of abortion law reform. Some liberal Protestants who read these stories insisted that the law needed to be changed to make abortion policy more "humane" for women seeking pregnancy terminations; this, in fact, was the *Christian Century*'s argument in 1961. But the liberal Protestant view that it was humane and compassionate to enable sinful behavior through more permissive laws was completely foreign to conservative evangelical thinking at the time. If sin had eternal consequences, it was never compassionate or humane to enable it or suggest in the law that it was acceptable. Evangelicals of the 1960s were unanimous in believing that all sex outside of marriage, including premarital sex, was sinful. Even as evangelicals debated a wide variety of moral issues, ranging from contraception to war to racial justice, they did not consider premarital sex or any other sexual activity outside of marriage to be a matter on which different moral opinions could legitimately be entertained. As long as abortion was portrayed in the press as an illegal activity that appealed only to women seeking to evade responsibility for a pregnancy that had occurred through illicit sexual activity, there was little chance that evangelicals would support it. What unmarried young women who died from botched abortions needed was not a safer way to terminate their pregnancies, but rather a gospel-produced deliverance from the power of sin. And what the nation's politics needed was not an abortion law reform movement but rather a wholesale evangelical campaign against pornographic magazines, which many conservative Christians (both Protestant and Catholic) blamed for the alleged decline in the nation's sexual morals.[15]

Evangelicals were predisposed to oppose abortion not only because they objected to the premarital or out-of-wedlock sex that preceded most abortions or because they believed that Christian couples had a divinely given duty to have children, but also because they had a reverence for fetal life as the creation of God, just as Rehwinkel's book had suggested. Clyde Narramore, one of the best-known evangelical Christian psychologists of the 1950s, included a lengthy section titled "Growth-Record of an Unborn Baby" in his 1956 book for teenagers, *Life and Love: A Christian View of Sex*, published by Zondervan. His purpose in this section was not to comment on abortion, which he addressed only in one short paragraph in an appendix to the book. His intention instead was to evoke a sense of wonder and awe in his readers as they contemplated the creative act of God in the formation of an embryo and fetus. After describing the process of fertilization in detail and the role of God's "divine plan" in shaping the chromosomal composition of each particular fertilized egg, he then described God's work in facilitating the embryo's rapid growth during the first month of pregnancy. "Could any mere man comprehend the amazing process by which this transformation takes place?" Narramore asked. "At work here is the intricate designing power of God! . . . After four weeks it is a very tiny being, about the size of a garden pea." And "by the second month the embryo is more clearly recognizable as human, though incredibly tiny to bear that resemblance. . . . Studies reveal that the heart and some other organs are functioning during the second month." Narramore, writing before abortion became a matter of political controversy, didn't engage in explicit speculation about exactly when the beginning of human personhood occurred or exactly what (if any) circumstances would justify the deliberate termination of fetal life, but it was clear from his lengthy description of the growth of an "unborn baby" that he viewed conception as the point at which God's divine plan for a human being began and that he saw the growth of human life from zygote to birth as a continuous, divinely guided process. There was no separate moment of ensoulment following conception nor any moment after conception when the embryo or fetus increased in value or suddenly acquired the quality of personhood. It was a unique individual from the moment of conception, and it belonged to its creator while also being fully dependent on its mother to sustain its life. "The baby is a separate being, even while living in direct dependence upon the mother's system in the uterus," Narramore said.[16]

For evangelicals who ascribed cosmic importance to the moment of conception and who viewed each stage of pregnancy as part of God's "divine plan" for both the couple who had conceived a child and for the "unborn baby" growing in embryonic form, the idea of deliberately terminating the pregnancy through an act of elective abortion didn't make sense. Indeed, Narramore's only reference to abortion came in an appendix to the book in which he briefly noted that "induced abortion" could be "criminally induced" or "therapeutic." This was standard Protestant thinking in the 1950s; elective abortion was "criminal," since it was illegal in every state, but abortions that occurred by a licensed physician in cases of medical necessity were "therapeutic." Like other evangelicals at the time, Narramore didn't get into the question that some doctors were debating about whether abortions could be legitimately performed for health reasons that went beyond strictly saving a woman's physical life in cases in which an unterminated pregnancy would likely result in her death. Some Catholic physicians were paying close attention to this debate in the 1950s, but evangelical writers were not. For them, it was sufficient to say that even in its embryonic stages, every human life was part of God's divine plan and was therefore worthy of reverence and awe, and that abortions not medically necessary were "criminal."[17]

But what about abortions deemed medically necessary? Evangelicals in the 1950s hardly ever commented on abortions performed by licensed physicians in hospitals. But in 1962 a national news story about therapeutic abortion forced people who had not thought very much about the ethics of the matter to decide what they believed. The abortion case was that of children's television star Sherri Chessen Finkbine, a married mother of four, who sought a pregnancy termination in 1962 because she suspected that the thalidomide-based tranquilizer that she had taken during the first few weeks of her pregnancy might have damaged the fetus she was carrying, and she did not want to risk bringing a severely deformed child into her family. A wave of press coverage during the next few years promoted the idea that the abortion laws should be modernized to allow women to obtain medically necessary abortions—that is, abortions in cases of rape, incest, suspected fetal deformity, or dangers to a woman's health.

EVANGELICALS' CAUTIOUS ACCEPTANCE OF THERAPEUTIC ABORTION

Finkbine's case appears to have caught evangelicals off guard. *Christianity Today* said nothing about it at the time. No polling of specifically *evangelical* Protestant public opinion exists from 1962 (that would not start until 1980), but a Gallup poll from 1962 shows that 56 percent of Protestants in general said that Finkbine did the "right thing" in getting an abortion; only 27 percent said she did the "wrong thing."[18]

The media's framing of the story as a medically advisable abortion for a middle-class, married, white woman who wanted more children in her family and who had the support of her husband in making the decision that they believed would be best for their other children meant that it didn't fit any of the categories in which evangelicals had previously placed abortion on the rare occasions when they had discussed it. Finkbine wasn't doing business with an unlicensed abortionist operating outside the boundaries of the law. She wasn't trying to cover up an out-of-wedlock pregnancy or an adulterous affair. She wasn't even trying to evade the duties of motherhood; on the contrary, she *wanted* more children.

A decade earlier, in 1952, a social science researcher had asked the pastor of the University Baptist Church of Charlottesville, Virginia, about his denomination's position on what was called "therapeutic abortion" as part of a study he was conducting on religious opinion on abortion. Therapeutic abortion was the type of pregnancy termination that Finkbine was seeking—that is, an abortion in a case that was deemed medically necessary, whether for physical or psychological reasons—but in 1952 there was so little public discussion of therapeutic abortion that the question caught the pastor off guard. His congregation belonged to the Southern

Baptist Convention (SBC), which had never addressed abortion in any of its resolutions. Nor, apparently, had the pastor discussed the matter in seminary or in any other church setting. He wrote to the head of the SBC's Social Service Commission for guidance in answering the question, but received little substantive help. Apparently, the SBC's denominational administrators had given no more thought to abortion than the Charlottesville pastor had. So, in response to the researcher's question, the pastor issued this statement: "Even though the Southern Baptist Convention has never made a public statement concerning its position on therapeutic abortion, I believe that the majority of our people feel that the advice of the physician should be followed. We believe this to be primarily a medical problem and that the theological implications can be trusted to our omniscient Heavenly Father."[19]

Not every pastor in Charlottesville had the same reaction to the social science survey question. A few ministers—especially a Lutheran pastor—expressed grave reservations about taking the life of a fetus, even when a doctor deemed it medically necessary. But most Protestant pastors who were surveyed reacted similarly to the minister of the University Baptist Church; they believed that this type of difficult medical decision was outside their direct purview and had to be left up to doctors, not the church, to resolve.

This attitude probably explained the decision of *Christianity Today* editors not to weigh in on the Finkbine case, despite the coverage that therapeutic abortion was receiving in the media and in the liberal Protestant journal *Christian Century*. But as public pressure for a revision in abortion law mounted over the next few years, evangelical magazines decided they needed to speak out on the issue.

In 1967, three states—Colorado, California, and North Carolina— became the first in the nation to legalize "therapeutic" abortion, which usually meant a doctor-advised abortion in a case of rape or incest, dangers to a woman's health, or suspected fetal deformity. Leaders in the Lutheran Church—Missouri Synod (LCMS) reacted with a swift condemnation of these liberalization measures. In March 1967, the *Lutheran News* published an article condemning all abortions, including ones done for therapeutic reasons.[20] The *Baptist Bible Tribune* (the newspaper of the Baptist Bible Fellowship, an association of fundamentalist independent Baptist churches to which Jerry Falwell's Thomas Road Baptist Church in Lynchburg, Virginia, belonged) called abortion "mass murder" in September 1967. "There is no difference between murder of life in the womb and murder of life in the crib," said Noel Smith, the *Baptist Bible Tribune* editor. He held out little hope that this trend could be stopped. "This country being what it is today, there is no doubt that we are going to become a nation of scientific mass murder, a nation of murderers and murderesses," Smith wrote. "And there is no doubt that an outraged Holy God is going to judge us — now, down here on this earth."[21]

But most evangelicals did not follow fundamentalists or conservative Lutherans in taking such an absolutist position, nor were they quite so apocalyptic in their expectations of an imminent judgment for something that the Bible never even directly condemned. In a reflection of a more widely held mainstream evangelical opinion, *Christianity Today* began issuing cautious endorsements of very modest abortion law reform efforts that would legalize abortion in a few specific situations, including rape, incest, and suspected fetal deformity, and also cases in which a doctor believed that a pregnancy termination was needed to protect a patient's health.

Evangelicals still viewed abortion as morally problematic for multiple reasons. If widely available, it would probably encourage premarital sex and allow unmarried people to avoid taking responsibility for their actions. Even if used only by married people, it raised troubling ethical questions, and not simply because it could be used as a form of casual birth control. Fundamentalists of the 1930s and 1940s had been sure that abortion was murder, and many evangelicals of the 1960s still thought they might have been right. But the Bible says nothing directly about abortion, they realized. Evangelicals who were less than a decade removed from their movement's change of mind on contraception did not want to make the same mistake with abortion that they had made with birth control; they did not want to declare that a matter on which the Bible was silent was inherently sinful. When they examined the biblical evidence, they decided that it was considerably more ambiguous than previous evangelical denunciations of abortion might have suggested. The question of when human life began was particularly unclear. Some biblical passages seemed to suggest that human personhood began long before birth, but there were other passages that seemed to indicate that whatever value a fetus had was subordinate to that of the pregnant woman. "Many Protestants find it difficult to take a solid stand because they see no clear New Testament teaching on the subject," *Christianity Today* stated in one of its first articles on abortion, published in 1967.[22]

For evangelicals who thought that the New Testament offered no clear guidance on abortion, the Old Testament passages that related to the subject offered little additional clarity. Exodus 21:22–25—the passage Jewish rabbinical scholars had used for centuries to argue for the permissibility of abortion in some cases—was a favorite of evangelicals who believed that the Catholic absolutist position of opposition to all abortions was too strict, but they had to concede that the passage was obscure, at least when interpreted according to the hermeneutics that evangelicals generally employed at the time. It was in the middle of the Torah—which was not where most evangelicals focused most of their theological attention—and its wording was far from clear, especially in the King James Version's rendering: "If men strive, and hurt a woman with child, so that her fruit depart from her, and yet no mischief follow: he shall be surely punished, according as the woman's husband will lay upon him; and he shall pay as the judges determine. And if any mischief follow, then thou shalt give life for life, eye for eye, tooth for tooth, hand for hand, foot for foot, burning for burning, wound for wound, stripe for stripe." Evangelicals debated whether the phrase "her fruit depart from her" indicated a miscarriage (as Jewish scholars believed) or merely a premature birth in which the child survived (as John Calvin had argued). If the passage was describing a miscarriage, it seemed to suggest that injuries to the pregnant woman would be punished to the full extent of the law (as befit attacks on a human person), but injuries to the fetus would be punished only with a potential fine, a distinction that seemed to some to imply the lesser value of the fetus. *Christian Life* magazine declared in 1967, in a reflection of this latter interpretation of the Exodus passage, "The Bible definitely pinpoints a difference in the value of a fetus and an adult."[23] And if that was the case, it was hard to argue against abortion in at least a few extreme cases. At the very least, abortion should be legal when a pregnancy endangered a woman's life, and it should probably be legal in a few other cases of medical necessity, evangelicals decided.

A few evangelicals used Genesis 2:7 (the verse from the Genesis creation account that said, "And the LORD God formed man of the dust of the ground, and breathed into his nostrils the breath of life; and man became a living soul") to argue that human life began only at birth, when a baby took its first breath. This appears to have been the view of the conservative SBC president W. A. Criswell, and although most evangelicals rejected this interpretation, it was popular among some Baptists who believed it reflected the most literal reading of the scriptural text. The interpretation was based on the premise that full human personhood began only when God created a soul or spirit within a person at some point subsequent to the formation of a physical body. When exactly ensoulment occurred had been a topic of debate among medieval scholastics and early modern Catholic theologians. Many had placed this moment at some point after conception, but they had not generally placed it as late as the moment of birth. But to at least a few Bible-believing Baptists, this appeared to be what Genesis 2:7 implied, and if that was the case, it was hard to get too upset about abortion, at least in cases when it was not connected to sexual sin.[24]

But a significant number of evangelical theologians (including some who were Baptist) rejected the idea that ensoulment occurred subsequent to the formation of a body. Twentieth-century neo-orthodox theologians, such as Karl Barth, rejected the view that the human body could exist without the soul or spirit or that the soul or spirit would exist apart from the body; God's intention was always for the complete integration of soul and body, which was why Christians believed in the resurrection of the body, not the escape of the soul from the body, as the Gnostics had said. Most evangelicals were not fully neo-orthodox in their theology, but the neo-orthodox arguments against soul/body dualism appealed to some of them. Southern Baptist Theological Seminary professor Frank Stagg, a coeditor of his denomination's Broadman commentary series, wrote in 1973 that the terms "body," "soul," and "spirit" in scripture did "not imply a dichotomous or partitive view of man. Man does not have a body; he is a body. . . . The New Testament knows of no disembodied soul or spirit. Wherever envisioned, in this life or the next, man is always in a body. As to the next life, the Biblical doctrine is resurrection, not immortality of the soul. . . . It is important to note that body belongs essentially to what man is. It is not a tomb or prison for the soul. It is not a part that can be shed. Man is a body, in creation, in sin, in redemption, in life beyond death."[25] If it were the case that the body and soul were inseparably interconnected, one could not point to a moment when a human body existed (even in embryonic form) and assume that it lacked a soul and was not yet a person. Stagg was not writing about abortion; indeed, he was probably not even thinking about the question of when human life begins when he wrote his strong rejection of soul/body dualism. But evangelicals who accepted the idea that the body, soul, and spirit were inseparably connected for eternity and that one could not destroy the body without destroying the image of God found it easy to imagine that the human body was of incomparable worth even in its embryonic form; one could never say that a human body — even a human body that was a zygote or an embryo — lacked a soul or that it was not an image-bearer of God.

This was the view of John Warwick Montgomery, a Lutheran theologian and apologist who was a leading evangelical pro-life voice in the late 1960s. "The intimate connection of soul and body in scripture establishes a predisposition against the idea of a divine 'superadding' of the soul to an already existent body," he wrote in 1968. Although soul and body were "ontologically distinct," they functioned so closely together, according to scripture, that it was not likely that there was ever a moment in time when a human body existed without a soul. And in Montgomery's view, the question of when a human body began to exist could be answered by science. The zygote that formed at the moment of conception had a unique chromosomal identity that was distinct from either of its parents, and if its growth was not interrupted, it would continue to develop into an embryo, a fetus, and then a newborn baby. The existence and development of the human body therefore began at conception, and if the body existed at that moment, so did the soul. True, the zygote could not yet do anything, but humans were valuable not because of what they could do but because of who they were in relation to God, a relationship that he insisted began at the moment that "God brought about his psycho-physical [that is, soul/body] existence in the miracle of conception." "For the biblical writers, personhood in the most genuine sense begins no later than conception," Montgomery wrote. "Subsequent human acts illustrate this personhood, they do not create it."[26]

Even some evangelicals who believed that the moment of ensoulment likely occurred after conception did not think that Genesis 2:7 taught that it could be identified so precisely with the point at which an infant took its first breath outside the womb. "The ancient Hebrews associated life in a unique way, not only with the breath, but also with the blood," Fuller Seminary professor Paul Jewett wrote in 1968. "'The blood is the living being,' we are told in Deut. 12:23, 24. . . . If one were to press this teaching about blood, as literal science, it would yield the result that the human fetus is informed with the soul, not at the moment the first breath is drawn, but when the blood system develops." One should realize, Jewett argued, that ensoulment and the divine image should not be narrowly identified with either breath or blood or with a particular stage in fetal development. "The fact that man's likeness to God, which is the ground of reverence for his life, is qualitatively distinct from the physiological basis of his life, means that all efforts to identify the presence of the human soul in terms of some stage of physiological development must prove frustrating," Jewett wrote.[27]

Jewett's conclusion was probably the mainstream evangelical theological position in the late 1960s — scripture did not say exactly when or how ensoulment took place. Most evangelicals who took this position believed that this uncertainty should lead to greater caution about taking life at its earliest embryonic stages rather than less. Kenneth Kantzer, a dean at Trinity Evangelical Divinity School, said that even if "Scripture may not tell us how to recognize the functions of a truly human and immortal soul" (in the sense of telling us how to recognize whether an embryo or fetus has a soul, and if so, at what exact stage of gestation this ensoulment occurs), this did not mean that one was free to abort an embryo or fetus. "From conception, the fetus is of immeasurable value because of its potential humanity," Kantzer said, because what gave the fetus worth was not primarily that it had a soul at a particular moment in time, but rather that it was, at the very least, "potential human life in process of becoming a human being." "The *culminating* decisive factor in *constituting* the human person is God's decision and purpose," he wrote. In other words, whether or not the fetus had a soul at a particular moment of gestation, one must assume that it was God's purpose for that particular fetus to develop into a full human being, and that God's purpose alone was enough to give infinite worth to the developing person in embryonic form. People did not have the right to terminate the development of an image-bearer of God, because the creation of such an image-bearer was God's work, not theirs. The fetus belonged to God, not to either of its parents. "Scripture does teach us that a human fetus is of immeasurable value because of its potential, in spite of the fact that it is not yet fully human," Kantzer said. "And Scripture demands, accordingly, that the human fetus be treated as of such immeasurable value by man."[28]

Most evangelicals in the late 1960s seem to have taken a view similar to Kantzer's. Even if ensoulment did not begin at conception, and even if a fetus was not a full human person, it was clear from scripture that the fetus was a potential human created by God for an eternal destiny, and destroying it was therefore a grave evil in most instances. With this theology, one could theoretically support the availability of abortion for a few carefully defined medical reasons, but elective abortion would be a bridge too far.

However, some evangelicals (such as John Warwick Montgomery) thought they could go even further and say that the fetus was not only "potential" life in the process of formation but an actual ensouled human person from the moment of conception. In addition to arguing that scripture did not teach that the creation of the soul was separate from the creation of the body, they also argued that there were several scriptures that suggested that fetuses in the womb were full human persons who were capable of being filled with the Holy Spirit or bearing the guilt of sin. The Gospel of Luke's description of the preborn John the Baptist's behavior offered especially compelling evidence of fetal personhood, they thought. In Luke 1:15, John the Baptist's father is told by an angel that the son his wife will conceive will "be filled with the Holy Spirit from his mother's womb" (KJV). The conservative evangelical New American Standard Bible (1971) made this verse's reference to prenatal life even more obvious: "He will be filled with the Holy Spirit *while still in* his mother's womb" (emphasis mine). The New American Standard Bible may have stretched the meaning of the Greek in this case; the more literal translation is "from" or "out of" his mother's womb. Nevertheless, it seems clear from the larger context of the narrative that the phrase referred to fetal movement at the end of the second trimester of pregnancy that Elizabeth, John the Baptist's mother, interpreted as a sign that her unborn baby was praising the preborn Christ. "As soon as the voice of thy salutation sounded in mine ears, the babe leaped in my womb for joy," Elizabeth tells Mary (Luke 1:44, KJV). For some evangelicals, this verse alone was enough to clinch the argument for fetal personhood, because the Greek word, *brephos*, translated as "babe" or "baby," was the same word used for newborn babies and young children elsewhere in scripture. Luke, it seemed, did not make any differentiation between a second-trimester fetus and an infant or young child; both were capable of being filled with the Spirit, both were capable of experiencing joy, both were capable of acknowledging Jesus, and, most importantly, both were designated with the same Greek word, which suggested to these evangelicals that they had the same ontological value. And if Luke, the inspired Gospel writer, made no differentiation between human life before and after birth, evangelicals who believed in biblical inerrancy should not either, they argued. But there were also a few other biblical passages they cited in support of their position that full human personhood began from the moment of conception. Psalm 51:5, Psalm 58:3, Psalm 139:13–16, and Jeremiah 1:5 spoke of God's creative work in a person's life beginning long before birth and of inclinations being formed in the womb. They seemed to speak of a continuity of personality and existence from conception through birth, childhood, and adulthood.

To evangelicals who believed in prenatal personhood, these verses were compelling, but they were sufficiently vague that evangelicals who did not believe in prenatal personhood found them fairly easy to dismiss. In the late 1960s, most evangelical theologians who wrote about abortion did not yet believe that any of these verses taught what Christian pro-life activists said they did, namely, that human personhood began at conception. In some cases, evangelicals who shied away from an absolutist stance on abortion believed that these passages were poetic descriptions whose metaphorical language should not be pressed too closely. In their view, the absence of biblical condemnations of abortion, combined with the Exodus 21 passage (or, for a few evangelicals, Genesis 2:7), offered clearer evidence of the Bible's position. But the most common evangelical position on abortion in the late 1960s did not rely on scriptural proof texts for evidence of when ensoulment or personhood began. Instead, it relied on what evangelicals believed were biblical principles about sex and the value of human life. Those principles, they thought, indicated that abortion was wrong most of the time, but that there were nevertheless extraordinary situations in which an abortion could legitimately be performed.

At the first major evangelical conference on abortion—the Protestant Symposium on the Control of Human Reproduction (August 1968)—the twenty-five Christian physicians, theologians, and college professors who gathered to discuss a response to the abortion law liberalization movement could not agree on exactly which situations justified an abortion, but they did reach a general consensus that abortion should neither be entirely prohibited nor permissively encouraged: "The Christian physician will advise induced abortion only to safeguard greater values sanctioned by Scripture."[29] *Christianity Today* adopted a similar position. Abortion should be allowed only on "substantial medical and other grounds that are biblically licit," said the magazine in 1969; it should not be available "merely on demand or for convenience."[30] The nation's other evangelical magazines, such as *Eternity* and *Christian Life*, concurred.

Evangelicals who took this view did not always agree on all of the theological nuances regarding the precise moment about the beginning of human personhood, but they could unite on the practical political application of those principles. Those who believed that the Bible differentiated between the value of fetal life and the lives of adult humans nevertheless believed that fetal life was "sacred" on the grounds that it was, at the very least, potential life that God was in the process of forming into a person bearing the divine image. Robert Visscher, an advocate of legalized therapeutic abortion, stated in *Christianity Today* in 1968 that if one believed that "the embryo, which is in the process of becoming a human being, under certain circumstances does not have the same rights as a viable fetus or the mother herself . . . this conclusion should not obscure the fact that the embryo is a human life and therefore is sacred." Even if it was doubtful whether the embryo had a soul, it was undeniably human life that God was in the process of making into a "human being," Visscher said, and as such, anyone who respected God's creative authority would refrain from destroying this human life unless it was medically necessary. Only someone who believed in an "existential" or "situation ethics" approach to morality would have no qualms about making abortion a matter of individual choice, Visscher said.[31] And since evangelicals did believe in moral absolutes and in God's sovereignty over human life, they would oppose elective abortion.

Similarly, even some of the evangelicals who believed that human life began at conception and favored enshrining this concept into the civil law code nevertheless thought that the cases of rape and incest, suspected fetal deformity, and dangers to a woman's physical health or life were so challenging for a person to bear that it would be wrong to use the force of law to require a woman in those situations to carry a pregnancy to term. Evangelicals could therefore disagree with each other on when exactly human personhood began, but nevertheless unite around the principle that abortion was a highly problematic termination of human life that might be acceptable in some very narrowly defined circumstances. In the late 1960s and early 1970s, there was therefore no evangelical magazine or evangelical leader that publicly advocated the legalization of elective abortion. But until the 1970s, very few publicly called for a complete ban on all abortions. With the exception of a small number of conservative Protestant groups—such as Missouri Synod Lutherans, who spoke alongside

Catholics in opposition to California's therapeutic abortion bill in 1967 — evangelicals decided not to campaign against therapeutic abortion laws that allowed for abortion in a few specific cases, such as rape and incest, dangers to a woman's life or health, and suspected fetal deformity.[32] In fact, many even endorsed such laws as a welcome alternative to "abortion on demand."

In the late 1960s, support for the legalization of therapeutic abortion was especially strong in the socially conservative, largely evangelical South. In northern and western states, legislative debates over abortion were often bitterly divisive, with Catholic opponents of abortion arrayed against liberal Protestants or Jews who supported abortion legalization. But in southern states where Catholics, Jews, and liberal Protestants were in the minority, an evangelical consensus in favor of limited "therapeutic" abortion laws quickly emerged. Between 1967 and 1970, the South was the region most likely to legalize abortion for limited medical reasons, with Georgia, Arkansas, Virginia, North Carolina, and South Carolina adopting legislation that allowed abortion in cases of rape and incest, suspected fetal deformity, or dangers to a woman's health.

In 1970, the Presbyterian Church in the United States (PCUS), a southern denomination that would merge with the Presbyterian Church (USA) in 1983 but that in the early 1970s was still more socially conservative than its northern mainline counterpart, passed a resolution endorsing the principle behind therapeutic abortion laws.[33] Abortion was the "willful destruction of the fetus," stated the PCUS resolution, but it could nevertheless "on occasion be morally justifiable" in cases such as "medical indications of physical or mental deformity, conception as a result of rape or incest, conditions under which the physical or mental health of either mother or child would be gravely threatened, or the socio-economic condition of the family."[34] Most evangelical commentary on abortion had not listed the "socio-economic condition of the family" as a legitimate reason for abortion, but all of the other exceptional cases listed in the resolution were standard phrases from therapeutic abortion laws and evangelical articles on abortion.

Southern Baptists shared their Southern Presbyterian neighbors' support for therapeutic abortion laws and opposition to elective abortion. In Texas, the head of the state Baptist convention's Christian Life Commission, Phil Strickland, campaigned for a liberalization of the state's abortion law, which at the time allowed for abortion only in cases when it was necessary to preserve a woman's life. In April 1969, the Texas *Baptist Standard* polled its readers on their attitude toward abortion law reform in Texas and found that 90 percent of respondents wanted the Texas law to be made "more humane."[35] Perhaps if Strickland and the Texas Baptists had succeeded in getting the Texas legislature to liberalize the state abortion law in 1969 to allow for abortions in cases of rape, the *Roe v. Wade* case would never have originated in Texas, since it was based on the claim that Texas did not allow "Jane Roe" (Norma McCorvey) to terminate a pregnancy that she alleged had resulted from rape. In reality, of course, Texas did not liberalize its law along the lines that Texas Baptists wanted, and the Supreme Court in 1973 not only struck down Texas's highly restrictive abortion law but also the more moderate therapeutic abortion laws that Baptists had helped to create in other southern states.

Before *Roe v. Wade*, though, these therapeutic abortion laws enjoyed widespread Baptist support, not only in Texas but across the South. A nationwide 1970 *Baptist Viewpoint* poll showed that 71 percent of Southern Baptist pastors and Sunday school teachers believed that abortion should be legal in cases of rape and incest, and 70 percent favored legalizing it for cases in which a pregnancy endangered a woman's health. But only 13 percent of Southern Baptist pastors and 19 percent of Southern Baptist Sunday school teachers approved of legalizing elective abortion in the first trimester of pregnancy, while a somewhat higher number (20 percent of pastors and 15 percent of Sunday school teachers) favored making nearly all abortion illegal, even in cases when a pregnancy endangered a woman's health.[36] In 1970, both the pro-choice position (legalization of elective abortion in the first trimester) and the pro-life position (prohibitions on all abortions, with possible exceptions in case of rape or incest, or to save a woman's life) were small minority positions among Southern

Baptist ministers, but of those two positions, the pro-life view was more common than the pro-choice. But support for either of those positions paled in comparison to the overwhelming consensus in favor of legalizing abortion for therapeutic reasons while keeping elective abortion illegal.

The SBC's first official position on abortion, adopted in 1971, reflected this consensus. Southern Baptists should work for "legislation that will allow the possibility of abortion under such conditions as rape, incest, clear evidence of severe fetal deformity, and carefully ascertained evidence of the likelihood of damage to the emotional, mental, and physical health of the mother," the SBC stated, while opposing the removal of all restrictions on abortion as inconsistent with its "high view of the sanctity of human life, including fetal life."[37]

EVANGELICALS BECOME MORE CONSERVATIVE ON ABORTION

The SBC intended this resolution as a moderate position in the growing national polarization over abortion—an alternative to both conservative Catholic absolute opposition to abortion and the emerging liberal Protestant consensus in favor of full abortion legalization. By the time the SBC adopted this resolution, in June 1971, four states (New York, Washington, Alaska, and Hawaii) had already legalized elective abortion, and many more were considering doing so. The SBC's resolution was as much a rejection of this move as it was a repudiation of the absolutism of the Catholic-dominated pro-life movement. But by the time it was issued, a growing number of evangelicals in both the North and the South had already decided that the approach outlined in the SBC resolution was not restrictive enough. When the resolution was brought to the floor for a vote at the 1971 convention, messengers (delegates) at the convention introduced two different amendments to weaken the resolution's affirmation of therapeutic abortion laws. Both amendment proposals were defeated, but the fact that they were introduced at all—and that no competing amendments were introduced to make the resolution more supportive of abortion legalization—showed that even in 1971, some Southern Baptists wanted the convention to adopt a more restrictive stance on abortion and avoid giving support to the therapeutic abortion laws that a number of evangelicals were already beginning to view as too permissive.[38]

Christianity Today, which as late as 1969 had endorsed a position very similar to the one the SBC adopted in 1971, began publishing anti-abortion editorials in 1970 saying that abortion was the taking of human life and that more forceful opposition to it was necessary. In "The War on the Womb," a two-page editorial published in June 1970, *Christianity Today*'s editors endorsed the view of the conservative Lutheran theologian John Warwick Montgomery that human life begins at conception and that Christians have a duty to defend the unborn in the political sphere. "For the biblical writers personhood in the most genuine sense begins no later than conception," Montgomery wrote.[39] Carl F. H. Henry, a former editor of *Christianity Today* and one of the leading evangelical theologians of this era, published an equally strong denunciation of abortion in *Eternity* magazine in 1971. The next year, Billy Graham declared that he was opposed to abortion in all cases except when it was necessary to save a woman's life and in instances of rape or incest.[40] The National Association of Evangelicals (NAE) adopted a position that was generally in line with this, but it also left the door open for abortions in cases when a pregnancy endangered a woman's health. "Neither the life of the unborn child nor the mother may be lightly taken," the NAE stated in 1971. "We believe that God, Himself, in Scripture, has conferred divine blessing upon unborn infants and has provided penalties for actions which result in the death of the unborn." Abortion therefore should be legally prohibited except in cases when it was necessary to "safeguard the health or the life of the mother" or in cases of rape or incest, but even then, the NAE cautioned, an abortion decision should be made "only after there has been medical, psychological and religious counseling of the most sensitive kind."[41]

The NAE resolution conspicuously omitted suspected fetal deformity in its list of potentially acceptable reasons for an abortion. And Graham was willing to restrict the grounds for therapeutic abortion even further, allowing it only in cases of rape and incest and in situations in which pregnancy endangered a woman's life. Evangelicals' list of potentially acceptable reasons for therapeutic abortion was beginning to narrow, even as they still held onto the general idea that there might be a few extreme cases in which abortion was possibly legitimate. But regardless of their willingness to allow abortion in a few exceptional cases, it was clear to many of them that "abortion on demand" had to be opposed. "Are modern exponents of abortion-on-request less barbaric than their Roman counterparts because they approve a more sophisticated discarding of infant life with the medical trash?" Carl Henry asked the audience at a seminar sponsored by the Christian Medical Society at Philadelphia's Tenth Presbyterian Church in November 1970. He hastened to add that churches needed to provide a "compassionate" response to women who were considering abortion in a case of rape or incest or in the case of a "seriously defective fetus," and that abortions might be permissible in such situations, even though he acknowledged that determining the moral course in such challenging circumstances was "not easy." But in the case of elective abortion, there was no moral ambiguity: abortion was "barbaric."[42]

A few evangelical denominations—mostly from the Lutheran and Reformed wings of evangelicalism—were willing to go further and say that all abortions were evil except possibly those that there were necessary to save a woman's life. In 1971, the Lutheran Church—Missouri Synod (LCMS), the largest conservative Lutheran denomination in the United States, adopted a resolution urging Lutherans to "regard willful abortion as contrary to the will of God."[43] In a longer report on abortion that the denomination adopted that year, the LCMS explained that "life and death belong to the province of God" and that "life is a gift of God" that must be gratefully received, not destroyed. Even fetal abnormalities or the prospect of economic distress did not justify an abortion, the LCMS report stated, because "fulfillment is often found in sacrifice for another human being and in trusting the God for whom no price came too high in the task of redeeming mankind by His Son. . . . Even very grave psychiatric considerations do not of themselves offer a justifiable ground for deciding on an abortion."[44]

The Orthodox Presbyterian Church's (OPC) 1971 report on abortion, which was largely the creation of Westminster Theological Seminary professor John Frame, made similar arguments and arrived at similar conclusions, but with a much more thorough review of scripture. In keeping with its identity as a very conservative Calvinist denomination committed to a high view of scriptural authority, the OPC centered its report on a comprehensive survey of the Bible's treatment of prenatal human life. The entire Bible treated barrenness as a curse and children as a blessing, the OPC report said. Several scriptures (such as Psalm 51, Psalm 139, and Luke 1) seemed to describe human personhood as beginning well before birth, since they spoke of human life in the womb as being known by God, inheriting sinful proclivities, and being filled with the Holy Spirit. The Bible strongly prohibited people from taking human life under any circumstances that were not directly authorized by God, said Frame in the OPC report. Since there was no direct authorization for the taking of human life in the womb, it was therefore sinful. Even Exodus 21:22–25, the passage that evangelical opponents of an absolute antiabortion stance most commonly cited in support of their position, could not justify abortion, the report said. At most, if this passage meant exactly what the evangelical opponents of the strong antiabortion stance said it meant, it suggested that unborn human life had at least enough value that even its *accidental* destruction should be punished by a fine, which hardly suggested that the *deliberate* destruction of unborn human life through abortion was acceptable. But in fact, this was not what that passage meant, Frame argued. Like Calvin, he suggested that the verse was referring primarily to a premature birth in which the child survived, not a miscarriage that resulted in the fetus's death, and if that interpretation was correct, the passage seemed to assign just as much value to the child (both before and after birth) as it did to the mother. On this reading, Exodus 21:22–25 became one of the most strongly antiabortion passages in the Bible.[45]

This antiabortion interpretation of the passage — which had been posited in the Reformation but was rejected by many evangelical biblical scholars in the late 1960s and early 1970s — soon became near universal among evangelical biblical scholars again. Whereas the Revised Standard Version (1952) and the New Revised Standard Version (1989)—the most popular translations in mainline Protestant churches—rendered the disputed word in Exodus 21 "miscarriage," several of the most popular late twentieth-century evangelical translations, including the New American Standard Bible (1971), the New International Version (1978), and the New King James Version (1983), translated it as "give birth prematurely."

But even if the passage in Exodus 21 were interpreted as the antiabortion evangelicals preferred, the evangelical opponents of abortion realized that the number of verses that seemed to clearly indicate the full personhood of previable fetuses was unusually low, certainly no more than half a dozen out of the entire Bible. And the interpretation of each of these in the abortion debate seemed to be open to question, as even John Frame conceded. Evangelical opponents of the antiabortion position pointed this out when arguing for liberty of conscience on the issue.[46] Yet for the most part, their voices did not win out, as the number of evangelical denominations adopting antiabortion resolutions continued to grow. In 1972, the Christian Reformed Church, the North American conservative Dutch Calvinist denomination associated with Calvin College, adopted a resolution opposing abortion in all cases except when a pregnancy endangered a woman's life.[47]

The Lutheran and Reformed denominations that passed resolutions against abortion before *Roe v. Wade* made up only a small fraction of American evangelicals, and in some ways they were not very representative. All three had strong ties to sixteenth-century Protestant Reformers (either Luther or Calvin) who had opposed abortion. All three had a strong view of God's sovereignty and affirmed a doctrine of predestination, which meant that the argument that God was sovereign over the life of the fetus and exercised ownership over each embryo made sense to them. All three had a very strong theology of original sin, and a belief in the "*imago Dei.*" Other evangelical denominations emphasized choice in conversion and focused their preaching on trying to get people to make a decision for Christ, but the three Protestant denominations that passed strong resolutions against abortion before *Roe v. Wade* practiced infant baptism and gave greater weight than many other evangelicals did to the possibility that God could sovereignly save infants or even preborn fetuses without a profession of faith on their part. It may have therefore been easier for them to adopt a theology of the infinite worth of fetal life than it was for other evangelicals. But even though these theological distinctions were significant, their importance should not be overstated, because even many evangelicals who were not part of a Lutheran or Reformed tradition had similar reservations about abortion. Carl Henry was part of the American Baptist Churches, Billy Graham was a Southern Baptist, and the National Association of Evangelicals was filled with many Wesleyan and charismatic denominations that rejected Reformed and Lutheran views of predestination and infant baptism, yet all of them adopted conservative positions on abortion before *Roe v. Wade*. One did not have to be a Lutheran or a Calvinist to oppose abortion from an evangelical perspective in 1971 or 1972. But the Lutheran and Calvinist denominations that passed resolutions against abortion in the early 1970s were able to provide a detailed theological rationale for that opposition that not all evangelicals who opposed abortion were yet able to do. By placing opposition to abortion in the context of the Bible's concern for human life at every stage—including not only before birth but perhaps even before conception, when a potential human being was already part of God's sovereign plans—conservative Lutherans and Calvinists created a countertheology to the liberal Protestant theology of existential individual moral choice that had led them to embrace the "right to choose." Evangelicals who were not part of Lutheran or Reformed churches would draw on these Lutheran and Calvinist insights a few years later when articulating their own biblical and theological reasons for opposing abortion.

Each of the denominational resolutions against abortion also encouraged Christians to advocate for restrictive abortion laws, just as the evangelical magazine articles had. Christians who adopted these positions on abortion were fully aware of the political context of the abortion debate and realized that in weighing in on this question, they were not merely telling congregants what options they had in cases of a crisis pregnancy; they were taking a stand in a contemporary political controversy and an emerging culture war. It was the presence of this culture war that emboldened them to take a firm stance on a matter that all of them realized had not been spelled out in scripture or in their church confessions with the specificity they might have liked.

Liberal Protestants also wrestled with a lack of clarity on abortion, because they could not say with definitiveness that the fetus was *not* a human life. That troubled many of them, because of their deep concern for human life in other contexts. But they arrived at a general pro-choice consensus partly because of their sympathy for the feminist cause and the rights of women, and partly because of their strong belief in the right and responsibility of the individual — not the church or the state — to follow their own conscience in making moral decisions. Abortion was too important and personal a decision to be made the subject of state law or church mandates.

Conservative evangelical Protestants arrived at the opposite conclusion because of their opposite inclinations on these questions. They believed in moral absolutes, so the more that liberal Protestants emphasized the moral relativity of the abortion question, the more evangelicals were determined to find a divinely dictated, unchanging moral principle on the issue. They were not interested in pragmatic arguments that suggested that the legalization of abortion would reduce the number of women who died each year from dangerous illegal abortions; such arguments, which were grounded in utilitarianism or in broadly based appeals to the social good, might have resonated with believers in the Social Gospel, but they had no appeal for people who believed that God had given unchanging moral laws for the governance of individual behavior. Evangelicals were also opposed to the second-wave feminist movement's emphasis on personal bodily autonomy, because they believed that this threatened the family and compromised divine mandates about sexual behavior and gender roles. As the abortion rights campaign moved beyond its origins as a medical debate and became identified with the feminist movement's campaign for women's rights — as it did at the end of the 1960s — conservative evangelicals who had strong reservations about both second-wave feminism and the sexual revolution became more antipathetic to it. As the relatively conservative abortion law liberalization campaign transformed into a movement to repeal all restrictions on abortion—and as it became clear that this movement had the support of second-wave feminist organizations, such as the National Organization for Women (NOW), and supporters of the sexual revolution, such as *Playboy* magazine—evangelicals had every incentive to interpret ambiguous passages of scripture through an antiabortion hermeneutic.[48]

Women joined men in making this argument, but in the evangelical circles of the late 1960s, the vast majority of those commenting on the morality of abortion were men. Even as the abortion debate became closely intertwined with debates about feminism, public discussions of abortion in evangelicalism continued to be male-dominated. The vast majority of articles on abortion published in evangelical magazines in the late 1960s and 1970s were written by men, and the denominational committees that formulated statements on abortion consisted mostly of men. The group of twenty-five evangelical scholars who attended the Protestant Symposium on Abortion in 1968 included only one woman—Sarah Finley, an assistant professor of pediatrics at the Medical College of Alabama in Birmingham.

The almost complete absence of women in the evangelical conversation on abortion in this era was largely a reflection of the fact that nearly all of the evangelical professors of ethics and theology, and nationally known pastors, were men. Some leading evangelical seminaries that subscribed to a view that the pastoral office should be reserved for men did not even admit women. Dallas Theological Seminary, for instance, did not admit its first female students until 1975.[49] Even Fuller Theological Seminary, which would eventually become an advocate of gender equality, waited until the mid-1970s to hire its first tenure-track female faculty member or begin awarding master's of divinity degrees to women.[50] Women had long served as evangelists in Pentecostal and Wesleyan denominations (and even in some Baptist circles), but the moderately Reformed wing of evangelicalism that dominated evangelical discussions of abortion—that is, the wing that produced the leaders of such institutions as *Christianity Today* magazine, Wheaton College, and Fuller Seminary—was doing very little at the time to encourage women's theological scholarship or promote women's ministry, and some denominations in this orbit did not ordain women to pulpit ministry at all. But the nearly complete absence of female voices among evangelical theologians did not seem unusual at the time, because mainline Protestant seminaries were nearly as male-centric in this era as evangelical institutions were. In 1968, Princeton Theological Seminary's fifty-six faculty included only one woman (an assistant professor of Christian education).[51]

In the late 1960s, few of the male evangelical physicians and theologians who commented on abortion seemed disturbed by the absence of evangelical women's voices in the conversation, which perhaps was not too surprising for men who operated in largely male professional spaces. One of the few who did note the phenomenon was Fuller Seminary professor Paul Jewett, who in the mid-1970s became a leading proponent of evangelical gender egalitarianism and women's role in ministry. It was ironic, he noted in passing at the 1968 Protestant Symposium on Human Reproduction, that evangelical men who could not agree among themselves about which situations justified abortion expected that "women, who are the most immediately involved in the problem, can only ask [male authorities], and never decide what they ought to do." Perhaps, Jewett suggested, the complexity of the difficulties involved in deciding whether a particular form of therapeutic abortion was legitimate "should serve to humble the male of the species."[52]

But on the rare occasions when evangelical women did enter into male-dominated conversations about abortion, their perspectives closely echoed those of evangelical men. Nancy Hardesty, an advocate of women in ministry, who, along with Letha Scanzoni, became a leading voice of evangelical feminism in the 1970s, published an article in *Eternity* magazine in 1967 that argued strongly against elective abortion.[53] NOW endorsed abortion rights in 1967, but evangelical advocates of women's rights took the opposite position, because unlike many of their secular counterparts in the feminist movement, evangelical feminists opposed the sexual revolution and premarital sex and therefore did not see abortion legalization as a path to liberation for women. Like other evangelicals, evangelical feminists such as Hardesty believed in the high value of fetal life and believed that it needed to be protected in most circumstances, even if they also supported legalizing therapeutic abortion (as Hardesty did herself). And if that was true for a self-identified feminist such as Hardesty, it was even truer for the many evangelical women who may have opposed second-wave feminism.

June Webb, a registered nurse in Atlanta who was president of Christian Action for Life, used her position on an abortion subcommittee in the PCUS General Assembly in late 1972 to argue against abortion. For Webb, the case for saving unborn human life was both biblical and scientific. The letterhead for Christian Action for Life featured a long column of Bible verses that showed the humanity of the unborn, with one of pro-life activists' favorite passages, Psalm 139:13–20, prominently listed at the top. At the same time, though, Webb viewed the issue of abortion through the lens of her medical training; when she wanted to convince her fellow committee members that abortion was the taking of a human life, she showed up to the committee meeting with a set of slides that pro-lifers commonly used to show audiences what a fetus looked like, a technique that sometimes moved skeptics to reconsider their support for abortion, at least in the case of second-trimester pregnancies.[54]

And among fundamentalist independent Baptists, women spoke out against both abortion and women's liberation in the early 1970s, equating opposition to abortion with a defense of the traditional gender roles that they endorsed. In 1973, Nelda Walker, a thirty-four-year-old fundamentalist Baptist pastor's wife from Fort Smith, Arkansas, told the National Women's Auxiliary of the American Baptist Association that abortion was "nothing less than legalized murder of masses of human lives," and that women who supported abortion or who objected to the restrictions on women's leadership in the church that she said were given by Paul the apostle were guilty of "rebellion against the will and purpose of God in our lives." For her, the fight against abortion was both a fight against feticide and a campaign against liberal feminism; it was a countercultural refusal to follow the feminists of her own generation. She found it ironic that "women of our generation promote murder of our babies while they march in protest in the streets of our cities against murder on the battlefield."[55]

Given the unusually strong opposition to abortion among fundamentalist independent Baptists—a level of opposition that exceeded that of most other evangelical groups in the early 1970s—it was perhaps not surprising that the only evangelical Protestant (Judy Fink) serving on the board of the National Right to Life Committee in the pre-*Roe* era was an independent Baptist. To a greater degree than most other evangelical pastors in this era, pastors of independent Baptist or Bible churches, who tended to be strongly biblicist and antifeminist, issued many denunciations of abortion in the early 1970s. Donald Camp, pastor of Grace Baptist Church in Anderson, Indiana, gave a public address against all abortion in January 1971.[56] In February 1971, Robert J. Terrey, pastor of Plymouth Baptist Church in Minnesota, published an article in his church newsletter opposing any liberalization of the abortion law in Minnesota, saying that "liberalizing abortion" amounted to legalizing "murder."[57] John R. Rice, an independent Baptist who edited the nation's largest fundamentalist periodical (the *Sword of the Lord*), had long issued passing comments against abortion, but in 1971 he published an entire book on the subject: *The Murder of the Helpless Unborn—Abortion*.[58]

The fundamentalist pastors who issued scathing denunciations of abortion in the early 1970s were political and theological conservatives who viewed themselves as well to the right of the SBC. Their network included small Bible colleges and the strongly fundamentalist Bob Jones University. As the SBC debated abortion year after year, the fundamentalist independent Baptists lined up against all forms of abortion, and then used the SBC's comparatively moderate stance and debates on the issue as a foil against which to contrast their own clear position. They coupled their denunciations of abortion with equally scathing condemnations of feminism. An October 1973 issue of Terrey's *Plymouth Crusader*, for instance, coupled antiabortion articles, fetal photographs, and a reprint of "Diary of a Fetus" (which was originally the work of a Polish Catholic, but Terrey may not have been aware of that) with an article satirizing mothers who wanted to work outside the home.[59]

Even outside of fundamentalist Baptist circles, opposition to all abortion (or, at the very least, all elective abortion) became an identifying mark of theological conservatism. In the PCUS, the *Presbyterian Journal*, a publication of the southern denomination's most conservative faction—a faction that would split off in 1973 to form the Presbyterian Church in America—protested against the denomination's moderate stance on abortion and endorsement of therapeutic abortion laws by publishing several articles in the early 1970s that opposed all abortion. One published in 1971 labeled abortion "infanticide." That same year, opponents of abortion within the PCUS held a floor vote to overturn the moderate resolution on abortion that the denomination had approved the previous year, because they objected to the resolution's suggestion that abortion was "morally justifiable" in some cases. The motion failed, but it did so by only a 19-vote margin out of more than 300 ballots cast. The close vote signaled the strength of the pro-life cause among Southern Presbyterians, and among Christian conservatives more generally.[60] The journal of the fundamentalist American Council of Christian Churches (ACCC), which operated as a more conservative alternative to the National Association of Evangelicals, published an article in 1970 that argued that the Bible suggested that every abortion killed a human being with a soul, since ensoulment probably occurred at the moment of conception.[61] In late 1970, the Ohio Baptist Fellowship Churches passed a resolution denouncing liberalized abortion laws as "murderous practices."[62] And among fundamentalist Lutherans—the strongest opponents of abortion among conservative Protestants—the denunciations of abortion became even more direct. In October 1970, the fundamentalist Lutheran periodical *Christian News* published "The Healer Has Become the Murderer," which argued that Exodus 21 required the death penalty for anyone who caused the death of a fetus.[63]

The reason why evangelical denunciations of abortion became far more common in 1970 and 1971 than they were in the late 1960s was not hard to guess. In the late 1960s, every abortion reform law passed by a state legislature was a therapeutic abortion bill that permitted abortion for only a few narrowly defined medical or psychological reasons. A few conservative Protestants (mainly conservative Lutherans and a few fundamentalists) objected even to these modest abortion law reforms at the time, but the vast majority of Southern Baptists and northern evangelicals were willing to allow for abortion in these exceptional cases. To a twenty-first-century ear, some evangelical commentary on abortion from the late 1960s therefore may even sound "pro-choice," because it's not hard to find evangelical statements at the time that indicate that abortion should be legally available in some cases. But a closer reading of these quotations will show in almost every case that what evangelicals were advocating was not the legalization of elective abortion but rather of therapeutic abortion, and even then, some evangelicals worried that therapeutic abortion laws might be misused. In 1970, their worst fears were realized when four states legalized elective abortion, a move that greatly increased the number of legal abortions performed in the United States. In 1970, there were 193,491 reported legal abortions in the United States, an increase of more than 700 percent over the 27,512 abortions reported in 1969. In 1971, the number of reported legal abortions increased to 485,816, more than twice the number performed the previous year.[64] Such a rapid increase in the number of legal abortions disturbed most evangelicals, even those who believed that therapeutic abortion should be legal or who didn't think that human life began at conception. Some of them (including the editors of *Christianity Today*) became more critical of abortion. Others (especially among fundamentalists) who perhaps had opposed abortion all along became more vociferous in their denunciation of abortion. And some continued to try to steer a middle path, opposing elective abortion but also insisting that abortion for therapeutic reasons should be legal. Like the SBC, the Assemblies of God adopted a resolution in 1971 that allowed for abortion in cases of rape, incest, or threats to a pregnant woman's health, but said that "abortion for reasons of personal convenience, social adjustment, or economic advantage" was "morally wrong" and should not be legalized.[65] The Church of the Nazarene also took this position, passing a resolution in 1972 that opposed abortion "for personal convenience or population control," and stating that abortion was "permissible only on the basis of sound medical reasons affecting the life of the fetus and that of the mother."[66]

With most of the nation's legal abortions now falling under the elective rather than the therapeutic category—and with the vast majority performed on unmarried rather than married women—it was becoming increasingly easy for evangelicals to draw the connection between abortion legalization and the sexual revolution. There was therefore a hardening of evangelical opinion against abortion even before *Roe v. Wade*, even if some evangelical leaders and evangelical denominations (including the SBC) still insisted that abortion for therapeutic reasons was permissible. But the Supreme Court's decision in 1973 that elective abortion in the first two trimesters of pregnancy was a constitutional right accelerated the evangelical backlash against abortion and left the short-lived evangelical campaign for therapeutic abortion laws in shambles. A modest abortion law permitting pregnancy termination for only for a few specific medical reasons was not an option after *Roe v. Wade*. When faced with the choice to either accept the Court's decision and make peace with the new legalization of elective abortion or join a campaign to overturn *Roe* and ban abortions, it did not take long for most evangelicals to side with the opponents of abortion. In doing so, they would transform the politics of the pro-life movement and, to a certain extent, their own theological framework.

EVANGELICAL POLITICS BEFORE *ROE*

Before *Roe v. Wade*, evangelicals did not have a unified political program. After all, theirs was a religious—not a political—movement, and it was centered on an emphasis on gospel-produced individual transformation through Christian conversion and spiritual regeneration. Because of this emphasis on divine transformation of the individual through the gospel, evangelicals were generally skeptical of social transformation projects. Unlike many liberal Protestant ministers, most of them were bystanders in the civil rights movement. Even those who supported the cause of racial integration, as the National Association of Evangelicals officially did, were reluctant to support a movement that had adopted civil disobedience as its tactic. For the most part, white evangelicals—and especially the leadership of the evangelical movement that was identified with *Christianity Today* magazine, Fuller Seminary, and Billy Graham's evangelistic ministry—was moderately conservative and supportive of both Dwight Eisenhower and Richard Nixon. Evangelicals were much more likely than liberal Protestants to support the Vietnam War, largely because of their strong opposition to communism.

If there was one political principle that united nearly all white evangelicals in the 1950s and 60s, it was that communism must be opposed, because it violated religious freedom and impeded the propagation of the gospel. The NAE denounced the United Nations in 1950 as being too tolerant of communism and ushering in an era of "world socialism and dictatorship," and for the next decade it echoed the right wing of the Republican Party in its calls for aggressive efforts against communist subversives at home and communist nations abroad. Billy Graham also made communism a central target of his preaching. And his magazine, *Christianity Today*, allied itself with J. Edgar Hoover, publishing articles from the FBI director even though he was not an evangelical.[67]

Beyond their concerns about communism, evangelicals were also concerned about alcohol use, secularization, the sexual revolution, and an erosion of family life. From the 1940s through the early 1960s—and especially during the election of 1960, when Senator John F. Kennedy (D-MA), a Catholic, was running for president—many northern evangelicals and Southern Baptists warned about the threat of Catholic political influence, but by the late 1960s, such warnings became less frequent, as evangelicals turned their attention to the more immediate threat of societal moral decay. Graham's sermons warned about the dangers of urban race riots, sexual licentiousness, family breakdown, widespread illicit drug use, and moral decay. The SBC passed new resolutions about alcohol advertising and widespread alcohol use almost every year in the early 1970s. Evangelicals issued a spate of books about sexual behavior, marriage, and home life. Evangelical magazines also began publishing more articles about the problem of pornography.[68]

But in all of this, evangelicals did not yet have a comprehensive political philosophy. Their political concerns overlapped those of many conservative Catholics, yet they evinced little interest in the comprehensive social vision and "Christocentric humanism" that had shaped Vatican II. The criticism that some American bishops issued toward the Vietnam War did not appeal to them. They gave strong support to Nixon's reelection campaign in 1972—with more than 80 percent of evangelical voters casting their ballots for Nixon—because he promised "law and order" in the face of societal moral breakdown.[69] The Nixon campaign accused Senator George McGovern of South Dakota, the Democratic nominee for president, of being the candidate of "acid, amnesty, and abortion," and evangelicals accepted this line, but when they did so, the idea that abortion was the most dangerous threat to the nation's moral order, rather than merely one problem among many, had not yet occurred to them.

The editors of *Christianity Today* were therefore shocked when the Supreme Court, in an opinion written by one of the justices that Nixon had nominated, issued a ruling only two days after Nixon's second inauguration that eviscerated the abortion laws of forty-six states and declared elective abortion a constitutional right. "Christians should accustom themselves to the thought that the American state no longer supports, in any meaningful sense, the laws of God, and prepare themselves spiritually for the prospect that it may one day formally repudiate them and turn against those who seek to live by them," *Christianity Today* stated.[70]

For the editors of Graham's magazine, *Roe v. Wade* was about more than abortion. It was a repudiation of Christian moral standards, and it realigned the U.S. government in opposition to Christians who were trying to live by God's law. Evangelicals may not have had a cohesive political program before *Roe*—and they may not have even had a fully developed theology on abortion—but the Court's ruling on abortion would prompt some of them to begin thinking about one. Before the battle was over, evangelicals' theology and politics would be reshaped in opposition to *Roe*. But the change was not instantaneous. Before evangelicals could join the pro-life cause, they needed a new paradigm for viewing abortion, and the next few years would be critical in developing one.

CHAPTER 4

CATHOLICS AND EVANGELICALS AFTER *ROE*

The Making of a Pro-Life Alliance

Two days after the Supreme Court issued its decisions in *Roe v. Wade* and the companion Georgia case, *Doe v. Bolton*, the National Conference of Catholic Bishops' (NCCB) Committee for Pro-Life Affairs issued a thunderous denunciation of the rulings: "The sweeping judgment of the U.S. Supreme Court in the Texas and Georgia abortion cases is a flagrant rejection of the unborn child's right to life. . . . This is bad morality, bad medicine and bad public policy, and it cannot be harmonized with basic moral principles. . . . We have no choice but to urge that the Court's judgment be opposed and rejected."[1] If Catholic doctors, nurses, or hospitals were ever required to perform an abortion, they had no choice but to disobey the law, the bishops said.

This last piece of advice was unprecedented for the bishops. Many individual Catholics had engaged in civil disobedience for moral causes in the recent past, but the bishops had never before issued an official excoriation of a Supreme Court ruling or encouraged civil disobedience so directly. "Since the establishment of the American Roman Catholic hierarchy in 1789, the bishops have been virtual apostles of respect for civil law," a *Commonweal* editor wrote. The bishops' response to *Roe* was therefore "without precedent in American Catholic history."[2]

But if the bishops' statement was without parallel in the Catholic Church, it closely presaged the reaction of *Christianity Today*'s evangelical Protestant editors only a few days later. "This decision runs counter not merely to the moral teachings of Christianity through the ages but also to the moral sense of the American people," *Christianity Today* said in February 1973. "Christians should accustom themselves to the thought that the American state no longer supports, in any meaningful sense, the laws of God, and prepare themselves spiritually for the prospect that it may one day formally repudiate them and turn against those who seek to live by them."[3]

Christianity Today's framing of *Roe* as a sign that the Supreme Court had repudiated Christianity and the "laws of God" became evangelicals' preferred interpretation of *Roe* by the end of the 1970s, just as it was the preferred interpretation of most pro-life Catholics. In evangelicals' view, *Roe* was no longer merely about abortion, as significant as that issue was. Most of all, it was a demonstration of the frightening consequences that resulted from the Court's rejection of God's moral standards. And it was only a harbinger of greater horrors to come. "Make no mistake: the logic of the high court could be used with like—in some cases with greater—force to justify infanticide for unwanted or undesirable infants," said *Christianity Today*. "The expression, 'capability of meaningful life' could cover a multitude of evils and will, unless this development is stopped now."[4] This was exactly what many pro-life Catholics had been saying for several years, and now some evangelicals were beginning to say it, too. The solution, the *Christianity Today* editorial seemed to indicate, was not merely greater restrictions on abortion but a change in the Court's philosophy and a return to a Christian standard of moral and legal reasoning.

During the 1970s, both Catholics and conservative evangelicals quickly moved toward an interpretation of the abortion issue that connected pro-life activism to a larger quest to return the nation to an explicitly Christian legal framework. This new understanding of the pro-life campaign as a quest to restore Christian values in the nation's law had not been nearly as prominent in discussions of the issue before 1973, and its introduction immediately after *Roe* changed the politics of the abortion issue in the churches. For some politically conservative Christians, this was a welcome development, but for others, it was a difficult adjustment and a source of debate in both the Catholic Church and the Southern Baptist Convention.

THE ABORTION ISSUE IN THE CATHOLIC CHURCH

Although many Catholic bishops in the United States had given tacit acceptance to differences of opinion on contraception among Catholics, they made clear immediately after *Roe* that there was no room for similar private judgment on abortion. The bishops reminded Catholics that any member of their church who obtained or performed an abortion would be excommunicated. This was a reiteration of existing canon law—not a new practice on the part of the bishops—but their bold reminder of the principle signaled that they intended to take abortion seriously and that there was no room in the Catholic Church for divergent interpretations of this doctrine. Catholics might be able to follow their own consciences on contraception and still be able to take Communion even while violating papal encyclicals on the subject, but the same would not be true of abortion. But it was not the reiteration of existing ecclesiastical penalties for abortion or even the bishops' discussion of the possibility of civil disobedience that had the greatest effect on the nation's political discussions of abortion. It was instead the bishops' decision to become more directly involved in policy debates on abortion.

The bishops quickly concluded that a constitutional amendment offered the best path to reversing *Roe v. Wade* and protecting unborn human life, so in November 1973 they launched the National Committee for a

Human Life Amendment to lobby for one.[5] There were numerous pro-life organizations already in existence—including the National Right to Life Committee, which had started in the office of the NCCB's Family Life Bureau five years earlier—but the bishops thought that an additional one was needed in order to provide some degree of church control over the effort. The bishops planned to allocate to the committee one cent for every Catholic in the United States, which would give the committee $500,000 to work with in its first year. For those who wondered whether this was an inappropriate use of church monies for political lobbying or an inappropriate intrusion of a sectarian religious organization into the political affairs of a pluralistic nation, the first president of the committee, Robert Lynch, had a ready response: "The human rights issue [that is, the right to life for the unborn] transcends any question of the morality espoused by any given church and strikes at the very heart of the principles upon which this nation was founded."[6]

In March 1974, several of the nation's leading archbishops arrived in Washington, DC, to testify in favor of a Human Life Amendment at a Senate subcommittee hearing. Mindful that bishops in the past had eschewed direct engagement in congressional committee hearings and that many would wonder whether the presence of the bishops inappropriately crossed the line separating church from state, Cardinal John Krol, the president of the NCCB, addressed the issue directly in his testimony by grounding his arguments in the language of human rights, which by this point was standard practice for church officials whenever they discussed abortion policy. "We do not propose to advocate sectarian doctrine but to defend human rights, and specifically, the most fundamental of all rights, the right to life itself," Krol said. "We reject any suggestion that we are attempting to impose 'our' morality on others. . . . The right to life is not an invention of the Catholic Church or any other church. It is a basic human right which must undergird any civilized society."[7]

The Senate did not act on the amendment proposal, but that did not deter the bishops. They received renewed impetus for their campaign from the Vatican when the Sacred Congregation for the Doctrine of the Faith issued another statement on abortion in 1974, *Declaration on Pro-*

cured Abortion. That document reiterated church teaching on abortion and refuted arguments that this doctrine dated back only to the nineteenth century, as some critics of the Catholic position argued. It was actually the unchanging teaching of the church stretching back to the earliest days of Christianity, the Vatican argued. But in addition, the Vatican declaration also made clear that opposition to abortion could not merely be a personal moral belief when abortion policies were at stake; Catholics had to use the civil law to protect unborn human life. "It is at all times the task of the State to preserve each person's rights and to protect the weakest," the Vatican said. "It is the task of law to pursue a reform of society and of conditions of life in all milieux, starting with the most deprived, so that always and everywhere it may be possible to give every child coming into this world a welcome worthy of a person." That did not mean that every abortion law necessarily had to impose penalties, the Vatican said. "Human law can abstain from punishment, but it cannot declare to be right what would be opposed to the natural law." If the law permitted abortion, that would be wrong. Catholics should not "take part in a propaganda campaign in favor of such a law, or vote for it." Clearly, abortion restrictions—or, to put it more positively, legal protections of the human rights of the unborn—were important to the Catholic Church. Yet at the same time, the church emphasized that restrictions alone were not enough. Like several earlier declarations from the church on the topic, the Vatican's declaration of 1974 reiterated the importance of "help for families and for unmarried mothers, assured grants for children, a statute for illegitimate children and reasonable arrangements for adoption." "A whole positive policy must be put into force so that there will always be a concrete, honorable and possible alternative to abortion."[8]

In November 1975, the NCCB committed the Catholic Church in the United States to a political lobbying campaign for the Human Life Amendment by issuing the "Pastoral Plan for Pro-Life Activities." The Pastoral Plan committed the bishops to organize pro-life groups at the parish level and committed the church to pro-life activism, which would include the defense of human life at every stage but would be especially focused on the issue of abortion. Although the document went beyond previous episcopal commitments in its declaration of the specific church-sponsored pro-life educational and political work that would be required to enact legal protections for the unborn, most of this merely built on the foundation that the Vatican and the bishops' Family Life Bureau had already laid in their previous pronouncements on the topic. Yet the document also signaled a subtle shift in the framework for this pro-life organizing — a shift toward an explicitly Christian framework for antiabortion policies.

As recently as 1974, when Cardinal Krol had testified at Senate subcommittee hearings on a Human Life Amendment, the nation's Catholic bishops had insisted that opposition to abortion was not a religious, but a moral, principle that stemmed from human rights ideology and natural law. The "Pastoral Plan for Pro-Life Activities" did not abandon that claim altogether, but it shifted its emphasis away from attempting to win the battle using secular arguments with universal appeal — which apparently had not worked — to conceding that the strongest arguments against abortion were "theological and moral." That was not because one needed direct revelation from God or an ecclesiastical teaching to know that human life began at the moment of conception, the bishops said; science offered compelling biological reasons to accept that fact. It was rather because only Christian theology offered a clear rationale for why all human life — including the life of the tiniest zygote — had eternal value and should be protected at all costs: "Respect for life must be seen in the context of God's love for mankind reflected in creation and redemption and man's relationship to God and to other members of the human family." This was not a novel teaching, of course; Vatican II had said very similar things. But until that point, most of the church's pro-life lobbying had not emphasized the explicitly Christian theological rationale for the pro-life movement's major argument. Cognizant of the American tradition of separation of church and state — and the long-standing suspicion of many Protestants that the Catholic Church did not sufficiently respect that separation — Catholic bishops had gone out of their way in the late 1960s and early 1970s to demonstrate that they did respect church–state separation and that their political lobbying against abortion had nothing to do with religion. Now the bishops were changing their approach and explicitly arguing that the human rights framework in which they had grounded their opposition to abortion was directly linked with Christianity.

"The Church's opposition to abortion," the bishops stated, was based both on the "Christian teaching of the dignity of the human person" and "the responsibility to proclaim and defend basic human rights, especially the right to life." "The maintenance and protection of human rights are primary purposes of law." But rather than say that human rights could be separated from the church's teaching about creation and redemption, the bishops' Pastoral Plan instead argued that U.S. law and its framework for the protection of human rights had historically been Christian. "As our founding fathers believed, we hold that all law is ultimately based on Divine Law, and that a just system of law cannot conflict with the law of God," the bishops said.[9] Although the bishops may not have fully realized it at the time, their new effort to ground pro-life activism in the claim that the founding fathers had intended the country to base its laws on the unchanging "law of God" made their cause much more attractive to conservative evangelical Protestants, who were developing a similar view of the relationship between the founding and divine law.

Conservative evangelical Protestants could also take comfort in the bishops' insistence that the foundation for their position on human life was not specifically Catholic but was instead broadly Christian. "Though I speak as the representative of a particular Church, the concern that I raise is not that of one particular denomination," Archbishop Joseph Bernardin said in a sermon on abortion in January 1977, the fourth anniversary of *Roe v. Wade*. "The issue is far more basic than that. It is a question of the value that we as a society place on human life. It is a question of whether we accept human life as a God-given gift or as a mere material object to be manipulated or destroyed at will."[10] This was a theistic framing of the issue that appealed to both Catholics and evangelicals who were mobilizing against secularism. If the position that people took on abortion reflected whether they saw human life as divinely created or a "mere material object" that was the product of natural forces and human manipulation, theologically conservative Catholics and evangelicals wanted to be on the theistic side of that divide.

THE POLITICAL DEBATES OVER ABORTION AMONG SOUTHERN BAPTISTS

Before 1973, the debate about abortion among evangelicals (including Southern Baptists) was primarily a debate about fetal personhood and the interpretation of biblical texts that might provide some clues as to when human life began. After 1973, the debate became inseparable from the question of the Christian identity of the nation and an unchanging, divinely given standard of morality. Those in the evangelical coalition who were the strongest advocates of church–state separation and religious liberty were the most reticent to denounce *Roe*, while those who were most worried about secularization and the moral decline of the nation were the first to lambaste the Supreme Court decision and join the pro-life movement, just as *Christianity Today* had. The debate about *Roe* and abortion among evangelicals thus became inseparable from a much larger contentious discussion about the future political direction of the evangelical movement. Nowhere was this discussion more heated and acrimonious than among Baptists. Baptists had taken the lead in championing church–state separation since Roger Williams's opposition to the Puritan establishment in Massachusetts in the seventeenth century, and many in the mid-twentieth century wanted to continue that tradition. But many Baptists were also conservative evangelicals who believed in using the power of the law to regulate vice and who worried about the sexual revolution and the secularization of the country.

In the early 1970s, the Southern Baptist Convention (SBC) was simultaneously an advocate for moral regulation and a defender of religious liberty. In 1971, Southern Baptists signaled their equal devotion to both causes by passing both a resolution urging Congress to enact legislation prohibiting the advertisement of alcohol on television and radio and another resolution declaring that prayer must be "voluntary and uncoerced by governmental or ecclesiastical authorities," a resolution designed to convey the SBC's antipathy to constitutional amendment proposals to reverse the Supreme Court's school prayer decision in *Engel v. Vitale* (1962) and restore classroom prayer in public schools. Neither resolution was in any way surprising, because Southern Baptists had for many decades lobbied for legal restrictions on alcohol while also opposing any hint of religious establishment, since they viewed themselves as the nation's staunchest defenders of religious liberty. Their 1971 resolution on prayer declared, "Baptists have made a major contribution to the world by insisting on religious liberty for all and by emphasizing that a genuine religious experience is a voluntary response to God."[11] Baptists prided themselves on being part of a tradition that emphasized the "priesthood of all believers" and freedom of conscience. Moral regulation was appropriate, therefore, only when it stemmed from concerns that were not merely religious, since religion, they believed, had to be voluntary. Their most prominent political cause of the mid-twentieth century—alcohol regulation—was grounded in scientific principles, not religiously sectarian doctrine, they believed. They argued that the U.S. government should restrict alcohol advertising not because the Bible condemned drunkenness (though they knew, of course, that it did) but because statistical evidence conclusively showed that alcohol was a leading contributor to car accident fatalities, national health problems, and crime.[12]

In taking this stance, they found themselves directly at odds with Catholics, who had long championed the innocent pleasures of wine (and use in the Mass) and taken a dim view of evangelical Protestants' prohibitionist inclinations. In the view of many pro-life Catholics, the Baptists' zeal for alcohol regulation was a religiously sectarian rather than scientifically grounded cause. On the other hand, they believed that their own defense of unborn human life was grounded in the scientific evidence about fetal development and the unique genetic composition of each embryo. "When human life begins is not a doctrine of the Catholic Church, or of any church. It is a biological fact," the NCCB said in 1981 in a reiteration of an argument they had been making for years. "When the chromosomes of the human sperm and ovum fuse, a new human being with a unique genetic make-up comes into existence."[13] For that reason, "abortion is not a 'private and individual issue,' nor is it a sectarian, denominational issue," Archbishop Joseph Bernardin said. "Abortion is a question of human and civil rights. Any Church body has a right, as does any and every group, to speak out when it feels that human rights are being violated." "The leadership of the Catholic Church is not attempting to force its opinion on anyone," Bernardin said, in a rebuke to the many people who viewed the church's pro-life activism as a dangerous violation of church–state separation. "It is simply exercising its responsibility in informing the public of the seriousness of the issue in question, and the ultimate consequences of the faulty logic upon which the abortion decision is based. The issue will ultimately be decided by the democratic process."[14]

But many Baptists took the opposite view. The Catholic Church's insistence that a zygote, embryo, or fetus was a full human person from the moment of conception and that abortion was always wrong was a theological position that could not be defended apart from church dogma. In the Baptists' view, personhood was inseparable from ensoulment, and since science could not answer the question of when a soul entered a human body—and since the Bible did not clearly answer that question, they thought—the question of the exact point a zygote, embryo, or fetus became a full person by obtaining a soul was a matter of theological speculation and therefore fell into the category of individual liberty of conscience. It could not be answered merely by repeating the pro-life movement's favorite argument that every zygote had a unique genetic identity from the moment of conception. Abortion might be morally questionable in many cases, and it was probably a good idea to try to reduce its incidence as much as possible, but it was wrong for a religious organization to use a theological interpretation that could not be firmly defended on either scientific or biblical grounds to deprive women of the ability to get a legal abortion even when a pregnancy severely threatened their health. At that point, the Catholic Church was threatening not only other people's liberties but other people's health and safety, and that had to be stopped.

The Baptist Joint Committee on Public Affairs (BJPCA), an interdenominational agency that drew support at the time from both the SBC and the northern-based American Baptist Churches USA, opposed the proposed Human Life Amendment on the grounds that a constitutional amendment protecting human life from the moment of conception violated individuals' religious liberty to make decisions in an area in which there was no theological consensus. *Roe v. Wade* "seems to be best for our pluralistic society," Elizabeth Miller, the secretary of issue development for the National Ministries of the American Baptist Churches USA, explained in 1976. "The decision of the Supreme Court does not determine whether abortion or any other act is moral or immoral. It simply defines the area in which the state has a legitimate interest and, therefore, the right to legislate."[15] The one state Southern Baptist periodical that endorsed the Court's *Roe* decision, the Virginia *Religious Recorder*, also did so on the grounds that the decision was an affirmation of the principles of religious liberty. So did *Baptist Press* Washington bureau chief W. Barry Garrett, a former associate director of the BJCPA. "Religious liberty, human equality and justice are advanced by the Supreme Court abortion decision," he wrote immediately after the Court issued its decision in *Roe*.[16] Most Southern Baptists who commented on abortion in the 1970s did not fully endorse *Roe*, but those who did invariably cited religious liberty as their reason for doing so – not gender equality, bodily autonomy, or women's rights. The BJCPA refused to comment on the morality of abortion itself, believing that this was a matter for churches and individual Christians—not an interdenominational political lobbying agency—to decide on the basis of scripture and theological principles.[17] But when it came to the government's role, the matter was clear: If the government restricted abortion on the basis of a particular religious tradition's understanding of fetal life, it would violate the religious liberty of those who disagreed and erode the separation between church and state.

This view was more common among members of the American Baptist Churches USA than it was among Southern Baptists, but it did appeal to a few Southern Baptist seminary faculty, such as Paul D. Simmons, a professor of Christian ethics at the Southern Baptist Theological Seminary. It also found a champion in the head of the SBC's Christian Life Commission, Foy Valentine. As the leader of the denomination's official political agency, Valentine tried to steer a moderately liberal course on matters of political controversy and gave greater emphasis to fighting poverty and racism than engaging in culture war campaigns to fight the sexual revolution. His ethical compass had been shaped by the civil rights movement and by fighting the fundamentalists in the denomination who did not share his view of racial justice. But though he was more liberal than some of these theological conservatives on the issue of abortion, he never went as far as the New York Baptist pastor Howard Moody, whose liberal views on civil rights and social justice had led him to found the Clergy Consultation Service on Abortion. To a much greater extent than Moody, Valentine had moral reservations about abortion; he said that he did not support "abortion on demand." One of Valentine's staff members at the Christian Life Commission characterized his views on abortion as "basically conservative."[18] At the same time, though, Valentine believed that therapeutic abortion could be legitimate, and he thought that Christians who joined the campaign to prohibit all abortions were inappropriately imposing a religiously sectarian view of human life on those who had good reasons for rejecting that absolutist position. His strong interest in defending the separation of church and state, which he viewed as a bedrock Baptist principle, made him suspicious of the antiabortion cause. Even though he said that *Roe* went further than he would have liked, Valentine decided that if he was faced with the choice of siding with anti-abortion absolutists or pro-choice activists who wanted to keep abortion legal, he would side with the pro-choice activists as the lesser of the two evils. Over the course of the 1970s, he found himself pushed closer to the pro-choice camp because of his strong suspicion that pro-life activists were going to violate the sacred principles of liberty of conscience and church–state separation.

Valentine's views were typical of an emerging faction in the SBC that in the late 1970s became known as "moderates." Moderates held generally conservative views on the Bible (even if they were more hesitant than the SBC's conservatives to claim that the scriptures were fully "inerrant"), but they resisted what they considered "fundamentalism," and they did not want to become involved in culture war politics. They were strong advocates of church–state separation, which they considered a long-standing Baptist hallmark. For most of the 1970s, moderates held all the major leadership positions in the SBC, from the presidency of the denomination to the top administrative posts at the various Southern Baptist agencies and denominational seminaries. On abortion, moderates such as Valentine did their best to retain the denomination's pre-*Roe*, middle-of-the-road position that allowed for therapeutic abortion but opposed "abortion on demand."[19]

But other Southern Baptist pastors who did not align with the moderates were convinced that abortion was murder and that laws needed to be passed against it on the same grounds that Southern Baptists had long called for legal prohibitions on other moral evils, such as alcohol. Immediately after *Roe v. Wade*, Texas Baptist pastor Robert Holbrook started Baptists for Life, with the intention of using the organization to lobby for a stronger antiabortion resolution from the SBC. Calling the legalization of abortion "one of the gravest moral crises of our time," he implored his fellow Baptists to "take part in whatever legal measures are proposed from Austin and Washington to reverse the Supreme Court decision which spells doom for untold thousands of unborn children." Baptists who thought that pro-life activism would violate the principle of church–state separation were strangely inconsistent, he thought, since the SBC had repeatedly taken stances on public policies on alcohol and gambling. "Surely the killing of the unborn is a more pressing matter than 'betting on a horse,'" Holbrook wrote. He believed that the reason Baptists had been slow to embrace the right-to-life cause was because they did not really believe that the fetus was a full human being, but in his view, the position of many Southern Baptist moderates that the fetus was not a full person and was instead only a "potential" or "developing" life made no sense from either a scientific or a biblical perspective. In May 1973, he published an article in the Texas *Baptist Standard* that recited the same scientific arguments that pro-life Catholics had made for years and paired them with the biblical verses about unborn human life (such as Psalm 139:13–16) that were quickly becoming popular with many pro-life evangelicals. "The testimony of medical science is that human life begins at conception," Holbrook said, and "the biblical evidence allows no place for the argument that the fetus' life has a developing value. Scripture asserts that the fetus is life and does not sophisticate the question by asking when it becomes 'human.'"[20]

All of these arguments could have been made the previous year or the year before, but Holbrook had not challenged the SBC's moderate stance on abortion in either 1971 or 1972. For him—as for many other evangelicals who enlisted in the pro-life cause—it was only *Roe v. Wade* that made it imperative to speak out. The Court ruling, he predicted, would result in 1.6 million abortions during the next year. The actual number turned out to be under 1 million in the immediate aftermath of *Roe*, but it rose to more than 1.5 million per year by the end of the decade. Catholics had seen the legalization of abortion at the state level in the late 1960s and early 1970s as a problem, but most evangelicals, especially among Southern Baptists, had not seen the urgency of the issue until *Roe* and the ensuing rise in the number of legal abortions. Perhaps that was partly because no state in the South (where most Southern Baptists lived) had legalized elective abortion until *Roe* compelled them to do so. *Roe* brought the issue into their own communities and forced them to confront the reality of legalized elective abortion. But it also challenged their view of the nation's institutions, forcing them to acknowledge the discrepancy between the Court's opinion and God's moral law.

Holbrook and his allies made their first attempt to challenge the SBC's moderate stance on abortion and put the denomination on record as categorically opposed to abortion at the convention's annual meeting in Dallas in June 1974. Hugo Lindquist, a fifty-year-old pastor from Oklahoma, introduced a resolution calling on "all Southern Baptist pastors and church congregations to preach and teach against the crime of abortion." The convention should "go on record as being opposed to abortion for any reason," Lindquist said, and it should also "go on record as favoring an amendment to the United States Constitution forbidding abortion."[21] This went too far for many Southern Baptists, and the motion was defeated by a wide margin. Following Valentine's lead, the convention instead adopted a motion that reaffirmed the SBC's endorsement of therapeutic abortion laws as a "middle ground between the extreme of abortion on demand and the opposite extreme of all abortion as murder." At the same convention, the SBC adopted a resolution opposing the "distribution of pornographic materials" and calling on Southern Baptists to "continue the fight until these items are removed from our midst."[22] Pornography was a clear social danger, they thought, and laws against pornography did not violate the principle of religious liberty. But abortion was another matter, many Southern Baptists believed. Those who still thought that abortion could be legitimate in a few therapeutic cases tended to see the pro-life movement as a religiously sectarian, "extreme" campaign. One article in the Texas *Baptist Standard* explained in July 1974 that "Christians should never claim that induced abortion is right. However, under certain circumstances it might carry fewer tragic, painful consequences than other possible courses of action." The article cited the favorite biblical passage of abortion moderates among evangelicals—Exodus 21:22–25—to argue that there was a difference in value between fetal life and maternal life.[23] And if that was the case, the type of resolution that Holbrook wanted went well beyond what the Bible warranted, even if abortion was morally problematic.

But Holbrook's battle had only just begun. After losing his fight for a stronger antiabortion resolution at the 1974 annual meeting of the SBC, he introduced the same antiabortion resolution again in 1975. The resolutions committee responded by choosing not to bring the resolution to a floor vote. The convention had already demonstrated its concern about "the widespread and irresponsible use of abortion," the resolutions committee noted, and that was why it had passed resolutions on abortion in 1971 and 1974, both of which expressed a "high view of human life, including fetal life," in the opinion of the resolutions committee.[24] No further action was needed, in their view. But abortion opinion among evangelicals in general and Southern Baptists in particular was rapidly shifting to the right. As the number of abortions in the country continued to increase each year and as the connection between the sexual revolution and abortion became more obvious to some conservative evangelicals, the long-standing view among some Southern Baptists that Exodus 21 suggested a lesser value for fetal life no longer seemed so persuasive, and the pro-life advocates' alternative explanation of this passage and their interpretations of their own oft-cited Bible verses (such as Psalm 139:13–16, Jeremiah 1:5, and Luke 1:40–44) started to look a lot more convincing.

In 1976, the SBC Resolutions Committee decided to revisit the abortion issue, and this time the denomination passed a much stronger antiabortion resolution that was closer to what Holbrook wanted.

"Every decision for an abortion, for whatever reason must necessarily involve the decision to terminate the life of an innocent human being," the 1976 resolution said. Because "the practice of abortion for selfish non-therapeutic reasons . . . destroys fetal life, dulls our society's moral sensitivity, and leads to a cheapening of all human life," the resolution urged Southern Baptists to "work to change those attitudes and conditions which encourage many people to turn to abortion as a means of birth control." The resolution did not clearly state whether there were any situations that could justify an abortion. In 1971 and 1974, the convention had explicitly declared that there were. In 1976, by contrast, the convention clearly said that every abortion "terminate[d] the life of a human being" and that abortion for "selfish non-therapeutic reasons" was wrong, but it did not resolve the question of whether any therapeutic concerns might be serious enough to justify the taking of fetal life through an abortion. The final sentence of the resolution (which some messengers at the convention wanted to modify, but which was ultimately left intact) appeared to be a concession to those who wanted to avoid linking the SBC to the pro-life movement or to an absolutist stand against all abortions: "We also affirm our conviction about the limited role of government in dealing with matters relating to abortion, and support the right of expectant mothers to the full range of medical services and personal counseling for the preservation of life and health." Previously, the convention had said that the "preservation of life and health" justified abortion. Now, the convention simply said that "expectant mothers" facing issues of "life and health" were entitled to the "full range of medical services and personal counseling" in such situations, a clause that was vague enough to possibly include abortion for those who wanted to think that it did, yet sufficiently unclear to avoid any conflict with Holbrook's total opposition to abortion.[25]

If the resolution read like an awkwardly worded compromise between opposing forces, that was a reflection of the level of disagreement on the issue at the convention. Abortion was the "most hotly-debated issue" at the 1976 annual meeting of the SBC, the Baptist Press reported. Some Southern Baptists, such as Holbrook, wanted a more sweeping declaration opposing all abortion, but their proposed resolutions were defeated. Others, such as Valentine, wanted Southern Baptists to continue to affirm exceptions for abortion in the case of rape and incest and other therapeutic cases. In the end, the SBC did neither. What was clear was that the SBC was rapidly moving toward a more restrictive stance on abortion, and that by 1976, any allowance it made for abortion in therapeutic cases was ambiguous at best. But because of the continued presence of many moderates in leadership positions in the denomination, the SBC was not quite ready for an absolutist stance on the issue.[26] Valentine, in fact, went so far as to deny that Southern Baptists were part of the same wing of Christianity as the northern evangelicals who were passing resolutions against abortion in their denominations and mobilizing in the emerging culture wars on the issue. "We're not evangelicals," he insisted in 1976. "That's a Yankee word. . . . We don't share their politics or their fussy fundamentalism, and we don't want to get involved in their theological witch-hunts."[27]

But Valentine had less ability to keep northern evangelical political influences out of the SBC than he would have liked. Like many other evangelicals outside of the SBC, a growing number of Southern Baptists believed that their country was experiencing a rapid moral decline, especially on issues of sexuality. In 1975, the SBC passed resolutions affirming marital monogamy and deploring the depiction of violence on television for entertainment purposes. The next year, the convention passed resolutions against pornography and homosexuality in addition to reiterating Southern Baptists' long-standing opposition to alcohol.[28] With so many concerns about the sexual revolution and the protection of the traditional family in the air, it was hardly surprising that many Southern Baptists were joining with other evangelicals outside the SBC to defend the family and protest against national moral decline by denouncing abortion. Valentine might have wished that it were otherwise, but many Southern Baptists were, in fact, evangelicals, and they didn't seem to mind the conservative politics of their "Yankee" evangelical counterparts.

GROWING OPPOSITION TO ABORTION AMONG EVANGELICALS OUTSIDE OF THE SBC

From 1973 through 1976, evangelical opinion continued to harden against abortion. On the right wing of the movement, politically conservative fundamentalists kept up a steady drumbeat of denunciations of the practice. Noel Smith, the editor of the *Baptist Bible Tribune*, published a spate of editorials against abortion. Billy James Hargis, the anticommunist radio preacher who founded the Christian Crusade, launched a new organization called Americans against Abortion to focus specifically on the issue.[29] Bob Jones University's institutional magazine, *Faith for the Family*, also denounced abortion.[30] And in June 1973, the General Association of Regular Baptists, a northern-based fundamentalist Baptist denomination, adopted a resolution calling abortion "murder."[31]

Among evangelicals outside of Baptist circles, opposition to abortion also increased. In 1975, the conservative southern Presbyterian Ruth Bell Graham (the wife of evangelist Billy Graham) organized an evangelical pro-life conference attended by twenty-five leading Protestant ministers, including Robert Holbrook.[32] Also in the summer of 1975, Chicago-based Trinity Evangelical Divinity School professor Harold O. J. Brown teamed up with Philadelphia physician (and future surgeon general) C. Everett Koop to found the Christian Action Council, which billed itself as the first Protestant pro-life organization. The claim may have been a bit exaggerated, since both Holbrook's Baptists for Life and Hargis's Americans against Abortion were founded before the Christian Action Council. But Brown was correct in seeing the Christian Action Council as the first broadly based, interdenominational, mainstream evangelical pro-life organization. The group fought back against the widespread stereotype that the pro-life cause was a Catholic sectarian issue. It was not. "Virtually all Christians from the beginning have been against permissive abortion and for the protection of all human life," the Christian Action Council said. It therefore wanted "to make clear to lawmakers that abortion and related problems are not merely sectarian or 'doctrinal' issues but of fundamental importance to the whole of Western civilization."[33]

Brown explained the connection between legalized abortion and the moral decline of a society in more detail in his book *Death before Birth*. Although he was a professor at an evangelical Protestant seminary and an ordained minister in the evangelical wing of the Congregational Church, Brown's arguments were nearly identical to those that Catholic pro-life advocates had made a decade earlier. Because abortion killed human beings, it desensitized people to the value of human life, Brown wrote. In the process, it moved the nation away from its historic Christian foundation for human rights values. "The abortion system, then, consciously or unconsciously converts people from the 'Hippocratic' ethic (which is essentially the Judeo-Christian ethic) of the value of all human life to a utilitarian ethic that values life in terms of its convenience, usefulness, and cost," Brown wrote. "An unwanted baby is inconvenient, expensive, and not useful at all. With a utilitarian ethic there is no reason to protect it. Since *Roe v. Wade*, an unborn child in America has no protection."[34] *Roe v. Wade* was a "judicially mandated paganization of American law and mores" – that is, a rejection of Christian principles and a return to the morals of ancient pagan societies. This was destroying the United States, he believed; it was now a society whose violence against the innocent was more heinous than that of any other society since ancient Assyria, with the sole exception of Nazi Germany. A campaign against abortion, in Brown's view, was fundamentally a campaign to purify the United States from its bloodguilt; it was a campaign for the restoration of the nation. "Protestant Christians who have any concern at all for the land in which we live and the people among whom we dwell . . . simply cannot ignore this massive and increasing blood pollution," he wrote.[35] For Brown and for many other evangelicals, the campaign against abortion was thus not solely or even primarily about saving babies (though it was that in part); it was above all a campaign to save the nation.

Christianity Today adopted a similar message. For *Christianity Today*, the issue of abortion was significant not only because it deprived fetuses of their lives but because the relativistic, anti-Christian thinking behind *Roe v. Wade* would lead to other horrors, such as infanticide and euthanasia. "Abortion on demand is with us. Now we are being prepared for the idea that ordinary dying is 'passive' euthanasia; in time we will be asked to accept 'active' euthanasia, first 'voluntary,' then, perhaps, on the orders of 'competent authorities.' We are now being accustomed to the idea of 'disincentives' to large families; next on the agenda, one fears, are 'penalization,' 'controls,' sterilization, then 'forfeiting' of the right to live," a *Christianity Today* editorial predicted in the summer of 1974. "Have you ever wondered how Germany's Christians could have remained silent and indifferent when Hitler began his far-reaching scheme of racial 'improvement'? If you are not actively opposing what is going on in our own country, in the direction of total control of human life, you have the answer."[36]

This argument was very similar to what Catholic opponents of abortion had been saying for the past decade. Indeed, by the mid-1970s, it was becoming increasingly difficult at times to tell the difference between evangelical pro-life arguments and those presented by Catholics. In the view of an increasing number of evangelicals, abortion was not merely an evangelical concern or a Catholic concern, but a matter that was vitally important to anyone who cared about the future of the nation and its foundation in human rights. "The ethical questions posed by abortion focus on the most fundamental of human rights, the right to life," *Christianity Today* said in 1976. "It is a principle that is even more basic and important than the right to food currently being championed by Bread for the World."[37]

Once evangelicals accepted the Catholic framing of abortion as a human rights concern and a matter on which the future of "Western civilization" depended, the handful of Bible verses that had featured so prominently in evangelical discussions of abortion in the late 1960s and early 1970s no longer mattered as much. Evangelicals still discussed those verses in settings in which they needed to convince fellow evangelicals that the Bible really did protect human life. And for some evangelicals, a few Bible verses about prenatal life—especially Psalm 139:13–16 (which included the line, "You knit me together in my mother's womb," as the evangelical-produced New International Version rendered it)—were still important motivators for action and a reminder that concern for the unborn had scriptural support. But most of *Christianity Today*'s discussions of abortion in the mid-1970s no longer cited the Bible at all, which was a contrast with the magazine's earliest discussions of the abortion issue. In their view, what made abortion so horrendous was not that it was at odds with a few biblical passages but that it was a violation of the most fundamental human right, an assault on the basic principles of Christianity and of Western civilization, and a dangerous precursor to infanticide or euthanasia. This was exactly what Catholics had been saying since the mid-1960s. In the 1960s, most evangelicals had ignored the Catholic warnings, but by the mid-1970s they found them persuasive. The reason for the change in evangelical attitudes toward abortion had less to do with new understandings of the Bible than with new understandings of the nation's culture. After seeing the proliferation of pornography in the early 1970s, the rise of the gay rights movement, and a spike in the divorce rate, evangelicals of the mid-1970s were far more open to alarmist narratives of cultural decline than they had been only a decade earlier. The nation was in crisis, they believed, and they were desperate for a political solution to the nation's moral problems. The abortion issue fit that narrative better than any other issue, because it was connected to both the U.S. government's rejection of Christian values (as evidenced in the Court's ruling in *Roe v. Wade*) and the sexual revolution. In the mid-1970s, no evangelical did a better job connecting those dots than Francis Schaeffer.

FRANCIS SCHAEFFER

Schaeffer, a conservative American Presbyterian missionary in Switzerland, was already a best-selling evangelical Christian apologist when he turned his attention to the issue of abortion in the mid-1970s. Thousands of young Americans and Europeans — many of them evangelical Christians but others of whom were skeptics or spiritual seekers curious about Schaeffer's message — made their way to his Alpine home, where he welcomed all visitors and encouraged them to dialogue with him in evening discussions on the rationality of the Christian faith. All worldviews other than biblical Christianity were based on self-contradictions, logical inconsistencies, or wishful thinking, he argued. Christianity alone could adequately explain all of life and give a person a rational foundation for belief in unchanging truths. After delivering this message to the hikers and hippies who made the trek to his mountain retreat, he took the message to Christian colleges and churches in the United States on a lecture circuit, and then published it in several widely distributed books of apologetics, starting with *The God Who Is There* in 1968. Schaeffer's early books did not mention abortion, but in the mid-1970s, he became interested in the issue, because he became convinced that permissive abortion laws were a sign of moral relativism. He first gave the issue prominent attention in a book and documentary film series on the moral decline of the West that he released in 1976 under the title *How Should We Then Live?* After presenting a sweeping 2,000-year history of the rejection of objective moral standards in art, music, philosophy, and theology, *How Should We Then Live?* turned its focus to the recent legalization of abortion, which in Schaeffer's view was a prime exhibit of the frightening consequences of a societal rejection of divinely given moral absolutes.[38]

Although Schaeffer framed his historical analysis as a study of the Western world, it was, to a large degree, a history of a loss of Christian moral absolutes in the United States. That was especially true when it came to the issue of abortion, which he viewed as a moral barometer of the country's moral state. According to Schaeffer, the United States had been founded on biblical principles that reflected its original Protestant heritage, but in the twentieth century, it abandoned that framework. *Roe v. Wade* was an "arbitrary ruling," he said, based not on medical science or constitutional principles but simply the whims of the Court. It was "sociological law" that reflected changing social and cultural norms rather than fixed constitutional meaning. And, worst of all, there were no obvious limits on the Court's power to arbitrarily redefine moral norms, because the Court's rulings were no longer grounded in fixed principles. "In regard to the fetus, the courts have arbitrarily separated 'aliveness' from 'personhood,' and if this is so, why not arbitrarily do the same with the aged?" Schaeffer asked, in a repetition of an argument that pro-life Catholics had been making for years. "So the steps move along, and euthanasia may become increasingly acceptable. And if so, why not keep alive the bodies of the so-called neo-morts (persons in whom the brain wave is flat) to harvest from them body parts and blood, when the polls show this has become acceptable to the majority? . . . . Law has become a matter of averages, just as the culture's sexual mores have become only a matter of averages."[39]

How Should We Then Live? was an evangelical sensation. The book sold 40,000 copies in the first three months, but the accompanying film series, which sometimes drew audiences as large as 5,000 at some of the churches that screened it, reached many more people, some of whom found their lives changed by the experience. At Covenant Theological Seminary in St. Louis, some of the students who saw the film series began joining local pro-life demonstrations. In upstate New York, Randall Terry (who would later found Operation Rescue) was moved to tears by the film series's depiction of abortion, and he resolved to devote his life to the pro-life cause. Jerry Falwell cited Schaeffer as a major influence on his decision to launch the Moral Majority and ally with Catholics and other nonevangelicals in an attempt to reclaim America for God through politics.[40]

Before Schaeffer, many evangelicals had attempted to link abortion to the sexual revolution, and a large number had argued that it was killing. But no one had yet made an effective, systematic case that abortion represented the current nadir of national moral decline and the evils of a progressive Supreme Court that had abandoned moral absolutes. And although many Catholics had warned that abortion would soon lead to infanticide and euthanasia, this was not a common evangelical Protestant argument until Schaeffer publicized it. Schaeffer gave evangelicals the narrative framework in which to understand abortion as the greatest evil of their generation, and, for some, the greatest evil that Americans had ever experienced. Evangelicals found this persuasive partly because it seemed logical. If the unborn really were human beings—a case that suddenly started to look a lot more probable, now that they examined a few scriptures that spoke of God's creative work in the womb—it made sense that abortion was the greatest act of genocide the nation had ever permitted. And since they were already concerned about the sexual revolution and the loss of religious values and religious symbols in public life, it made sense that this was a product of a liberal rejection of Christian moral absolutes. And since many evangelicals already distrusted the Supreme Court as a liberal institution, it made sense to them that it was the Court that had perpetrated this evil on the American people, the same court that had ruled against school prayer and Bible reading and that had protected the rights of pornographers and criminals. Of course, this interpretation ignored the many abortions that had taken place both legally and illegally before *Roe*, but evangelicals had little interest in talking about those and soon forgot that they had even existed. For the next half century, evangelical narratives of abortion history nearly always began with *Roe*, because it was *Roe* that epitomized moral relativism and the country's rejection of God. Fighting abortion, therefore, meant one thing above all else: reversing *Roe*. This was to be a political campaign that would focus not primarily on reducing the national abortion rate but rather on restoring Christian values in public life by reversing *Roe*, protecting the unborn in public law, and ending the greatest moral threat to the nation.

Schaeffer followed up on the success of *How Should We Then Live?* with another book and documentary film devoted specifically to abortion and other life issues, including euthanasia and infanticide. *Whatever Happened to the Human Race?* (1979), which he coproduced with C. Everett Koop, reiterated the arguments of *How Should We Then Live?* but made the case for pro-life activism even more explicit. The book opened with a comparison between abortion and the Holocaust and then hammered home the point that Schaeffer had made in his previous documentary film series: Legalized abortion would lead to infanticide and other actions against human life, because the Supreme Court decision that had legalized abortion in the United States was a product of relativistic thinking that was constrained by no parameters other than social opinion. Schaeffer called this form of relativistic thinking "humanism," which he said was simply the West's latest attempt to replace a fixed, absolute divine standard of morality with an atheistic, relativistic philosophy that was human-derived and human-centered. "In one short generation we have moved from a generally high view of life to a very low one," Schaeffer wrote. "Why has our society changed? The answer is clear: The consensus of our society no longer rests on a Judeo-Christian base, but rather on a humanistic one."[41] The abortion issue was important, therefore, not merely because human life was at stake, but because the moral foundation of society was on the line. If Christians lost their battle to restore moral absolutes in abortion law and return the nation to its Christian foundations, they would lose their country, and no human rights would be guaranteed.

THE RELIGIOUS POLITICS OF ABORTION IN THE 1976 PRESIDENTIAL ELECTION

With both Catholics and evangelicals moving rapidly toward a more concerted pro-life effort, opposition to abortion was gaining ground in the lead-up to the 1976 presidential election. A majority of Americans wanted abortion to remain legal in some cases, but the public backlash against the new abortion clinics that were springing up in cities throughout the country in the aftermath of *Roe v. Wade* led some people who had not paid much attention to the pro-life movement before to begin identifying with the cause. *Roe* had forced forty-six of the fifty states to liberalize their abortion laws, and this prompted a backlash in some areas of the country, including heavily Catholic Rhode Island (which had banned nearly all abortions before *Roe*) and much of the evangelical-dominated South (which had legalized therapeutic abortion before *Roe* but had never legalized "abortion on demand"). As the numbers of legal abortions rapidly climbed, the pro-life movement's proposed constitutional amendment banning all abortions began to look more attractive to some people. Forty-five percent of all Americans—including 52 percent of Catholics and 45 percent of Protestants—supported a constitutional amendment prohibiting all abortions, according to a Gallup poll taken in March 1976. Voters in the two parties were evenly split on the issue; 48 percent of Democrats and 48 percent of Republicans supported the proposed constitutional amendment to ban all abortions nationwide.[42]

Yet most of the leading contenders for the Democratic Party's presidential nomination refrained from supporting the amendment. The

Democratic Party had not yet taken an official stand on abortion, and the party still had many members who were socially conservative Catholics or southern or midwestern evangelicals. But it also had a strong contingent of pro-choice feminists who were beginning to exert a powerful influence on the party. With the exception of George Wallace (the former Alabama governor whose campaign for the 1976 Democratic presidential nomination was based on his appeal to social conservatives) and Ellen McCormack (a New York right-to-life activist whose presidential campaign focused almost entirely on her opposition to abortion), none of the party's presidential aspirants wanted to risk offending the party's pro-choice feminists. Representative Mo Udall (D-AZ), a lapsed former member of the Church of Jesus Christ of Latter-Day Saints (LDS), endorsed abortion rights without equivocation. That stand was at odds with the position of the LDS Church (which permitted abortion only in cases of rape or incest or dangers to a woman's life), but so were several of Udall's other positions. Senator Birch Bayh (D-IN), a Methodist, expressed a few personal reservations about abortion, but used his position as chair of the Senate Subcommittee on the Constitution to block antiabortion constitutional amendment proposals.[43]

Senator Ted Kennedy (D-MA), who was widely expected to be the party favorite if he entered the race, ultimately decided not to run for the 1976 presidential nomination, but he nevertheless signaled the direction in which the party was moving on abortion by reversing his position on the issue in 1975 and endorsing abortion rights. From 1971 to 1975, he had opposed abortion legalization, just as many other Catholics in Massachusetts did, but in 1975 he announced that not only would he not support attempts to overturn *Roe* through a constitutional amendment but he would also support Medicaid funding for abortion. He still believed abortion was wrong, but he did not want the law to discriminate against the poor by denying them funding for a procedure that wealthier women were able to access.[44]

Kennedy's brother-in-law Sargent Shriver also backed away from his previous antiabortion stance during his campaign for the 1976 Democratic presidential nomination. Shriver was a devout Catholic who, along

Catholics and Evangelicals after *Roe* 161

with his wife, Eunice Kennedy Shriver, had once been a strong supporter of the pro-life movement. Eunice had even been a keynote speaker at right-to-life conferences before *Roe v. Wade*, and she had written defenses of antiabortion laws. But in 1975, both Eunice and Sargent announced that they did not support the pro-life movement's efforts to pass an antiabortion constitutional amendment, because it was highly unlikely to pass in Congress and was therefore a waste of political capital. It would be far better for the pro-life movement to focus on policies that would decrease the abortion rate, such as "life support centers" for women facing crisis pregnancies.[45]

This stance became the norm for Catholic (and some Protestant) Democrats with senatorial or presidential ambitions. In state legislatures and even in the U.S. House of Representatives, a substantial minority of Democrats remained in favor of restrictive abortion laws, which continued to be popular with many Democratic voters. But among Democratic senators, such pro-life views became increasingly rare after the mid-1970s, and among presidential aspirants they were rarer still. Faced with the choice between alienating the party's increasingly powerful pro-choice feminist wing or the party's pro-life constituency, Catholics such as Shriver and Kennedy attempted to split the difference by professing their personal opposition to abortion while at the same time pledging to protect its access for the sake of equality in a pluralistic society.

This attempt to move Catholic teachings on abortion out of the realm of public policy and into the area of personal conviction for the sake of protecting the values of a pluralistic society did not sit well with the nation's Catholic bishops, who viewed it as a violation of the social mandate of Vatican II. The church had a duty to be involved in political affairs for the sake of promoting justice, since "social injustice and the denial of human rights can often be remedied only through governmental action," the bishops said in February 1976. Abortion was perhaps the foremost of these issues. The bishops' official statement "Political Responsibility" in the 1976 election listed abortion as the first order of concern and stated that the bishops supported "passage of a constitutional amendment to restore the basic constitutional protection of the right to life for the unborn child." Nevertheless, the bishops knew that they were walking a fine line in advocating this specific policy solution, because in the same document they quoted approvingly their earlier statement in 1971 that "it does not belong to the Church, insofar as she is a religious and hierarchical community, to offer concrete solutions in the social, economic, and political spheres for justice in the world." By going beyond merely condemning abortion in the abstract and using their teaching office and church resources to endorse and lobby for a specific policy proposal—an antiabortion constitutional amendment—the bishops were moving dangerously close to linking the church with the "concrete [policy] solutions" that they said the church was not equipped to provide. Perhaps for that reason they suggested at times that the antiabortion constitutional amendment, as important as it was, could not be a political litmus test in itself, as pro-life organizations such as the National Right to Life Committee wanted to make it. They did not excommunicate Catholic politicians who opposed the amendment. Nor did they tell Catholics directly that they had a moral duty to vote only for candidates who pledged their support for antiabortion legislation. There should be no "religious voting bloc," the bishops said, and they had no desire to "instruct persons on how they should vote by endorsing candidates." And if there would be no bloc voting from Catholics or official endorsements from the bishops, there would be no single-issue voting either. "Rather, we hope that voters will examine the positions of candidates on the full range of issues as well as the person's integrity, philosophy, and performance."[46]

The bishops issued that statement in February 1976. At the time, the presidential race was still wide open, and neither party had yet taken an official position on abortion. Ellen McCormack, a Catholic pro-life activist from Long Island, New York, had entered the Democratic Party primary as a single-issue candidate who had no chance of winning the nomination but who intended to use her candidacy to gain publicity for the pro-life cause and prevent the Democratic Party from endorsing abortion rights. A few bishops were excited by her candidacy. The bishop of the Diocese of Covington, Kentucky, sent a letter to members of the diocese encouraging them to vote for candidates who "clearly and firmly declare themselves defenders of the right to life." In response, 30 percent of Democratic primary voters in Covington cast their ballots for McCormack.[47] But most bishops shied away from this single-issue voting strategy, and they made no effort to intervene in a presidential primary on behalf of a candidate who had no chance of winning. Instead, they waited anxiously as former Georgia governor Jimmy Carter, a moderately pro-choice candidate, racked up the votes needed for the nomination.

Carter's views on abortion aligned almost perfectly with those of the moderates in the SBC, which was not surprising, because he was an active Southern Baptist deacon and Sunday school teacher in the moderate mold himself. He was personally uncomfortable with abortion, saying at one point on the campaign trail, "I think abortion is wrong and that government ought not ever do anything to encourage abortion."[48] He opposed federal funding for abortion. He supported policies that he believed would reduce the abortion rate. But at the same time, as a strong advocate of freedom of conscience and church–state separation—which were first-order principles for Southern Baptist moderates—he did not support proposals for an antiabortion constitutional amendment, and he believed that as president he would be constitutionally bound to enforce the dictates of *Roe v. Wade*. This was exactly how Foy Valentine and other moderates in the SBC approached the abortion issue, and it was also reflective of a centrist political approach that had widespread bipartisan support. Although President Gerald Ford occasionally mentioned his willingness to support a constitutional amendment that would rescind *Roe v. Wade* and return the power of abortion regulation to the states, in practice his administration's abortion policies were no different than the ones Carter favored. Nor were they any different from the ones Sargent Shriver proposed. If anything, Carter's support for the Hyde Amendment, first approved in 1976, which prohibited Medicaid funding for most elective abortions, put him somewhat to the right of most of the other contenders for the Democratic presidential nomination. Carter's candidacy alone, therefore, did not alarm the nation's Catholic bishops. His position on abortion was not what they wanted, but it was not outside the mainstream.

What did alarm them, however, was the Democratic Party's decision to include an endorsement of abortion rights in its platform, making it the first major party platform in history to endorse the idea. Carter had tried hard to keep abortion out of the platform, because he knew it would be divisive.[49] But pro-choice feminist delegates at the convention insisted that the party needed to go on record in support of abortion rights, especially in view of the threat that *Roe* faced from antiabortion constitutional amendment proposals. The Carter campaign team pushed back a bit and succeeded in moderating the platform language, but in the end, the party still went on record in opposition to the antiabortion constitutional amendment that the nation's Catholic bishops had listed as a top political priority. "We fully recognize the religious and ethical nature of the concerns which many Americans have on the subject of abortion," the Democratic Party platform stated. "We feel, however, that it is undesirable to attempt to amend the U.S. Constitution to overturn the Supreme Court decision in this area."[50] By later standards, this wasn't a very strong endorsement of abortion rights. It did not declare that women had a "right to choose," and it did not say that abortion was health care that should be protected. Instead, it merely said that it was "undesirable" to amend the Constitution to reverse *Roe v. Wade.* But this was enough to shock the Catholic bishops, who sensed that the party had repudiated the most foundational value of the just society that they wanted to create. Because of its abortion plank, the Democratic Party's platform was "morally offensive in the extreme," said Archbishop Joseph Bernardin, the president of the NCCB.[51]

For most of his ecclesiastical career, Bernardin resisted the idea of single-issue voting. Earlier that spring, in fact, he had sent a letter to members of his diocese in Cincinnati discouraging them from making any single issue a litmus test for candidates, even as the bishop in the neighboring diocese of Covington, Kentucky, was issuing the opposite instruction.[52] But once the Democratic Party officially repudiated the pro-life constitutional amendment proposal that the bishops favored — and, what was worse, did so without consulting the Catholic bishops on the issue — he believed that he could not remain silent. When he led a delegation of bishops to meet with Carter, he pressed him on abortion. Carter backtracked slightly, saying that he did not fully agree with the platform's position and that if supporters of an antiabortion amendment tried to get one passed in Congress, he would not stand in their way. But Bernardin was not completely mollified. Carter's position was "deeply disturbing" and "inconsistent," he said.[53]

Sensing an opportunity to pick up some additional Catholic votes, the Ford campaign encouraged the Platform Committee at the Republican National Convention to include an endorsement of an antiabortion amendment in the party platform. There were still plenty of pro-choice Republicans in top leadership positions in the party (including First Lady Betty Ford, Vice President Nelson Rockefeller, and Republican National Committee chair Mary Louise Smith, among others), but the party nevertheless adopted its new plank on abortion with only mild internal dissent. Some pro-choice Republicans in Congress and the Ford administration may not have taken it very seriously, but the bishops did. They had a cordial meeting with Ford in which they told him that although they would have liked him to go further than merely supporting a states' rights amendment and instead endorse an amendment that would protect all human life from the moment of conception, they were still "encouraged" by his position, which they considered much better than Carter's. "The specific difference is an unwillingness, at this time, on the part of the Democratic candidate to support any kind of constitutional amendment and a willingness on the part of the Republican candidate to support an amendment," Bernardin explained to the press.[54]

The backlash against Bernardin's statements was swift. Many outside the Catholic Church were alarmed by the bishops' apparent endorsement of a political candidate, which went beyond what they had ever done before, and what they had stated only a few months before that they would never do. And some politically liberal Catholics were upset that Bernardin and his fellow bishops had made abortion the single focus of concern, evaluating the candidates on this issue alone. Abortion was undeniably an important issue for faithful Catholics, but it was hardly the only issue that Vatican II and recent papal encyclicals on social issues discussed, and until now it had never seemed to be the sole issue of political concern for the bishops either. Bernardin said that after his meetings with the candidates, he was deluged with mail, much of it critical. Timothy Healy, the Jesuit president of Georgetown University, warned that the church was in danger of being identified with a particular political party. *America* magazine noted that even though "indignation at the Democratic platform statement on abortion was widespread," that did not mean that Catholics would refrain from voting for Carter, especially since he had tried to distance himself from the platform statement. The Catholic position on abortion needed to be understood in the context of a "total reverence for life," *America* suggested, which meant that although the right to life for the unborn was important, Catholic voters could not ignore other life issues, such as the Ford administration's "indifference to the international food crisis." "The bishops have repeatedly insisted that Catholics cannot vote on a single issue alone," *America*'s editors reminded readers.[55]

Bernardin seemed to agree, and he tried to course-correct almost immediately. "It is not our job to endorse candidates or oppose candidates," he told the press. The church hierarchy would remain "absolutely neutral" in the presidential race, he promised. Catholics were therefore free to "vote as their conscience dictates," because the church would not suggest a particular ballot choice.[56] The leaders of national pro-life organizations, such as the National Right to Life Committee (NRLC) and American Citizens Concerned for Life, supported Ford because they had made an antiabortion constitutional amendment their single issue of concern. But the nation's Catholic bishops did not do this. They continued to lobby for a constitutional amendment to protect the unborn, but did not believe that it was appropriate for the church leadership to attempt to tip the scales in a presidential election by publicly supporting the party that had just endorsed this amendment proposal.

To at least a few Catholics in the pro-life movement, the bishops' stance was too moderate. Thirty-two percent of Catholics in 1975 wanted abortion to be illegal in all circumstances—compared to only 17 percent of Catholics who wanted abortion to be legal in all circumstances—and among those 32 percent were some who thought the church hierarchy was not speaking out forcefully enough on the issue.[57] During his time as president of the NCCB, Bernardin received letters of complaint from Catholics who urged him to take stronger action against abortion. Usually, their differences of opinion with Bernardin centered on whether abortion should be the church's primary issue of political concern or whether instead—as Bernardin and most of the other bishops believed— it made more sense to view it as inseparably linked to a much larger set of human life issues that could not be abandoned in the fight against abortion. For many pro-life activists, all other causes paled in comparison to the need to protect unborn human life, and they couldn't understand why the bishops didn't see things the same way. "There are many 'issues,' 'causes,' and 'concerns' in these times; some very worthy and others questionable," Mary Reed of Cincinnati told Bernardin in a letter in 1974, "*but* none can come close to the murdering of unborn babies." She couldn't understand why her priest read a letter from the bishop urging support for the plight of migrant farm workers but said nothing about an upcoming right-to-life rally. "We were encouraged to boycott the supermarkets which did not sell the right kind of lettuce," Reed said. "Why were we not encouraged to march for 'life'?" "What are you afraid of?" Mrs. Robert Meyer of Anna, Ohio, asked Bernardin that same year. "Why don't the bishops come out as boldly for life as they do for Cesar Chavez's union fighting another union?" In response to each of these letters, Bernardin explained that the bishops were doing as much as they could to get *Roe v. Wade* reversed. "I can assure you that I am doing everything possible to bring about a Constitutional Amendment which is the only solution to the problem," Bernardin told the Franciscan Sisters of the Poor at Saint Clare Convent, who had sent him a petition asking him to do more on the issue. But, he added, "in order to do this, a favorable climate will have to be established."[58] Establishing that "favorable climate" would require a holistic approach of education on the issue, lobbying for other "life" issues that went far beyond abortion, and working within the political system to gradually build support for the cause.

    This stance led to tension between the bishops and pro-life groups not affiliated with the church, such as the NRLC, which claimed more than 1 million members in the mid-1970s. Most NRLC members were Catholic, and an overwhelming majority of them were devout churchgoers; a poll taken in 1980 showed that 90 percent of them attended church at least once a week.[59] But in contrast to the bishops, the NRLC encouraged its members to treat abortion as a single-issue political litmus test and to vote against any political candidate who refused to endorse the Human Life Amendment. This was its stance in the 1976 election, but in 1977 the NRLC became even more overtly political when it formed a political action committee to raise money for pro-life candidates and target opponents for defeat. Pro-life activists began distributing campaign literature in Catholic church parking lots on Sunday morning to make sure the faithful knew about congressional candidates' stances on abortion and voted accordingly. But because the bishops advocated a gradualist, holistic approach to the issue that eschewed appeals for single-issue voting, church leaders sometimes found themselves at odds with local right-to-life organizations, despite their shared concerns about abortion. Right-to-life activists complained about the bishops' alleged lack of courage and unwillingness to act, and bishops in turn viewed the right-to-life tactics as counterproductive at times. When Cincinnati pro-life activist Jack Willke (who was vice president of the NRLC in the mid-1970s and would serve as president of the organization in the 1980s) asked his archdiocese for $30,000 to fund Ohio Right to Life, the Cincinnati archdiocesan pro-life coordinator, Fr. James Bramlage, recommended that Archbishop Bernardin deny the request. "It would be like paying someone to shoot at you," he said.[60]

The leaders of right-to-life organizations, such as the NRLC and March for Life, often preferred fiery priests who were single-mindedly committed to the antiabortion cause and who were not afraid to denounce their opponents without equivocation. To lead the invocation at the Ohio congressional breakfast at the 1979 March for Life in Washington, DC, they chose Fr. Roger Griese, who had filled the pages of his Dayton parish bulletin with scathing denunciations of pro-choice activists, who he said were worse than Herod and his slaughter of the Holy Innocents. Herod "was a 'piker' compared with this group and their allies, Planned Parenthood, ACLU, NOW, most of the ERA pushers, many members of the national administration, seven members of the 1973 Supreme Court, and both of our Ohio Senators," Griese wrote in September 1978. "Herod killed about 60 male babies. These people are responsible for the murder of *over one million per year since 1973!*" For his invocation at the March for Life event a few months later, Griese did not disappoint. He began with an ecumenical appeal to people of all faiths to join in the campaign for life, but then ended the prayer with imprecations against the movement's opponents couched in the language of spiritual warfare. "May we not grow fearful of the opposition of those who hate You and hate Your creation," Griese prayed. "Enlighten them, convert them—or, if by their own free choice they continue to oppose You, then defeat them, O Lord, as once You defeated the enemies of Your Chosen People." Bernardin was not impressed, especially after Griese published yet another fiercely worded antiabortion bulletin article, this time denouncing the local Episcopal bishop for his pro-choice activism. "I really believe, Roger, you went beyond the bounds of propriety in your bulletin," he told Griese two weeks after his return from the Washington March for Life. "I am as strongly opposed to abortion as you, but I do not believe we should be inflammatory or derogatory in our comments. I firmly believe such tactics are counterproductive."[61]

Bernardin took a similarly dim view of the willingness of a few pro-life activists to illegally block abortion clinic doors as an act of nonviolent civil disobedience. In the 1980s and 1990s, this would become a widespread tactic in the movement, when Operation Rescue mobilized tens of thousands of people who were willing to get arrested for their actions, but in the late 1970s, it was only just beginning to be embraced by a few Catholic young people who wanted to put their bodies on the line in the fight against abortion. Bernardin tried to discourage it. Even though nonviolent civil disobedience in order to save the unborn was "not morally wrong," it was unwise, he told Marge Kelly, a young Catholic woman who had faced arrest in Cincinnati because of her participation at an illegal sit-in at an abortion clinic in 1978. He admired her "sincerity and dedication to the cause of the unborn," he said, but he warned her that her actions of civil disobedience "would probably result in more alienation, possibly even more violence, without a compensatory betterment of the situation."[62]

Bernardin still held onto Vatican II's social vision of a Christocentric humanism for a pluralistic society, and he did not want the church's witness cheapened by taking sides in a partisan debate or allying with a cause that might create a political backlash against the Catholic Church's holistic pro-life campaign.

EVANGELICALS AND THE ABORTION ISSUE IN THE LATE 1970S

If the nation's Catholic bishops refused to make abortion a litmus-test issue in the 1976 presidential election, evangelicals didn't either, but for different reasons. For nearly all of the evangelicals who had enlisted in the pro-life campaign by 1976, abortion was not a stand-alone issue but was rather a symptom of the nation's larger moral decay, as manifested by the sexual revolution, a widespread perceived secularization, and the loss of the United States' standing in the world following the scandal of Watergate and the abandonment of the military effort in Vietnam. In January 1976, evangelical theologian (and former *Christianity Today* editor) Carl F. H. Henry set the tone for evangelicals' approach to the presidential election by publishing an "open letter to President Ford" in which he listed the nation's social ills, one of which was abortion. "The worst crime rate in civilizational history, the evident breakup of the American home, the selfish abortion of unwanted fetuses, the crippling curses of alcoholism, drug and cigarette-addiction, the flagrant schemes of welfare opportunists, the degrading moral permissiveness of visual and printed arts characterize a hell-bent if not hell-destined generation," Henry wrote. "Despite the tolerant mood of the times, these are not mere matters of private morality."[63] Henry, who had been an early leader in mobilizing conservative Protestants against abortion in the early 1970s, was certainly concerned about the issue in 1976, but the fact that he listed it only as one of a number of other related concerns about societal moral decay indicated that he (like nearly all other evangelicals at the time) thought that it could not be addressed apart from a much larger comprehensive moral program. Even Harold O. J. Brown, who had cofounded a Protestant pro-life organization and had done more than almost any other evangelical to mobilize his fellow Protestant Christians on the abortion issue, suggested that Christians did not necessarily need to make an antiabortion constitutional amendment a political litmus test when evaluating Jimmy Carter's candidacy, because if Carter was a true Christian, he would have to address the issue of abortion as part of a larger moral agenda. "Evangelicals concerned about abortion are not altogether dismayed by Democratic Presidential nominee Carter's statements to the effect that he does not favor a constitutional amendment to reverse *Roe v. Wade*," Brown wrote in September 1976. "If he is an evangelical, and thinks biblically, and if he has power, he will not long be able to remain altogether idle in the face of a judicially mandated paganization of American law and mores."[64] Evangelical magazines covering the 1976 presidential election thus devoted far more coverage to Carter's faith than to any of his specific policy stances, because in the view of many evangelical Christians, a born-again Christian who was guided by the Bible and the Holy Spirit would have to share their moral concerns, including their concern about abortion and all other evils stemming from the sexual revolution.

But Carter was a Southern Baptist moderate, not a northern evangelical, and he did not share the view of such evangelicals that the United States needed moral legislation to stop abortion and rescue the nation from sexual licentiousness. Like other Baptist moderates, he considered church–state separation a more important matter than moral legislation that he thought might erode the boundaries against religious establishment. Evangelicals such as Brown argued that the idea of church–state separation should be interpreted narrowly to mean merely a prohibition on an established church rather than a wall of separation guarding the government from religious influence.[65] But Baptist moderates interpreted this prohibition more broadly, and they were especially wary of Catholic attempts to make abortion prohibitions absolute, since they considered these efforts a violation of the principle of freedom of conscience and a threat to medically necessary abortions that they believed were morally acceptable.

Indeed, during the Carter administration, Foy Valentine became more vocal than ever in his support for abortion rights. Until then, he had championed the SBC's position of the early 1970s – that is, that elective abortion was morally problematic, but therapeutic abortion might be acceptable and should remain legal. But in 1977, a year after the SBC agreed to tighten its policy on abortion and move closer to a fully antiabortion position, Valentine signaled his opposition to this line of thinking by signing the Religious Coalition on Abortion Rights's "Call to Concern."

The Religious Coalition on Abortion Rights (RCAR), which was founded in late 1973, consisted primarily of liberal Protestant ministers (along with a few adherents of non-Christian faiths) who believed that abortion rights were rights for the liberty of conscience and should be defended, just as *Roe* had said. In the "Call to Concern," the ministers stated that the Catholic Church's antiabortion lobbying was a "serious threat to religious liberty and freedom of conscience," because it ignored the diversity of religious opinion on "when human personhood begins" and violated the principle affirmed in *Roe* that "the law ought not to compel the conscience of those who believe abortion to be in harmony with their moral convictions." This was exactly what many liberal Protestants had said in the early 1970s, and it was what they were still saying in 1977. In the early 1970s, Valentine had not aligned himself with the liberal Protestant position on the issue, but in 1977, he did. RCAR's "Call to Concern" endorsed *Roe* and called for a preservation of Medicaid funding of abortion, stances that went far beyond even the most liberal of the SBC's resolutions on abortion from the early 1970s. Valentine signed it anyway, as did a few other Southern Baptist moderates, including several professors from Southern Baptist Theological Seminary. The next year, Valentine accepted an invitation to join RCAR's board.[66]

When a South Carolina Baptist pastor questioned him about his actions, Valentine replied that he still held a "strong commitment" to the SBC's stand on the morality of abortion. It was "always wrong," he said, but "in some cases such as rape and incest it may be the lesser of two evils." This was an "essentially conservative" position, he said. It was certainly more conservative than the position of many other RCAR members who insisted that women considering a pregnancy termination had the right to determine the morality of abortion for themselves. But despite these differences, Valentine agreed to join RCAR's campaign because of his opposition to the Catholic bishops' Pastoral Plan. "The battle has been joined by the Roman Catholic Bishops, and I think it is imperative that we do not sit still to let American public policy be changed in favor of their particular interpretation of the matter," he wrote. He and other members of RCAR were "determined to resist the Roman Catholic hierarchy's efforts" to "enact into federal law the official Roman Catholic dogma concerning abortion."[67]

For evangelicals such as Harold O. J. Brown and pro-life Southern Baptists such as Robert Holbrook, there was a clear connection between the morality of abortion and public policy; if abortion was murder, it needed to be illegal, just as the Catholic bishops had declared. But for Baptist moderates such as Valentine and President Carter, liberty of conscience and the principles of *Roe* were such important principles that they had to be upheld at all costs, even if the cost was allowing the sin of abortion in a pluralistic society. Pro-life evangelicals such as Brown, Schaeffer, and a host of others had embraced the notion that the United States was founded on Christian principles that needed to be reclaimed through antiabortion laws, but Baptist moderates such as Valentine strongly resisted this idea. The United States was a pluralistic society where church and state must remain firmly separate. In church, Baptist moderates such as Valentine might still be moderate conservatives on abortion, saying that it should be used only in a very narrow range of therapeutic or medically necessary situations. But when it came to setting public policy in the secular sphere, they acted like liberal Protestants, saying that women and doctors should have the right to make their own choices on abortion, even when those choices were wrong.

RCAR said that its members had a diversity of views about the morality of abortion, but they were united in the belief that the "religious liberty" of individual consciences would be "threatened" if "the state enacts into law one particular religious viewpoint." "Coalition members believe that abortion is a highly personal decision that should be determined by an individual's own conscience, religious beliefs and medical situation — not by the dictates of the state," RCAR said in one of its publications from the late 1970s. In Valentine's view, this made RCAR an important ally in the defense of religious freedom. But in the view of an increasingly discontented conservative faction in the SBC, this put Valentine and other SBC leaders on the wrong side of the most important moral question of their time. "It is very serious to assert that the largest evangelical denomination, which is usually identified as conservative and Bible-believing, is associated on the abortion question with some of the most radical and liberal theological groups in their support of the infamous Supreme Court decision of 1973," Robert Holbrook wrote in a mass mailing titled "Is the Southern Baptist Convention Pro-Abortion?" "BUT THAT IS THE CASE!"[68]

Holbrook's charge struck a nerve, because popular evangelical sentiment against abortion was rapidly building in the late 1970s. In 1978, the Presbyterian Church in America (PCA), a new conservative evangelical denomination that had formed as a splinter from the southern-based Presbyterian Church in the United States (PCUS), adopted an unequivocal antiabortion resolution. "We are convinced Scripture forbids abortion," the PCA resolution declared. "Abortion is wrong; it is sin. . . . God in His Word speaks of the unborn child as a person and treats him as such, and so must we."[69] That same year, Jerry Falwell, a televangelist and fundamentalist Baptist megachurch pastor in Lynchburg, Virginia, began making abortion a central subject of his preaching, starting with a three-part sermon series on homosexuality, abortion, and pornography. He thought of each of these issues in national terms; they were a "cancer" destroying the United States. "The decision by the Supreme Court legalizing 'abortion-on-demand' did more to destroy our nation than any other decision it has made," he said in May 1978. "What is happening to our nation? Abortion is stripping us of the value of life. We are killing off the next generation and destroying our consciousness in the process."[70]

Like Schaeffer, Falwell focused solely on *Roe* when talking about the beginning of the abortion problem in the United States; he never mentioned the hundreds of thousands of abortions (both legal and illegal) each year in the United States before 1973. Because abortion was primarily a national and political sin — not merely a personal sin that could be dealt with through pastoral counseling or teaching in the local church — it required a national political solution. The remedy for *Roe v. Wade* was a reversal of the decision, either through a constitutional amendment (as pro-life activists advocated in the 1970s) or through a change in the composition of the Supreme Court (as they would begin advocating in the 1980s). A reversal of *Roe* would come about only if Christians voted in large numbers for candidates who shared their views on abortion policy. By the late 1970s, pro-life preaching in evangelical churches became inseparable from political efforts. Pastors who spoke out on abortion almost invariably did so in the context of decrying a national moral decline and rallying the faithful to resist this decline by voting for candidates who wanted to restore morality in the nation. The Catholic bishops had hesitated to become too overtly political in their pro-life messages, but Falwell had no such qualms. Neither did Schaeffer.

Schaeffer, in fact, directly encouraged Falwell to launch a political movement to restore morality in U.S. law, starting with abortion. As a fundamentalist Baptist, Falwell had long believed that it was wrong to ally with people who were not born-again Christians, which excluded most Catholics from consideration in his thinking at the time. But in a telephone conversation with Falwell, Schaeffer told the Baptist pastor that it was okay to ally with "co-belligerents" who shared his views on abortion but disagreed with him on theology; this was not a compromise with religious error, he said, because the alliance was moral or political rather than religious.[71] Falwell accepted the advice. He agreed to meet with New Right activists Howard Phillips, Richard Viguerie, and Paul Weyrich, who urged him to begin mobilizing a "moral majority" of evangelical voters. Catholics played an outsize role in creating the New Right, a populist conservative movement of the late 1970s that wanted to shift power in the Republican Party from the "blue bloods" to blue-collar voters who were social conservatives opposed to the cultural liberalism of the educational and political establishment. Weyrich, a conservative Catholic who had founded the Heritage Foundation and a few other right-wing political organizations, correctly believed that evangelicals shared most of these concerns—including his concern about abortion—and he hoped that Falwell could be the New Right's liaison in mobilizing evangelical voters. Falwell agreed. In June 1979, he launched the Moral Majority to register Christian voters and alert them to the urgency of key moral issues in the public square. Saving the country from moral destruction was so important, he believed, that he now said that pastors should "register people to vote," "explain the issues to them," and "endorse candidates, right there in church on Sunday morning."[72] If they did not, he expected God's imminent judgment on a nation that had exchanged its Christian heritage for the liberal values of secular humanism.

Falwell's fundraising letters for the Moral Majority mentioned the evils of abortion, but they never addressed it as an isolated issue. Instead, they treated abortion as part of a larger constellation of evils that included homosexuality, pornography, and other threats to the family. Above all, his letters focused on saving the nation by bringing the law into alignment with God's principles in order to avert God's judgment. "Without sacrifice, this old nation is going to go down the drain," he warned in a direct mailing from the Moral Majority in August 1979. "God has not given up on us yet, but how long will He put up with Christians being silent?"[73]

This same anxiety about national moral decline influenced the conservative faction in the SBC, which succeeded in ousting the moderate leadership and electing one of its own—Memphis Bellevue Baptist Church pastor Adrian Rogers—as president in 1979. In the years leading up to the conservative takeover, the grassroots antiabortion campaign within the SBC had been growing, and it was closely connected to political demands, because pro-life activists within the SBC thought of their campaign primarily as part of a larger political movement to ban abortion through civil law. Christians for Life, an organization of Southern Baptists that Missouri Baptist pastor John Wilder started out of the Tower Grove Baptist Church in St. Louis, had one central goal: convincing messengers at the 1977 SBC's annual meeting to vote for an official denominational endorsement of the Human Life Amendment. Wilder's effort failed that year, but it succeeded in 1980, a year after the conservative takeover of the SBC.

In 1980, the SBC adopted a series of resolutions on a bevy of culture war issues, including pornography, the Equal Rights Amendment, and school prayer. The convention called for a day of prayer and fasting to beseech God for the spiritual renewal of the nation. And, as part of that larger culture war package, the convention passed a new resolution on abortion that endorsed "appropriate legislation and/or a constitutional amendment prohibiting abortion except to save the life of the mother."[74] The SBC was now officially in support of the antiabortion constitutional amendment that Wilder, Holbrook, and the larger pro-life movement favored. By that point, this was the view of the overwhelming majority of Southern Baptist pastors; one survey showed that 75 percent of SBC pastors in 1980 supported a constitutional amendment to ban abortion.[75]

By passing such a resolution, the SBC set itself on a culturally conservative political trajectory that linked abortion with related concerns about national moral decline and that ensured that its pro-life commitment would be primarily expressed as a political cause, not merely a teaching about personal behavior regarding abortion, as Valentine wanted. The Baptist moderates had lost. So had self-described theological conservatives at the 1980 convention who wanted to preserve an exception for rape and incest, as the editors of the Virginia Baptist Convention's *Religious Herald* suggested, and as many prominent evangelicals, including Billy Graham and Carl F. H. Henry, had long advocated.[76] But by adopting a resolution that favored a total ban on abortions except when necessary to save a mother's life, the SBC aligned itself with the anticipated language of an antiabortion constitutional amendment and with the broader pro-life movement. This was not primarily an ethical directive, but rather a political resolution with a legislative goal. Like the Moral Majority, the leadership of the SBC would now be officially committed to the political project of saving the nation from moral destruction, with activism on abortion playing a central role in that project.

On the surface, the stance seemed very close to the position of the NCCB, which had been lobbying for a Human Life Amendment since 1973. But there was a key difference: the SBC, Falwell's Moral Majority, and other conservative evangelicals grounded their antiabortion activism in a larger concern about national moral decline and liberal attacks on the family, while the Catholic bishops wanted instead to make the pro-life cause part of a larger campaign for the protection of human life against the evils of war, poverty, and capital punishment. Before there could be complete unity between evangelicals and Catholics in the pro-life campaign, the two groups would have to agree not only on the need to oppose abortion but also on the larger political and social framing of their defense of the unborn. By 1980, evangelicals and Catholics could mostly agree on the first point: abortion was wrong. But it would require another decade of debate to sort out their differences on the second point. At the heart of that debate was the Catholic-inspired consistent life ethic.

CHAPTER 5

THE RISE AND FALL OF A CONSISTENT LIFE ETHIC

In October 1979, the Catholic bishops of the United States released a guide to political issues in the 1980 election titled "Political Responsibility: Choices for the 1980s." Four years earlier, the bishops had released a guide to the presidential election of 1976 that gave prime consideration to abortion, but this time, the bishops charted a somewhat different course. Although the 1980 political guide began with the issue of abortion (as the 1976 guide had), it then diverged markedly by offering a detailed discussion of several issues that the bishops had not even mentioned in 1976: arms buildup, the dangers of nuclear war, and the evils of the apartheid system in South Africa, among other matters. With the exception of abortion, nearly all of the political opinions the bishops' document expressed corresponded to the positions of politicians on the left rather than the right, and all of them were supported with an appeal to the concept of "human dignity" or "human rights," the same principles that the bishops had used as a foundation for their pro-life stance. "Our national economic life must reflect broad values of social justice and human rights," the bishops said. "Above all, the economy must serve the human needs of our people. It is important to call attention to the fact that millions of Americans are still poor, jobless, hungry and inadequately housed and that vast disparities of income and wealth remain within our nation. These conditions are intolerable and must be persistently challenged so that the economy will reflect a fundamental respect for the human dignity and basic needs of all."[1]

The bishops were not abandoning their fight against abortion, but they were making a concerted effort to avoid linking the pro-life cause to the political right. The key to avoiding a right-wing co-option of the pro-life cause, they thought, was to link the church's opposition to abortion with the church's broader social program, or, in a phrase that became a central part of the church's political vision in the 1980s, a "consistent life ethic." If the church showed as much concern for the prisoners on death row as it did for fetuses in the womb, and if the church gave the same priority to the alleviation of poverty as it did to the campaign for the rights of the unborn, it would avoid the wrong sort of political entanglements that had threatened to tarnish the bishops' political influence during the Ford versus Carter contest in 1976. In 1980, the bishops were so eager to avoid any hint of an alliance with the political right that some of them were even willing to distance themselves from pro-life organizations if that was what it took to keep the church out of the Republican Party's orbit and protect the values of human dignity that Vatican II had endorsed for both the born and the unborn. "There are many in the prolife movement who do not share the bishops' broad application of the respect-life principle," wrote Msgr. George Higgins, who had worked for the National Conference of Catholic Bishops (NCCB) for decades and had established a reputation as a politically progressive priest who strongly supported labor unions, in September 1980. "Instead they apply the principle selectively—to the unborn child, but not to prisoners on death row, nor to the poverty-stricken family in the inner city, nor to the starving child in the Sahel. . . . We cannot wait until a Human Life Amendment is passed to face the problems of massive poverty and starvation, of high unemployment and severely inadequate housing. While some threats to human life are obviously more serious than others, none can be adequately dealt with in isolation. To suggest otherwise is to promote the kind of moral and political naivete that will ultimately hinder the struggle for human dignity."[2]

But the NCCB's vision of a nonpartisan consistent life ethic that gave as much attention to fighting poverty and capital punishment as it did to the campaign against abortion proved to be short-lived. By 1984, some of the nation's leading bishops were already moving away from it, because they believed it was inadequate to stop what they considered an abortion holocaust. This debate was directly related to the Republican and Democratic realignment on abortion. For much of the 1970s, abortion had not been a partisan issue, but by the 1980s it was. The NCCB's internal debate about how to frame their campaign against abortion therefore had national partisan ramifications that would reshape the politics of the Catholic Church in the United States.

CATHOLICS' HESITANCY TO JOIN THE CONSERVATIVE CULTURE WARS

On most political issues, the Catholic clergy of the late 1970s identified more with the political left than the political right. Most of the young priests who were ordained in the immediate wake of Vatican II (from the late 1960s through the mid-1970s) were political progressives whose views had been shaped by civil rights advocacy, opposition to the Vietnam War, and support for expanded social welfare programs to help the poor. The bishops too, though perhaps not quite as liberal as the younger parish priests, were also supportive of the principles of human rights, alleviation of poverty, and international peace advocacy, principles central to Vatican II and some of the papal encyclicals of the 1960s, such as John XXIII's *Pacem in Terris* (1963). They still considered abortion a grave evil and a nonnegotiable issue. But as they saw the parties beginning to diverge on abortion, they decided that rather than denounce the Democrats and risk alienating a party that shared their views on many other issues, they would attempt to persuade Catholics that the pro-life cause was a central component of a broader progressive human rights agenda that had much in common with the principles that many liberal Democrats shared.

Under the leadership of San Francisco archbishop John Raphael Quinn, who served as president of the NCCB from 1977 to 1980, the nation's bishops moved even further away from Republican-leaning pronouncements than they had under the leadership of Archbishop Joseph Bernardin, who had also been wary about inadvertently signaling approval for the political right. Quinn, whom the *New York Times* described as "very conservative when it comes to doctrine" but "progressive on social issues," already had a long record campaigning against the death penalty, and he led the bishops to give greater priority to that issue and to the dangers of arms buildup and nuclear war.[3]

These were somewhat new stances for the Catholic Church in the United States. In the 1960s and early 1970s, there had been no consensus among the nation's bishops on capital punishment; some bishops opposed the death penalty, but others said that it was necessary to protect innocent human life. Pro-life activists, like the nation's bishops, were also divided on the death penalty, with many saying that although they were categorically opposed to the destruction of "innocent life" in every circumstance (including abortion), they did not have the same moral reservations about taking the lives of those who were not innocent (such as criminals) when doing so was necessary to save the lives of others, as was presumably the case in both just war and the death penalty for murderers. But in 1974, two years after the Supreme Court restricted the death penalty in *Furman v. Georgia* (1972), the NCCB issued a short statement declaring their categorical opposition to the death penalty, the first time that they had gone on record against capital punishment. The Supreme Court authorized the limited reinstatement of the death penalty in 1976 in *Gregg v. Georgia*, but the bishops doubled down on their opposition to it, even as conservative politicians argued that it was necessary. In 1980, the bishops issued a lengthy statement that offered rebuttals to each of the common arguments in favor of capital punishment and provided evidence that the death penalty was never necessary. Its use was an affront to Christian values, they argued. To a large extent, the bishops' new quest to end capital punishment was a logical outgrowth of their campaign against abortion, or, at least, that was the way they saw it. With so much of their political effort focused on protecting life from the moment of conception, it seemed incongruous to them that they would be silent when human life was threatened by the reinstatement of the death penalty. "Abolition of capital punishment is also a manifestation of our belief in the unique worth and dignity of each person from the moment of conception, a creature made in the image and likeness of God," the bishops said.[4]

CONSISTENT LIFE ADVOCACY AMONG PROGRESSIVE EVANGELICALS AND CATHOLICS

This message had particular appeal to a number of younger Catholics who believed in the church's moral authority and the value of unborn human life, but who also identified with the social justice causes of the left. This was the case for Juli Loesch Wiley, who, in 1979, at the age of twenty-eight, founded Prolifers for Survival as an organization dedicated to (in her words) "pushing a moral critique of war and the nuclear arms race within the pro-life community." Wiley had distanced herself for a short time from the church's teachings on sexuality when she was a committed feminist in her mid-twenties, but at the end of the 1970s, she began to see that "the whole 'sexual revolution' failed to live up to its claims." It hurt women, she decided. She returned to the church and welcomed its teaching on the "solidarity of woman and embryonic child," because she thought that it was more consistent with her politically progressive, ecofeminist values than anything she heard from the secular left. It was the United States Catholic Conference that was consistently "lobbying against the death penalty, strip mining, *and abortion*," she said; it was the American cardinals who were testifying in Congress against both "funding the MX missile *and abortion*." "At their most dogmatic, this Church's teachings *are* consistently against murder, the bomb, abortion, or a baseball bat,"

Wiley wrote. "The Church gave me a coherent ethical position on life-and-death questions, for which I was grateful; but, much more than that, the Church is a community with the heart of Jesus at heart. . . . Now, I saw, with a flow of wonder, the identification of God Almighty with the embryo. I saw also the outpouring of the Spirit on women, slaves and Gentiles, and children, born and unborn, as a revelation; don't cut us apart! We are one!"[5]

Wiley was dismayed that this egalitarian vision of God's concern for every person, born and unborn, caused her—a self-described "progressive"—to be lumped in with political conservatives simply because she wanted to the "replace the Sexual Revolution with Sexual Shalom" and "restore the traditional Christian vision of natural sex, sacred sex, at the service of the family, and bonding, and life."[6] Neither the left nor the right fully identified with her approach; only the Catholic Church did, she thought.

Wiley was not alone in this approach. In the early 1980s, a number of Catholic pacifists championed what they called a "consistent life ethic" that included opposition to war, abortion, and all other threats to human life. Jesuit priest Daniel Berrigan, who went to prison in 1970 for vandalizing a draft office and destroying draft files as part of a protest against the Vietnam War, was arrested again in 1991 for participating in an illegal sit-in to block an abortion clinic. To his allies on the left who were disturbed that a progressive antiwar activist would attempt to keep women from accessing abortion services, Berrigan explained that he had always been an advocate for all human life, from conception to old age.[7]

It was Catholic "consistent life" advocates such as Wiley and Berrigan who convinced evangelicals on the left to enlist in the antiabortion campaign. Although most white evangelicals were politically conservative, a minority of young antiwar progressives in northern evangelical colleges and seminaries created the organization Evangelicals for McGovern in 1972 and then spent the rest of the decade writing about justice for the poor in new magazines such as *Sojourners* and *The Other Side*. Because these progressive evangelicals were critical of alliances between Christianity and the state, they had no interest in the evangelical pro-life cause as long as evangelical opposition to abortion was closely tied to Francis Schaeffer's vision of restoring a Christian America and moral absolutes in civil law. They had been sharply critical of Billy Graham's alliance with Richard Nixon in the early 1970s, and they did not want to see the next iteration of this Christian nationalism play out in an alliance between pro-life evangelicals and Ronald Reagan. For most of the 1970s, therefore, they said almost nothing about abortion; some were even pro-choice. But they found the pro-life advocacy of peace activists such as Wiley much more appealing. It was centered on a critique of American materialism and individualism and a celebration of communal values and concern for the poor and marginalized that closely accorded with their own ethic. When they encountered this alternative framing of the pro-life cause, they quickly converted to it. In 1980, *Sojourners* devoted an entire issue to the need to oppose abortion with a "consistent life" ethic.[8]

Although *Sojourners* was an evangelical Protestant publication, several of the articles for this special issue came from the Catholic peace movement; Wiley herself wrote one of the pieces. Conservative Southern Baptists and Christian Right activists took their cues on abortion from advocates of pro-family politics affiliated with the New Right, but progressive evangelicals found their inspiration from Catholics on the left who framed opposition to abortion as part of a consistent life ethic. Both groups of evangelicals were working more closely with Catholics than they had a decade before, and both were becoming more strongly insistent on the need to campaign against abortion, even though their social visions were different. Among evangelicals, the culturally conservative group was by far the larger entity; *Sojourners*' progressive evangelical readership was fairly small in comparison. Among Catholics, by contrast, the advocates of a consistent life ethic had greater influence, at least in the church hierarchy.

For the Catholic bishops, the trend toward a consistent life ethic reached its height in 1983, when the NCCB issued a sixty-four-page pastoral letter titled "The Challenge of Peace." Written largely under Archbishop Bernardin's leadership, "The Challenge of Peace" was both a condemnation of nuclear arms buildup (a policy that the Reagan administration was then pursuing) and of abortion. The bishops were clear: Being pro-life meant being consistently pro-life, or what Bernardin called a "seamless garment" that covered a defense of human life in every area.[9] Pro-life peace activists such as Wiley were delighted, as were progressive evangelicals. In 1986, "consistent life" advocates among both evangelicals and Catholics formed the JustLife PAC to promote the political campaigns of congressional candidates who favored "consistent life" principles. And in 1987, one of the most prominent progressive evangelicals—Ronald Sider, an Eastern University sociology professor who had written the widely influential *Rich Christians in an Age of Hunger* a decade earlier—published *Completely Pro-Life: Building a Consistent Stance*, which argued that Christians needed to couple opposition to abortion with opposition to capital punishment, nuclear arms buildup, and other threats to life. That same year, Sider's organization, Evangelicals for Social Action, joined the Seamless Garment Network that members of Wiley's Prolifers for Survival founded to promote Bernardin's consistent life ethic.[10]

Many of the Catholics and evangelicals who advocated a consistent life ethic believed that on issues other than abortion, they were more likely to receive support from the political left than the political right. It bothered them that their natural allies on most human life issues parted ways with them on what they considered the most important issue of human life: abortion. The bishops were still just as committed as ever to lobbying for an antiabortion constitutional amendment; indeed, in 1983, they devoted considerable lobbying effort to supporting the Hatch amendment, a constitutional amendment proposal to rescind *Roe*. In their campaign for this amendment, they had to work mostly with Republicans (including many who supported the Reagan administration's nuclear arms buildup), but that was not necessarily the bishops' preference. In "The Challenge of Peace," they begged pro-choice, antiwar liberals to see the light and join the church's stand against abortion. "If you wish peace, defend life," the bishops wrote, quoting the late Pope Paul VI. "We plead with all who would work to end the scourge of war to begin by defending life at its most defenseless, the life of the unborn."[11]

THE RELIGIOUS DEBATE OVER ABORTION IN THE 1984 PRESIDENTIAL ELECTION

The Democratic Party did not heed the call. Instead, the 1984 Democratic presidential nominee, former vice president Walter Mondale (D-MN), selected as his running mate a pro-choice Catholic, Representative Geraldine Ferraro (D-NY) from Queens. Described by the press as a "devout" Roman Catholic, Ferraro said that she did not "believe in abortion," but added that she could not "impose" her belief on others.[12] This was becoming an increasingly common stance among Catholic Democrats. By 1984, Senator Ted Kennedy (D-MA) had been pro-choice for nearly a decade, and so had many other prominent Catholics in the party. Governor Mario Cuomo (D-NY) took a nearly identical stance of being pro-choice but personally opposed to abortion.

But to the Catholic bishops of New York, a politician's profession of personal opposition to abortion meant nothing if it was accompanied with a pro-choice policy stance. In April 1984 — three months before Ferraro joined the Democratic ticket — the bishops of New York signaled the direction that the bishops would take in the election: "We fail to see the logic of those who contend, 'I am personally opposed to abortion, but I will not impose my personal views on others.'" In June, the archbishop of New York, John O'Connor, reiterated that stance: "I don't see how a Catholic in good conscience can vote for a candidate who explicitly supports abortion."[13] The statement should not have been a surprise to anyone who knew O'Connor, who at that point had been in his post as New York archbishop for only a few months. The previous August, when he was bishop of Scranton, he had sent his diocese a pastoral letter: "I will give no support, by word or action, that could be in any way construed in favor of any politician, of any political party, who professes either a specific pro-abortion position or takes refuge in a so-called pro-choice position. I categorically reject the evasion: 'I am personally opposed to abortion, but this is a pluralistic society, and I must respect the rights of those who disagree with me.'"[14] But whether expected or not, O'Connor's statement in New York in June struck some of the Catholic Democratic pro-choice politicians in the state as fighting words. "The church has never been this aggressively involved," Cuomo said. Instead of using a politician's position on abortion as a single-issue litmus test, voters should look at the entire party platform and ask themselves which set of policies best represented Christian principles, the governor argued. In his view, the Democratic Party was far more Christian in its policies toward the poor than the Republican Party was, regardless of the abortion issue.[15]

The conflict between the bishops and pro-choice Catholic Democrats heated up after Ferraro became the Democratic Party's vice presidential nominee. On most social and political issues, Ferraro agreed with the bishops. Of the sixty issues that the NCCB highlighted in its political guide for the faithful in 1984, Ferraro accepted the bishops' position on forty-four. (By contrast, the Republican platform lined up with the bishops on only sixteen of the sixty issues).[16] But on abortion, Ferraro did not agree with the bishops, and that led her into conflict with her church's hierarchy. Unlike both pro-life activists and the Catholic bishops, Ferraro described her personal opposition to abortion only as a matter of faith, not as a matter of moral reasoning based on scientific evidence or natural law. "As a Catholic, I accept the premise that a fertilized ovum is a baby," she said. But she then explained: "I have been blessed with the gift of faith; but others have not. I have no right to impose my beliefs on them."[17] But, as one pro-life advocate pointed out in a letter to the *New York Times*, "opposition to abortion is not a religious belief." It was instead a moral issue that did not depend on revelation or personal faith. Just as the Catholic Church's opposition to nuclear war was a matter of morality rather than revealed dogma, so its position on abortion was a matter of morality, which meant that, contra Ferraro, it was perfectly appropriate to "impose" this moral stand on others through policy.[18]

At the local level in New York, Catholic clergy had debated this issue with Ferraro ever since she first ran for Congress in 1978. While preparing for her first congressional campaign, she met with Msgr. Anthony Bevilacqua of Brooklyn and explained her position of being pro-choice and personally opposed to abortion, a position she thought at the time she could square with the teaching of the Catholic Church, just as

John F. Kennedy had insisted that he could uphold church–state separation as a faithful Catholic. The monsignor disagreed. "Gerry, you're wrong," he told her, according to Ferraro's recollection. "That is not the Church's teaching." But Ferraro refused to back down. "I feel my position is right in not imposing my views on anyone else," she told Bevilacqua. She "felt very, very strongly about the separation of church and state," and if opposition to abortion was a religious position, as she insisted it was, it was inappropriate to enshrine it in law, regardless of what the bishops said.[19]

In September 1984, Governor Cuomo offered a more detailed defense of a Catholic pro-choice position. Speaking at the University of Notre Dame to a packed room full of Catholic theologians, other faculty, and students, Cuomo acknowledged that the church's teaching on abortion was based not merely on a religious idea but on a moral principle. Unlike Ferraro, he suggested that Catholics who attempted to enshrine that moral principle in law were not necessarily violating the separation of church and state. But he disagreed with the New York bishops' view that Catholics had a moral duty to do so. "My church and my conscience require me to believe certain things about divorce, birth control and abortion," Cuomo said. But "my church does not order me—under pain of sin or expulsion—to pursue my salvific mission according to a precisely defined political plan." The Catholic Church in the United States was no longer engaged in a political campaign to rescind no-fault divorce laws or restrict contraceptive access, he pointed out. In both of those cases, he said, Catholic bishops rightly calculated that a political campaign on their part might do more harm than good. Divorce and contraception might be sinful, but the people had made clear that they were here to stay. And on abortion, it was equally clear that a sizable percentage of morally conscious people who agreed with the bishops on other political issues disagreed with their view on abortion. "Those who endorse legalized abortions . . . aren't a ruthless, callous alliance of anti-Christians determined to overthrow our moral standards," Cuomo said. The advocates of abortion rights included mainline Protestant denominational leaders and Jewish rabbis who agreed with the Catholic bishops on the need to protect the rights of immigrants, stop nuclear arms buildup, and promote peace.

"In many cases, the proponents of legal abortion are the very people who have worked with Catholics to realize the goals of social justice set out in papal encyclicals," he said. And if that was the case, it was better to build bridges with these potential allies in the quest for a just society rather than use one's political power to force them to live under a restrictive abortion policy that they disagreed with. Social justice meant far more than anti-abortion laws, and if that was the case, the church should not demand that politicians support those laws, especially when doing so would threaten the political alliances needed to secure other important political objectives. "Approval or rejection of legal restrictions on abortion should not be the exclusive litmus test of Catholic loyalty," Cuomo said. "We should understand that whether abortion is outlawed or not, our work has barely begun: the work of creating a society where the right to life doesn't end at the moment of birth; where an infant isn't helped into a world that doesn't care if it's fed properly, housed decently, educated adequately; where the blind or retarded child isn't condemned to exist rather than empowered to live."[20]

Cuomo's speech demonstrated the difference between two groups of Catholics. On one side were those who believed in the pluralistic, liberal, social justice-oriented society that Vatican II and the NCCB had envisioned, but who also believed that in a society that disagreed on abortion, it was best to make political alliances with pro-choice people of good will who shared most of the tenets of that vision even if it meant distancing themselves from the pro-life movement. On the other side were those who believed that protecting the right to life for the innocent unborn was such a foundational principle that it was impossible to imagine a just society without it. For those people, abortion was the single most important issue, the sine qua non in every election.

Eventually, most Catholic Democratic politicians chose some variation of the path that Cuomo and Ferraro forged. Either they insisted that abortion was strictly a religious personal issue that would be wrong to impose on others in a society that separated church and state or they argued, as Cuomo did, that in a society with a diverse range of moral views on abortion, it was best to make the pragmatic choice and pursue a Catholic social vision by making alliances with those who shared many of the bishops' political priorities, even if they did not agree on abortion.

CATHOLICS FOR CHOICE

Some Catholics went further and argued that the pro-choice position was not merely strategic or a temporal necessity in a pluralistic society but was an authentically Catholic, morally right position. On October 7, 1984, an organization called Catholics for a Free Choice published a full-page advertisement in the *New York Times* that stated, "A diversity of opinions regarding abortion exists among committed Catholics." The view that recent papal statements against abortion reflected the "only legitimate Catholic position" was "mistaken," Catholics for a Free Choice said; "a large number of Catholic theologians hold that even direct abortion, though tragic, can sometimes be a moral choice." Catholic politicians, priests, theologians, and educators needed the freedom to dissent from the church hierarchy's views on abortion, the ad stated; they should not be penalized for advocating for a pro-choice position or even for saying that in some cases, abortion could be moral. The advertisement was signed by ninety-seven Catholic professors, priests, and nuns.[21]

This may have been the first time that many Americans had heard of Catholics for a Free Choice, which had no more than 5,000 members at the time. The organization had started more than a decade earlier, in 1973, when Patricia McQuillan—a Catholic mother, stockbroker, and member of the National Organization for Women who was dismayed at her church's teachings on abortion and who wanted to find a way to reconcile second-wave feminism with her faith—joined with several other pro-choice Catholic women to launch an organization to protest the church hierarchy's opposition to abortion and especially protest the bishops' use of church resources to fund an antiabortion campaign. At the time, McQuillan's opposition to all abortion restrictions was a minority position among Catholics, as was her strong feminist opposition to the church hierarchy. McQuillan believed that the bishops and pope had lost their right to speak for the church because they had long practiced misogyny by, among other things, excluding women from the clergy and from the bishops' councils. An all-male hierarchy did not constitute the church, she said; only the total number of people of God did, and that certainly included women. On the first anniversary of *Roe v. Wade*, McQuillan made headlines by walking up the steps of St. Patrick's Cathedral in New York City with a few female friends, a bishop's miter and vestments in hand, then donning the miter and proclaiming herself "Her Holiness Pope Patricia the First." The church's stance on abortion was "strictly political and has nothing to do with 'religion' as taught by Jesus," she told the assembled crowd. She and other Catholic women would "no longer accept the erroneous dictates of the magisterium or the 'teaching authority' of the church regarding women." It was time for women to follow their own consciences on the matter and for both the church and the law to stay out of women's private decisions.[22]

For the first few years of its existence, Catholics for a Free Choice was a small and relatively uninfluential organization, but it represented the views of a much larger number of Catholics than those who paid membership dues and formally joined the organization. Part of the reason for that was the increased willingness of many Catholics to dissent from church teaching. Even by the early 1970s, a majority of married Catholics of childbearing age were not following church teaching on contraception, and a near majority of Catholics of all ages were skipping church; 71 percent of Catholics in 1964 reported in a Gallup survey that they had been to church within the last seven days, but that number dropped to 54 percent by 1975 and then to 50 percent by the mid-1980s.[23] Dissent from the church's teaching on abortion seemed to closely track with declining Mass attendance rates. Only 17 percent of Catholics who frequently attended church in the late 1980s said that elective abortion (that is, abortion for "any reason") should be legal, compared to 46 percent of those who characterized their church attendance as "not high."[24]

But to a greater degree even than church attendance, what divided pro-choice Catholics from those who were pro-life was a different locus of authority. Catholics for a Free Choice insisted that the hierarchy was not the church and could not speak unilaterally for the church; the church instead was the whole people of God, as Vatican II had said. But although Vatican II had indeed emphasized this point, it had not suggested that this broad understanding of the definition of the church in any way ended the authority of the magisterium. Catholics for a Free Choice, by contrast, believed that the laity often knew better than the hierarchy, and they viewed their campaign as a needed challenge to an all-male church hierarchy that they considered antidemocratic and misogynistic. On issues of sexuality, especially, they believed that lay Catholics who were in sexual relationships were far better authorities than celibate clergy. On abortion, women who could become pregnant knew better than male bishops. "The laity are again, along with the theologians, leading the church on the moral freedom to practice contraception and to use abortion when necessary as a backup," said Marquette University ethics professor Daniel Maguire, a leader in Catholics for a Free Choice. "Perhaps if the hierarchy were married with families, they could follow the wisdom of the laity in this at a faster pace. It would be a shame if it took a century or two for them to respect the conscience of the laity, graced and grounded as that conscience is in the lived experience of marriage and children."[25] When John Paul II insisted that the church's teaching on abortion was unchangeable and must be enforced by quelling dissent on abortion from Catholic theologians, Maguire and other pro-choice Catholics responded that this was wrong and an abuse of the hierarchy's power, which had no legitimacy in Christianity. "The Vatican's effort to claim a monopod authority is heretical to the best in the Jesus movement," Maguire wrote. Besides, Catholics for a Free Choice argued, the church's theological tradition on abortion was inconsistent and unpersuasive. Many revered Catholic thinkers of the past, including Thomas Aquinas, believed that ensoulment occurred well after conception, which is why the Catholic Church had not always viewed early abortions as homicides. Because the Catholic Church's understanding of fetal life and abortion had changed over time, lay theologians and even individual Catholics who were not professional theologians had the right to reinterpret the tradition for themselves and reach their own conclusions.

But ultimately, Catholics for a Free Choice argued, the supreme moral authority in these questions should not be historical investigation or theological inquiry; it should be individual conscience. *Conscience* was the title of Catholics for a Free Choice's official magazine; it was also the fundamental basis of its moral claims. Frances Kissling, who served as president of Catholics for a Free Choice from 1982 to 2007, argued that because the Catholic Church had never infallibly defined when fetal personhood began, the Catholic concept of probabilism meant that individual Catholics must decide this matter for themselves, using their own conscience as a guide. "The absolute prohibition on abortion by the church is not infallible," she said. "Only the woman herself can make the abortion decision."[26] After Kissling stepped down as president, subsequent presidents of Catholics for a Free Choice (which changed its name to Catholics for Choice in the twenty-first century) continued making this argument. "As Catholics, we are called by our faith to follow our conscience in all matters of moral decision-making and respect the right of others to do the same," Catholics for Choice president Jamie Manson declared. "This includes the right to make decisions about abortion and reproductive healthcare."[27] The Vatican disagreed in 2002: "A well-formed Christian conscience does not permit one to vote for a political program or an individual law which contradicts the fundamental contents of faith and morals."[28] Catholics for a Free Choice did not accurately represent Catholic doctrine, the Vatican said.

The bishops responded to Catholics for a Free Choice's 1984 *New York Times* ad with a clear denunciation. The statements in the ad "contradict the clear and constant teaching of the church about abortion, a teaching which they as Catholics are obliged to accept," the NCCB said in November 1984. Probabilism did not apply in the matter of abortion, because "Catholic theology does not allow the application of the theory of probabilism in cases which contradict Church teaching or where the risk of taking life is present." In the case of abortion, both caveats applied: Catholics for a Free Choice's statements contradicted church teaching and they led to the taking of life. A few days after the NCCB issued this statement, the Vatican's Sacred Congregation for Religious and Secular Institutes sent letters to the nuns, priests, and monks who had signed the advertisement from Catholics for a Free Choice demanding that they recant or be dismissed from their orders or clerical positions. Theologians teaching at institutions who were not under Vatican control faced less direct pressure. In some cases, their diocesan bishops requested a meeting with them. In other cases, Catholic colleges rescinded their lecture invitations. Daniel Maguire, who had several summer speaking engagements canceled because of his support for the ad, called it "a blacklisting like during the McCarthy period in the '50s." In Catholics for a Free Choice's view, the actions of the Vatican and the U.S. bishops were an attack on "free speech" and an abuse of power, but in the view of many pro-life Catholics, these were necessary commonsense measures to draw the line on one of the clearest issues of Catholic moral teaching and enforce the authority of the magisterium against the moral anarchy of individual opinion.[29]

Most Catholics, it turned out, took a position somewhere between the magisterium and Catholics for a Free Choice. One survey from 1989 showed that 63 percent of Catholics (compared to only 57 percent of white Protestants) said that abortion was "murder." Yet this same survey also showed that only 25 percent of Catholics wanted to ban abortion altogether. Seventy-five percent agreed with the statement, "I personally feel that abortion is morally wrong, but I also feel that whether or not to have an abortion is a decision that has to be made by every woman herself."[30] It appeared that the pope and the bishops had succeeded in convincing a majority of Catholics that abortion killed innocent unborn babies, but they had not succeeded in convincing all of them that this moral stance should be translated into public law. Instead, many Catholics insisted that their own moral views on such matters were not objective universal dictates that could form the foundation of a Christian society but were rather personal matters of conscience. In other words, the overwhelming majority of Catholics took positions that closely reflected the positions of pro-choice Democrats, such as Mario Cuomo, regardless of how strongly the bishops stated that this was wrong.

Although the bishops were united in opposing Catholics for a Free Choice's stance and even the more moderate position of pro-choice Democrats, such as Cuomo, they were sharply divided among themselves about whether to frame the abortion issue as part of a consistent-life seamless garment or instead as a unique, stand-alone issue that could serve as a political litmus test. Archbishop O'Connor clearly favored the latter course of action, but in a protest against that move, twenty-three bishops affiliated with the peace organization Pax Christi signed a statement declaring that "one cannot examine abortion as though it were the only moral issue facing our people.... As bishops we are gravely concerned that the threat of nuclear war is being neglected in the current examination of moral issues in the public order." Archbishop Bernardin, now a cardinal, continued to insist that both abortion and opposition to nuclear war were equally important issues, and that the church must be just as outspoken on both parts of the seamless garment. Indeed, he said, the best way to ensure the passage of antiabortion legislation was to be consistent in defending the entirety of the church's social justice teaching, since "the credibility of our advocacy of every unborn child's right to life will be enhanced by a consistent concern for the plight of the homeless, the hungry and helpless in our nation, as well as the poor of the world."[31]

But if there were bishops who supported Bernardin's view, there were also many others who supported O'Connor's. Seventeen New England bishops signed a letter in the fall of 1984 declaring that abortion was "the critical issue in this campaign."[32] Because of their belief that they should avoid direct political endorsements, they did not tell Catholics to vote Republican. And because of their belief that it was better to influence the faithful through teaching rather than coercion, they did not deny Communion to Ferraro or Cuomo, as some bishops in the twenty-first century would do to other pro-choice Catholic politicians, such as Democratic presidential candidate John Kerry (D-MA) in 2004. But the 1984 presidential campaign was still a watershed moment for abortion politics in the Catholic Church. From that moment on, the number of bishops who pushed for a progressive seamless garment life ethic gradually diminished, while those who shared O'Connor's position that abortion must take first priority in the church's list of social concerns continued to increase. Ever since the mid-1970s, the pro-life movement had wanted the bishops to make the abortion issue a single-issue litmus test of the highest priority rather than merely a piece of a seamless garment, and now they were finally getting their wish. Whereas Bernardin had worked hard to get the church to communicate its pro-life stance as the foundation of a larger consistent life ethic, O'Connor used his position as the country's most powerful Catholic prelate (as the archbishop of New York was) to move the church toward making it a political litmus test. "I simply don't see the rationale for saying that a politician is for better housing, a lower rate of unemployment, a more rational foreign policy—and the only thing wrong is he supports abortion, so it's okay to vote for him," O'Connor said. "You have to go back to the basic question: What is abortion? Do you think it's the taking of innocent human life or don't you?"[33] Of course, Bernardin and the other bishops who had endorsed the consistent-life ethic shared O'Connor's belief that abortion was the "taking of innocent human life"; they just said that because other issues (such as nuclear arms buildup) also had the potential to take innocent human lives, those issues also had to matter in voters' choices. What mattered most was the holistic vision of a just society, and that society was not likely to be created if voters narrowly focused only on abortion and ignored all the other social principles that Vatican II had endorsed. But in the view of O'Connor and other pro-life advocates, abortion involved such massive destruction of so many innocent lives that it made all other assaults on human life pale in comparison. It had to be stopped. This had been O'Connor's conviction from the beginning of his episcopal career. When he was named bishop of Scranton in 1983, he vowed to discuss the value of unborn human life in every public address he ever gave, a promise he continued to cite the next year as archbishop of New York.[34] In this, he had the strong support of John Paul II, who was dedicated to a similar project on a global scale.

Whether because of the pope or because of O'Connor, opposition to abortion became central to the ideological identity of faithful conservative Catholics by the late 1980s, and a dividing line between nominal Catholics and devout churchgoers. According to a 1987 New York Times/CBS News poll, 61 percent of all American Catholics believed that abortion was "the equivalent of murdering a child."[35] This view was even more widely held among the most devout. A 1989 New York Times/CBS News poll showed that the majority of nominal Catholics who said that religion was not very important in their own lives favored keeping abortion legally available, but only 28 percent of Catholics who said that religion was "very" or "extremely" important to them wanted abortion to remain legal.[36] Even as Catholics dissented from the church's teachings on contraception and divorce, opposition to abortion unified most of the faithful, at least those who attended Mass regularly and considered their faith an important part of their lives.

CONSERVATIVE CATHOLICS AND THE POLITICS OF THE FAMILY

Some of the devout Catholics who strongly opposed abortion welcomed the move by conservative bishops such as John O'Connor to downplay the consistent life ethic, because they wanted to make the fight against abortion not part of a larger campaign for an expanded social safety net but rather the central component of a campaign to protect the family, which they saw as the foundation of society. Politically liberal Catholic bishops saw Reagan's social policies as threats to a humane society, but conservative Catholics who identified with the New Right viewed Reagan as a champion of their vision of a family-centered society that protected parental rights while limiting the power of the state. When it came to politics, the majority of U.S. bishops were "truly ignorant," Paul Weyrich, founder of the Heritage Foundation and a leading figure in the New Right, told a *Washington Post* reporter in 1981. His colleague Richard Viguerie agreed: "The Catholic hierarchy in America is becoming synonymous with liberal politics."[37]

Both Weyrich and Viguerie were Catholics, but instead of deferring to the bishops' guidance on political questions, they launched their own "pro-family" campaign that in their view was more authentically Catholic in its values than the bishops' political program. One of Weyrich's associates at the Heritage Foundation, Onalee McGraw, published a book about secular humanism in the same year (1976) that Francis Schaeffer addressed the subject in his best-selling book *How Should We Then Live?* But McGraw's book, *Secular Humanism and the Schools: The Issue Whose Time Has Come*, focused more specifically on parental rights in education, an issue that was a central concern for Catholics in the New Right and that would soon become a major issue for conservative evangelicals. Another Heritage Foundation associate, Connie Marshner, who worked closely with Weyrich, got her political start by supporting a campaign for parental rights in education in Kanawha County, West Virginia, in 1974, and then wrote *Blackboard Tyranny* to argue against the public school system and encourage the growth of private Christian schools. In 1979, she helped write the Family Protection Act, an attempt to protect parental rights in education that did not pass in a Democratic-controlled U.S. House but served as a precursor to social conservatives' legislative priorities in the Reagan administration and beyond. Marshner's husband, William Marshner, was a charter faculty member at Christendom College, a New Right-oriented traditional Catholic institution formed around the dream of Catholic-based cultural renewal and a revival of "Christendom" in Western society. A network of conservative Catholic institutions, such as *Triumph* magazine (edited by William F. Buckley Jr.'s brother-in-law L. Brent Bozell), the *Wanderer*, the University of Dallas, Christendom College, and some of Weyrich's organizations, promoted a vision of society that was skeptical of both liberal government programs and libertarian rejections of moral regulation. Instead of the expanded government programs that the bishops wanted, Catholic New Right activists pushed for a pro-family approach that envisioned an expansion of parental rights and traditional Catholic teaching about the home as central to a recovery of Christian values.[38]

Because their twin enemies were secularism and the sexual revolution—the same movements against which conservative evangelical Protestants were mobilizing—many of these traditional Catholics made common cause with evangelicals, just as Weyrich had when he helped recruit Jerry Falwell to found the Moral Majority. Indeed, their political and social commentary was at times almost indistinguishable from that of conservative evangelical Protestants. All these conservative Catholics strongly opposed abortion, which they viewed as the greatest challenge to human life and Christian values that the country faced. Bozell was a veteran of pro-life organizations. The *Wanderer* had been publishing articles against abortion for decades. Weyrich provided the office space for Judie Brown's American Life Lobby. In campaigning against abortion, they believed that they were not only campaigning for human life but were also battling secular humanism, assaults on parental rights, and challenges to the traditional Christian sexual ethic.

The conservative Catholics who campaigned for parental rights and who viewed the liberal state as a threat to their Christian values also included plenty of opponents of second-wave feminism who connected pro-choice feminists' advocacy of abortion rights to what they believed was their larger disrespect for the family and their willingness to use the power of the state to protect individual autonomy at the expense of children's well-being, or, in the case of abortion, their lives. From the beginning of the 1970s, the pro-life movement had some members who called themselves feminists. It even had a handful of members who had once been members of the National Organization for Women (NOW), as were Feminists for Life cofounders Pat Goltz and Catherine Callaghan before they were expelled from a Columbus, Ohio, chapter of NOW because of their opposition to abortion. But by the end of the 1970s, far more pro-life activists were persuaded by conservative Catholic Phyllis Schlafly's STOP-ERA campaign that the Equal Rights Amendment (ERA) (and likely the larger second-wave feminist movement itself) threatened the family and would be used to expand abortion rights. In 1980, only 9 percent of National Right to Life Committee (NRLC) members said they supported the ERA.[39]

If pro-life activists were conservative on matters of gender, they were equally so on matters of sex. Ninety-six percent of NRLC members in 1980 believed that homosexuality was "always or almost always wrong," and 87 percent said the same about premarital heterosexual sex. Since 70 percent of NRLC members were Catholic at the time, these survey results indicated that the Catholics who were most likely to participate in an organized pro-life campaign were likely to hold conservative values on sex, gender, and the family that were very similar to those of many conservative evangelical Protestants.[40] It was thus not too surprising that some of them followed Weyrich's and Viguerie's lead in ignoring the liberal-leaning political pronouncements of the Catholic bishops and voted for candidates who wanted to expand parental rights to exempt their children from sex education classes or who promised to reduce government regulation of private Christian or parochial schools. The church could best pursue its mission to help the poor not by supporting federal poverty relief programs, as the bishops thought, but instead by reducing the tax burden on families and empowering faith-based private charitable organizations. The New Right, along with the leaders of most of the nation's pro-life organizations, supported Ronald Reagan's presidential candidacy in 1980, even as the bishops went out of their way to avoid any hint of approval for the GOP platform.

Conservative Catholics who grounded their political vision in a defense of the family and conservative views on sex found inspiration in the social teaching of John Paul II, who became pope in 1978. During John Paul II's first visit to the United States in October 1979, he repeatedly spoke about threats to the family that emerged from ignoring the church's teaching on abortion and marriage. He devoted the homily in his Mass on the Washington Mall—a rock-star-like celebration that drew nearly 200,000 attendees—to a discussion of the evils of abortion and cultural liberalism's attack on the church's teachings on sexuality: "If a person's right to life is violated at the moment in which he is first conceived in his mother's womb, an indirect blow is struck also at the whole of the moral order, which serves to ensure the inviolable goods of man. Among those goods, life occupies the first place." In itself, this was hardly a surprising statement; Catholics had been issuing similar warnings for decades. But many of those earlier warnings had suggested that an acceptance of abortion would lead to a general disregard for human life at other stages. Though by no means denying this connection, the pope largely ignored it in his homily and instead focused on the more urgent matter of marriage, sexuality, and the family. The Catholic teaching on abortion was inseparable from a larger concern for marriage and the family, he suggested. In Philadelphia, where as many as 500,000 people greeted him, the pope said,

"There can be no true freedom without respect for the truth regarding the nature of human sexuality and marriage. In today's society, we see so many disturbing tendencies and so much laxity regarding the Christian view on sexuality that have all one thing in common: recourse to the concept of freedom to justify any behavior that is no longer consonant with the true moral order and the teaching for the church."[41]

At the beginning of John Paul II's papacy, many bishops and priests gave greater emphasis to promoting a liberal social vision than to defending conservative values in the area of sexuality. But by the mid-1980s, that was beginning to change, as conservative bishops that John Paul II had appointed (such as John O'Connor) gained greater influence.

EVANGELICALS

The Catholic bishops' decision in 1984 to treat abortion as a more important political matter than nuclear arms buildup or other social justice issues brought them into closer alliance with evangelicals. The minority of evangelicals who were progressive Democrats (a group that was only 20 to 25 percent of white evangelical voters, at most) lauded the bishops' consistent life ethic, but the bishops' stances on nuclear arms, capital punishment, and antipoverty programs were at odds with those of most white evangelicals. Jerry Falwell and his Moral Majority strongly supported Reagan's nuclear arms buildup. Reagan also found some other evangelical allies for his arms policy when he promoted it in a speech at the National Association of Evangelicals' annual meeting in 1983. White evangelicals also endorsed capital punishment.[42] For evangelicals, these stances were consistent with their faith. After all, the Old Testament mandated capital punishment for murder (and a number of other crimes), and the New Testament spoke of the government's duty to use the power of the "sword," a passage that many evangelicals interpreted as support for both just war and capital punishment. The Catholic bishops may have viewed nuclear arms buildup as immoral, but many evangelicals saw it as a necessary deterrent in the fight against international communism. As long as the Catholic bishops insisted on treating abortion as part of a consistent life ethic, there would be tension between the political priorities of the bishops and those of the evangelical Christian Right. But by treating abortion as a single-issue political litmus test, the bishops erased those differences. Both conservative Catholics and conservative evangelicals could unite in a campaign to stop abortion.

Like conservative Catholics, evangelicals were also beginning to treat abortion as the single most important political issue. In 1980, the Moral Majority and the rest of the Christian Right had treated abortion as a foundational issue in their campaign against the sexual revolution and secularization, but they had not yet made it their single most important priority. By 1984, they were ready to do so. The more they talked about abortion, the more heinous the sin appeared. A few years earlier, preachers such as Falwell had paired sermons on abortion with excoriations of pornography and homosexuality, but the more that they talked about these issues, the clearer it seemed that "baby killing" was even worse than sexual sins, as bad as those were. The Christian Right's message to its supporters in 1984 was thus more directly focused on abortion than it had been in 1980; it was *the* central issue in the presidential election, as far as they were concerned. In 1980, they had not paid much attention to the power that the president had to reverse *Roe v. Wade* through appointing the right judicial nominees to the Supreme Court, but after the pro-life movement identified this as a key strategy in 1983, the Christian Right picked up on the idea and highlighted it in their 1984 campaign messages. "There is no doubt that the future of our nation for the rest of this century and into the beginning of the 21st century rides on the outcome of this election," Moral Majority vice president Cal Thomas told Christian radio audiences in 1984. "Supreme Court judges will probably be chosen by the next President. Will they keep the abortion floodgates open or start to close them? It's up to you."[43]

In the 1980s, nearly all groups of evangelicals moved to the right on abortion. Those who had been silent on abortion or who had been willing to accept it under limited conditions began to insist that it was a terrible evil. And those who were already against abortion became even more strongly opposed. In 1981, Francis Schaeffer suggested for the first time that Christians might have a duty to "disobey the state" if they could not restore Christian values and pro-life principles by working through the courts and the regular political process.[44] In 1986, Randall Terry's Operation Rescue began putting that principle into practice by mobilizing evangelicals to illegally block abortion clinics and face arrest for their actions, just as a few Catholics had done in the late 1970s and early 1980s.

Operation Rescue was the largest (and most fully ecumenical) grassroots fusion of Catholic and evangelical pro-life efforts, and it was led largely by charismatics and Pentecostals, who had initially been slower than many Reformed, Lutheran, and fundamentalist Baptist denominations to join the pro-life cause. Pentecostals had traditionally been less interested than other evangelicals in efforts to transform the nation's culture through politics, but by the 1980s, under the influence of the charismatic religious broadcaster Pat Robertson, whose television program *The 700 Club* had a widespread following among Pentecostal Christians, many Pentecostals and other charismatic evangelicals began wholeheartedly embracing the culture-war rhetoric of Schaeffer and the apocalyptic worldview of Tim LaHaye, a Baptist pastor who was deeply concerned about a secular humanist conspiracy in political, legal, and educational institutions. When Terry, a twenty-nine-year-old Pentecostal minister in upstate New York, teamed up with Catholic pro-life practitioners of civil disobedience to block abortion clinics, he succeeded in mobilizing tens of thousands of evangelicals and Catholics for the cause. By 1992, 40,000 Operation Rescue volunteers (both evangelical and Catholic) had been arrested.[45]

Many denominational leaders were hesitant to endorse Operation Rescue's strategy. The Catholic priest who was most closely associated with Operation Rescue's direct-action tactics—Fr. Frank Pavone, founder of Priests for Life—experienced constant conflict with his episcopal superiors, and in 2022, he was removed from the priesthood for his insubordination and for desecrating an altar by placing a fetus on it.[46] Many evangelical leaders—including those who were strongly opposed to abortion—were cool toward Operation Rescue. Charles Stanley, who served as president of the SBC in the mid-1980s and was also on the board of Moral Majority, said that he could not endorse Operation Rescue's practice of civil disobedience, which he believed was a violation of scripture.[47] But even if evangelical denominations did not necessarily countenance everything that Operation Rescue did, the organization's success in mobilizing many of their members for the cause kept the abortion issue at the forefront of evangelical and conservative Catholic attention in the late 1980s and pushed evangelical denominations to do more for the pro-life cause. Operation Rescue successfully fused the language and techniques of civil rights activism with apocalyptic conservative culture-war rhetoric that predicted the coming wrath of God against the United States unless the abortion holocaust ended. This rhetoric entered Christian music, Christian television and radio preaching, and Christian magazines, along with the Sunday sermons at many churches.[48] In most of these cases, the message was distinctly political: It focused on saving the nation by saving unborn babies. And it was also fused with a conservative message on sexuality, and with a distinctly Christian message about God and salvation. By the mid-1980s, most evangelical denominations found this message impossible to ignore, and they responded by strengthening their commitment to the pro-life effort, which they almost invariably depicted primarily as a political effort to save the nation from abortion.

Under the SBC's new conservative leadership—and in response to pressure from strongly pro-life conservative evangelicals both inside and outside of the denomination—Southern Baptists began making the pro-life campaign their leading political cause. In a sign of the denomination's new direction, the SBC invited Schaeffer's son, Franky Schaeffer, who was known at the time as a strident pro-life activist who was even more militant on the issue than his father, to speak to the SBC's 1984 Pastors' Conference. Not surprisingly, Schaeffer used the opportunity to castigate Southern Baptists for their hesitancy in fully embracing the pro-life cause. It was time to "make abortion a priority," Schaeffer told the Southern Baptist pastors. "The fact that you have not done it and know that you should means you will stand in judgment for not using your resources." The assembled pastors responded to Schaeffer's hard-hitting exhortation with a standing ovation.[49] The SBC was already an officially pro-life denomination, since it had adopted a resolution in 1980 opposing abortion in all cases except when a pregnancy endangered a woman's life. In 1982, the SBC passed a resolution declaring that "both medical science and biblical references indicate that human life begins at conception" and urging Southern Baptists once again to work for a constitutional amendment banning abortion except when necessary to "save the physical life of the mother," a resolution that the SBC reaffirmed in 1984.[50] But Southern Baptists for Life, which formed in 1984, pushed the SBC to do more, just as Schaeffer advocated. In January 1986, the SBC began an annual tradition of celebrating Human Life Sunday by encouraging pastors to preach a sermon against abortion on the anniversary of *Roe v. Wade*. "We stand very strongly against abortion," SBC president Charles Stanley said in October 1985, while speaking on behalf of the denomination, "and agree that it is murder except for the preservation of the physical life of the mother."[51]

Social survey data supported Stanley's description of Southern Baptist sentiment. A nationwide poll of Southern Baptist pastors and lay church leaders taken in 1985 indicated that only 10 percent were pro-choice. By contrast, 40 percent said that abortion should be illegal in all circumstances or should be allowed only when a woman's life was in danger, and another 50 percent were willing to allow for abortion only in cases of rape or incest or when necessary to save a woman's life.[52]

After Foy Valentine, the last of the leading SBC moderates, retired as president of the Christian Life Commission (CLC) in 1987 and was replaced by the strongly pro-life Richard Land, the SBC began engaging in political lobbying on behalf of the pro-life cause to an even greater extent. The CLC's magazine *Light* published articles against abortion in nearly every issue in 1987. The SBC began reaffirming its strong antiabortion stance with new resolutions on abortion nearly every year.[53] In the early 1970s, the SBC had done something similar regarding alcohol, passing new resolutions each year to decry the liquor industry and reaffirm its stance of total abstinence. At the end of the 1980s, abortion replaced alcohol as the SBC's primary political target. The CLC voted in March 1990 to request that its executive director not invite anyone who held pro-choice views to speak at any meeting or event sponsored by the CLC. This was a more stringent litmus test than the SBC applied to any other political or social issue, but CLC commissioner Liz Minnick explained that "abortion is the benchmark issue . . . because this is life. The way you look at abortion colors the way you look at all issues."[54]

In a sign that total opposition to abortion was now an essential part of broader evangelical orthodoxy, Intervarsity Press withdrew D. Gareth Jones's work of evangelical bioethics, *Brave New People*, from circulation in 1984 after the Christian Action Council and Franky Schaeffer complained that the book allowed for abortion in cases of suspected fetal deformities. Jones, a New Zealand evangelical, was generally opposed to elective abortion, and only a few years earlier, his willingness to allow for abortion in a few exceptional cases probably would not have raised many eyebrows among most evangelicals in the United States.[55] But the ground had swiftly shifted among American evangelicals, and a stance that would have been fine in the 1970s was now unacceptable in the 1980s. "A consensus *is* developing," Presbyterian Church in America pastor Paul Fowler wrote in 1987. "Virtually everyone in the evangelical wing of the church is against abortion-on-demand. The prolife movement has drawn together such diverse groups as the Moral Majority and Evangelicals for Social Action, and found a voice in magazines such as *Moody Monthly* as well as *Sojourners*."[56] Indeed, abortion might have been the only political issue that progressive evangelicals and right-wing fundamentalists agreed on in the mid-to-late 1980s; they both believed it must be stopped, since it was baby-killing. And although progressive evangelicals on the left continued to champion a consistent life ethic in the late 1980s, most other pro-life evangelicals gave it no consideration at all, since for most evangelicals, it was a foreign concept that was never a part of their conceptualization of the pro-life campaign. For most conservative evangelicals (including Fowler), pro-life activism had nothing to do with nuclear arms policy, but instead meant denouncing abortion as murder and working through the political process to end it through restrictive legislation and the reversal of *Roe v. Wade*.

Fowler still thought that more needed to be done—churches needed to preach more firmly against abortion, and evangelicals who were still silent on the issue or who were still willing to countenance abortion in a few exceptional circumstances needed to understand how strongly the Bible proclaimed the value of unborn human life. But he rejoiced that pro-life evangelicals were winning the battle for their churches, and they were joining with Catholics to take their moral fervor on the issue into the political arena. Indeed, their influence on the issue was so strong that it was even beginning to affect liberal Protestant denominations that had once been firmly pro-choice.

CHAPTER 6

LIBERAL PROTESTANTS AFTER *ROE*

A Theology for a Pluralistic Nation

In 1988, the American Baptist Churches USA (ABCUSA) issued a new type of abortion resolution—a resolution acknowledging that members of the denomination could not agree on the subject. For the previous twenty years, Protestant denominations had issued resolutions on abortion that called for moral action of one sort or another. Twenty years earlier, the American Baptists had been at the forefront of that movement; they had passed resolutions in 1967 and 1968 calling for the legalization of abortion in at least some circumstances. They had been early members of the Religious Coalition for Abortion Rights, as was fitting, perhaps, for the denomination that was once the church home of Howard Moody, founder of the Clergy Consultation Service on Abortion. But by the late 1980s, some of the Protestant denominations that had once been leaders in the campaign for abortion rights were retreating from the cause, and those that had once been somewhat ambivalent on abortion were becoming stridently pro-life. In this climate, perhaps it was best to take no official position at all, the ABCUSA decided.

"Many American Baptists believe that, biblically, human life begins at conception, that abortion is immoral and a destruction of a human being created in God's image," the ABCUSA stated. But "many others" in the denomination believed that "while abortion is a regrettable reality, it can be a morally acceptable action and they choose to act on the biblical principles of compassion and justice." And if members of the denomination could not agree on whether abortion was murder or a "morally acceptable action," they were equally divided about whether it should remain legal or be prohibited by law. "Consequently, we acknowledge the freedom of each individual to advocate for a public policy on abortion that reflects his or her beliefs," the ABCUSA concluded. The resolution passed by a vote of 161 to 9.[1]

The ABCUSA's resolution was only the most forthright acknowledgment of a reality that was affecting nearly all pro-choice Protestant denominations in the 1980s: the presence of a growing pro-life sentiment within even some of the most liberal (and once most strongly pro-choice) denominations. Both the United Methodist Church and the Presbyterian Church (USA) moderated their official pro-choice stances in response to internal pro-life pressure, and several other liberal Protestant denominations debated whether to do so. In the early 1970s, many liberal pro-choice Protestants had insisted that organized opposition to abortion was confined to Catholics. By the end of the 1980s, it was obvious that that was no longer true; dissent over abortion was both a Catholic and a Protestant phenomenon that influenced nearly all denominations.

But supporters of the pro-life cause did not succeed in bringing all groups of Christians into the right-to-life camp. Instead, abortion remained a polarizing issue in the nation's churches. What the American Baptists stated about their own denomination in 1988 could have been said of Christianity in the country as a whole—there was still substantial disagreement on abortion, with no resolution in sight.

LIBERAL PROTESTANTS IN THE DECADE AFTER *ROE*

One might have expected that the liberal Protestants who had advocated liberalized abortion laws before *Roe* would have been jubilant when the Supreme Court gave them a decision in 1973 that codified what their denominational resolutions had been calling for. But instead, they adopted a somber tone that reflected their conviction that abortion was morally ambiguous. *Roe* was necessary, they believed, because abortion bans only made the situation worse. But abortion was never something to celebrate. And when abortion rates rapidly rose in the years after *Roe*, even the *Christian Century*, which had long been a persistent advocate for abortion legalization, sounded a note of warning. "*Roe v. Wade* opened the floodgates for thousands of thoughtless and unwarranted abortions," Kenneth Vaux wrote in the *Christian Century* in March 1975. It left people "morally dissatisfied."[2]

In the wake of *Roe*, liberal Protestants positioned themselves as moderates in the abortion debate who could bring a truce to the controversy by standing against proposed abortion bans while also convincing pro-choice activists not to push for more than they already had. Even government funding of abortion should be curtailed if it "violate[d] the ethical conscience of antiabortionists who do not want any of their tax money aiding in an act they consider to be murder," J. Claude Evans wrote in 1979.[3] Before *Roe*, Evans had been a leading pro-choice voice at the *Christian Century*, and he never reneged on his commitment to keeping abortion legal, but at the same time he considered conscience rights so inviolate that he wanted to protect the rights of those who opposed abortion on moral grounds.

Indeed, for liberal Protestants in the 1970s and early 1980s, the abortion rights campaign was primarily about religious freedom. Their main reason for championing *Roe* and supporting legal abortion, they said, was because they wanted to defend religious liberty against the attacks of Catholic bishops who, in their view, were trying to subvert the country's long-standing separation of church and state by enshrining their church's dogma into civil law. This was the framework that the Religious Coalition for Abortion Rights (RCAR) adopted when it formed in the fall of 1973 in order to lobby against the attempt of the Catholic bishops and the pro-life movement to pass an antiabortion constitutional amendment. Although the earliest public relations materials from RCAR briefly mentioned the health and socioeconomic inequities that would result if *Roe v. Wade* were rescinded, they focused mainly on the threat that an antiabortion constitutional amendment posed to individual Americans' freedom of conscience. "The Coalition members believe that abortion is a highly personal decision that should be determined by an individual's own conscience, not by the dictates of the state," a 1974 RCAR brochure stated. Because "there are widely differing viewpoints in the religious community on the abortion issue, in a pluralistic society, it is important that all religions have the right to practice their beliefs freely and that the state remain completely neutral."[4] RCAR thus framed itself primarily as an advocate for church–state separation and individual liberty of conscience; the morality of abortion itself was not something the organization wanted to discuss very much.

United Methodists took the lead in organizing RCAR. Of the thirty-three initial sponsors of the organization in 1974, nine were Methodist bishops, a much higher number than came from any other denomination. For nearly twenty years, RCAR located its offices in the United Methodist Building on Capitol Hill, across the street from the Supreme Court, and it dedicated itself to championing the *Roe v. Wade* decision that had been written by a liberal Methodist. But like most liberal Methodists, the leaders of RCAR attempted to be as broadly ecumenical as possible in their outreach to other religious groups. RCAR's other sponsors included representatives from Jewish organizations, mainline Presbyterians, Episcopalians, and denominational leaders in the United Church of Christ (UCC). Over the next few years, a number of American Baptists and Southern Baptists also joined, attracted by RCAR's focus on religious liberty.[5]

For an ecumenical lobbying organization whose members spanned the theological spectrum from Unitarians to American Baptists, a narrow focus on religious liberty made sense. It avoided the thorny theological issues that might have divided this coalition if RCAR had attempted to say anything more specific about abortion's morality or role in society. RCAR's focus was political, not pastoral or ecclesiastical; it did not tell churches how they should counsel their own members about abortion decisions or what pastors should say about abortion from the pulpit. Instead, it acted as a lobbying organization with one principal goal—ensuring that abortion would remain legally available so that everyone would have the freedom to make their own decisions on the issue.

But even when speaking for their own church organizations, where one might have expected a greater degree of theological specificity, liberal Protestant advocates of abortion rights often did no more than reiterate a version of RCAR's argument about the value of individual choice without state coercion, an argument that was largely a repetition of the Supreme Court's reasoning in *Roe v. Wade*. "The most important freedom of all is the freedom to exercise responsibility for one's life in all its phases," UCC president Avery Post said in January 1981 on the eighth anniversary of *Roe v. Wade*. The UCC, Post said, supported the right of every woman to "obey the dictates of her conscience with regard to her private life and the function of her body."[6] This was exactly what the previous UCC president, Robert Moss, had said in 1974: "We have not taken a position in favor of abortion. The issue is one of freedom—whether the woman and her physician in what is usually an unplanned emergency can make the decision as to what is God's will, without being dictated to by Government."[7]

These declarations reflected liberal Protestantism's emphasis since the early postwar years on freedom of conscience and the individual's right to make their own moral decisions without coercion from either church or state, but by the early 1980s, even some liberal Protestant theologians who wanted to keep abortion legal found the theological rationale for this stance uncompelling. The line of argument that liberal Protestants used to defend abortion rights "reflects individualism which derives from the Enlightenment and not from the Christian faith," said UCC minister and Union Theological Seminary professor Roger Shinn in March 1981. Shinn was thoroughly liberal in both his theology and politics, and he was no supporter of the pro-life movement, but he wanted the UCC to present a better argument on behalf of the denomination's abortion rights position. Other UCC leaders to the right of Shinn were even more adamant that liberal theological arguments for abortion were not working. "If freedom of the individual before God is to be the prime category for choice, what is the church saying in behalf of conscience and character formation and the responsible use of freedom?" UCC pastor Walter Krebs asked the denomination's general secretary for the Board of Homeland Ministries in a private letter in February 1981. He said that one couldn't simply assert the right of everyone to make their own moral decisions without engaging in some discussion of the appropriate criteria to use to guide one's conscience. That discussion, he thought, was noticeably absent in the area of abortion, where liberal Protestants were leaving people to make their own decisions without any guidance from the church or any attempt to provide a cohesive theological defense of the pro-choice position. "Insofar as I can discover, we herald freedom of conscience, whatever that may mean, and then toss in a few religious platitudes and call it theology," Krebs said.[8]

Despite the internal calls for liberal Protestants to develop a more persuasive theological defense of abortion rights, most of them did not change their arguments. As a result, they were blindsided by a revolt against their position in their own denominations.

Throughout the 1970s, liberal Protestants had insisted that nearly all of the organized opposition they faced came from the Catholic Church hierarchy. This was never really true, but it accorded well with liberal Protestants' belief that their own position of individual freedom represented majority opinion and that the campaign against abortion came not from the grassroots but from a church hierarchy they had long suspected was a potential threat to individual liberty, especially on issues of reproductive rights. Liberal Protestants' earlier battles with the Catholic bishops over birth control access were still relatively fresh in their memory, and they imagined that the abortion debate was simply the latest iteration of this long-standing battle between liberal Protestant defenders of freedom of conscience and Catholic hierarchs who were not. "There is no question that a major factor in this success [of the campaign to restrict abortion] has been the implementation of the Conference of Catholic Bishops 'Plan for Pro-

Life Activities,'" RCAR said in January 1979.[9] Secular pro-choice activists were sometimes even more adamant that their opposition came mainly from the Catholic Church. "Without the ecclesiastic, financial, and political support of the conservative Catholic hierarchy, we would have a skirmish on our hands, not a war," Cincinnati writer Eric Rockwell said in February 1979 when presenting the views of the Freedom of Choice Coalition.[10] But this was a misunderstanding of the situation. Even as early as the 1960s and early 1970s, much of the Catholic opposition to abortion came from grassroots lay activists, not the bishops, and by the late 1970s, there were so many conservative Protestants expressing opposition to abortion that Jim Castelli of the Catholic News Service estimated that "antiabortion sentiment is at least as strong among evangelicals—some 50 million of them—as it is among Catholics."[11] Because liberal Protestant pro-choice advocates were slow to recognize the growing connection between evangelicalism and antiabortion sentiment, they were unprepared for the groundswell of opposition to abortion that developed in their own churches in the 1980s.

DEBATING ABORTION AMONG MAINLINE PROTESTANTS IN THE 1980S AND 1990S

Nearly all the mainline Protestant denominations—including even some of the most liberal, such as the UCC—had substantial evangelical minorities. In the 1970s, those evangelical minorities had not raised much of an issue about abortion, because it was not yet a political priority for most conservative Protestants. The evangelicals in these denominations complained about many other policy stances of the liberal denominational leadership, and some became upset enough to leave these denominations altogether—as the Presbyterian Church in America did, for instance, in 1973, when it split from the southern mainline denomination Presbyterian Church in the United States—but in those divisions, abortion usually played only an incidental role. But in the early 1980s, evangelicals shifted from treating abortion as one of a number of important political issues to viewing it as *the* single foundational issue on which all others depended, just as conservative Catholics at the time did. When that happened, the evangelical minorities in the officially pro-choice mainline Protestant denominations did likewise. Many of them were tuning in to the same Christian pro-life broadcasts that evangelicals in the Southern Baptist Convention (SBC) or other conservative evangelical denominations listened to, so when James Dobson's *Focus on the Family* radio program encouraged them to take a stand against the evils of abortion, they found the message persuasive. They were alarmed about the same sexually licentious trends in society that disturbed other evangelicals. They had the same respect for the Bible that other evangelicals did. When they heard preachers on radio or television discussing Psalm 139 or Jeremiah 1:5 — some of the favorite verses for the evangelical pro-life cause — they found these passages compelling, especially when they reflected on the close association between abortion, sexual sin, and the moral decline of the nation. If both scripture and science indicated that abortion really was the destruction of a human person, it was difficult to see why they should not enlist in the defense of the unborn, starting in their own denominations. It was not a coincidence, therefore, that at the very moment when the Moral Majority and the SBC began making abortion their signature issue — and when the airwaves were filled with evangelical discussions of abortion — the first pro-life organizations in liberal Protestant denominations began forming. Presbyterians Pro-Life was organized in the Presbyterian Church (USA) in 1984. Lifewatch formed in 1987 to represent the views of abortion opponents in the United Methodist Church. By 1989, even the United Church of Christ had a pro-life group: UCC Friends for Life.

Because these organizations drew members mainly from the evangelical or theologically conservative wing of their denominations, they often paired statements against abortion with opposition to homosexuality or other defenses of a conservative Christian sexual ethic. They appealed to the Bible as their primary or sole moral authority in a way that pro-choice advocates in these denominations generally did not. Whereas liberal Protestants often held a subjective understanding of moral decision-making, believing that decisions about abortion were morally complicated and should not be subject to absolute dictates, their pro-life counterparts in these denominations insisted that moral absolutes did matter. Moral relativism, they thought, had brought about both the sexual revolution and the abortion rights movement, and the secular drift of the nation and an abandonment of the Bible as a final standard of authority. "Moral relativism regarding abortion is directly related to moral relativism regarding sex," Frederick W. Schroeder, emeritus president of Eden Seminary (a UCC institution), stated in 1981.[12] Liberal Protestant pro-choice advocates saw support for abortion rights as a way to protect the freedom of individual consciences from state coercion, but mainline Protestant pro-life advocates had a different understanding. Their primary goal was not to increase government power, but to reassert the authority of the Bible over individual consciences and then, as a secondary goal, to bring the nation's law into harmony with that standard — as was appropriate, they thought — if abortion was murder. The Bible, not the individual conscience, was the final moral authority. And in this case, they believed that the Bible had spoken clearly, even if their liberal counterparts disagreed.

The pro-life advocates were therefore fighting not merely for a change in denominational policy on abortion; they were making an all-out effort for the revival of conservative theological standards in their denominations in opposition to the liberal leadership in their churches. "The moral, spiritual, and theological decay in the mainline denominations, and particularly in our own PC(USA), has grown to the point where we can no longer hide it from our congregations," Timothy Bayly wrote in the Winter 1990 issue of *Presbyterians Pro-Life News*. Bayly's article, "Stand Fast; Defend the Faith," was typical for the periodical, which, along with articles against homosexuality and in defense of biblical authority, published pieces such as "The Presbyterian Church (USA) Needs Those Who Will Stay and Call the Denomination Back to Holiness" and "Presbyterians Face a Pastoral Crisis: Loss of Both Christian Heritage and Church Discipline."[13] Presbyterians Pro-Life pointed out that their denomination had been officially opposed to abortion in the early 1960s, but since then it had abandoned its pro-life stance and, in the opinion of the Presbyterian pro-life activists, its respect for biblical authority too.

"I find myself apologizing for my church," Presbyterians Pro-Life member Deborah Anderson told a *New York Times* reporter at the General Assembly of the Presbyterian Church (USA) in June 1985. "I say I believe in Jesus Christ, who gives life, but my church is saying it is O.K. to kill." At the Presbyterian General Assembly where Anderson was staffing a booth for Presbyterians Pro-Life, her organization was also showing continuous screenings of the new pro-life documentary *The Silent Scream*, which showed ultrasound images of an abortion that pro-life activists said depicted the second-trimester fetus screaming as its life was being terminated. Pro-life activists considered it one of the most powerful public relations tools for their campaign, which is why Presbyterians Pro-Life brought it to the meeting. But in an adjacent room at the convention, pro-choice Presbyterians were showing *Response to the Silent Scream*, a film production of Planned Parenthood of Seattle.[14] The two sides were engaged in a contest for the future of their denomination, with each group borrowing material from activist groups outside of Presbyterian circles.

Although the conservative pro-life organizations within the officially pro-choice mainline Protestant denominations, including the Presbyterian Church (USA), did not achieve either of their main goals—a complete reversal of their denominations' pro-choice stances and a recommitment of their denominations to a biblically based theological conservatism—they did succeed in moderating their denominations' pro-choice pronouncements, at least to a limited degree. Although they made biblically based arguments in their own publications, their general strategy in appealing to their denominations' liberal leadership was to highlight the humanitarian imperative to care for the unborn, a stance they argued was in keeping with the values of liberal Protestants. In 1988, pro-life advocates in the Presbyterian Church (USA) brought Mother Teresa to speak about abortion to the denomination's General Assembly. The Presbyterian Church (USA) did not immediately change its stance on abortion, but the General Assembly did agree to "restudy" the issue.[15] The study that this Presbyterian task force completed in 1992 shifted the denomination's stance on abortion in a markedly more conservative direction. Unlike earlier pro-choice resolutions, this report was grounded in a detailed analysis of scripture and an acknowledgment of scriptural authority. Although "there are no biblical texts that speak expressly to the topic of abortion," the report stated, "taken in their totality the Holy Scriptures are filled with messages that advocate respect for the woman and child before and after birth." Some on the task force believed that the scriptures indicated that human life began at conception; others did not. The denomination was therefore not going to take a firm antiabortion stance, but neither would it suggest that abortion was a morally neutral option. "By affirming the ability and responsibility of a woman to make good moral choices regarding problem pregnancies, the Presbyterian Church (U.S.A.) does not advocate abortion but instead acknowledges circumstances in a sinful world that may make abortion the least objectionable of difficult options," the report concluded.[16]

In the United Methodist Church (UMC), pro-life activists convinced the denomination's General Assembly in 1988 to add a qualifying sentence to its pro-choice position statement: "*We cannot affirm abortion as an* acceptable means of birth control, and we unconditionally reject it as a means of gender selection."[17] Lifewatch wanted the denomination to go much further, though. In 1990, it published the Durham Declaration, which urged the UMC to "practice and to teach a sexual ethic that adorns the Gospel," to resist the surrounding culture's belief in bodily autonomy, and to "teach our churches that the unborn child is created in the image of God and is one for whom the Son of God died."[18] The UMC did not adopt the statement, but pro-life Methodists continued to gain ground in the denomination until 2016, when the UMC voted to leave the Religious Coalition for Reproductive Choice (formerly known as the Religious Coalition for Abortion Rights, RCAR), the organization of which the UMC had been a founding member four decades earlier.[19]

The Episcopal Church, which had endorsed the cause of abortion law liberalization as early as 1967 and which had been at least moderately pro-choice ever since that time, also moved to the right on abortion in the late 1980s. In 1988, it adopted a resolution: "While we acknowledge that in this country it is the legal right of every woman to have a medically safe abortion, as Christians we believe strongly that if this right is exercised, it should be used only in extreme situations. We emphatically oppose abortion as a means of birth control, family planning, sex selection, or any reason of mere convenience."[20]

Even the UCC, arguably the most liberal of the mainline Protestant denominations, faced substantial pro-life pressure to modify its stance in support of abortion rights. Although the UCC's national general synod never retreated from its pro-choice position, several UCC regional conferences in socially conservative areas of the country did. In 1986, the UCC's Penn West conference passed a resolution affirming that the unborn were included among the "weak and defenseless" people that Christians were called to protect, and that churches should therefore develop "alternatives to abortion by providing ministries of Christian compassion to women and their babies." In 1990 the UCC's southern conference adopted a resolution confessing that it was "deeply divided" over "the rights of unborn human fetuses and the morality of freedom of choice."[21]

The acknowledgment of irreconcilable internal divisions on abortion, which shaped the ABCUSA's revised official position statement on abortion in 1988, was also at the heart of mainline Lutherans' new approach to the abortion issue. In 1991, the Evangelical Lutheran Church in America (ELCA) (which, despite its use of the name "evangelical," was thoroughly mainline and did not identify with the conservative evangelical movement associated with *Christianity Today* magazine and Billy Graham) issued a new social statement on abortion that began with the confession, "Induced abortion, the act of intentionally terminating a developing life in the womb, is one of the issues about which members of the Evangelical Lutheran Church in America have serious differences."[22]

Twenty-one years earlier, the ELCA's predecessor denomination, the Lutheran Church in America, had issued a much more strongly pro-choice resolution. Acknowledging that the fetus was the "organic beginning of human life" and that the "termination of its development" was "always a serious matter," the resolution nonetheless drew a clear distinction in value between the life of the fetus and the life of a pregnant woman who "is in living relationship with God and other human beings." "A woman or couple may decide responsibly to seek an abortion," the Lutheran Church in America concluded in 1970.[23]

In 1991, some mainline Lutherans still believed this, but as the ELCA's social statement acknowledged, many did not. Some believed that abortion killed a human being and that the law should prohibit all abortions except those necessary to save a woman's life, the evangelical consensus position of that time. In attempting to navigate the deep divisions between these individual beliefs within their own denomination, members of the ELCA drew up a lengthy compromise resolution that affirmed both the "value of unborn life" and the "value of the woman and her other relationships." "A developing life in the womb does not have an absolute right to be born, nor does a pregnant woman have an absolute right to terminate a pregnancy," the ELCA asserted. "Abortion should be an option only of last resort," mainline Lutherans said. "Because of the Christian presumption to preserve and protect life, this church, in most circumstances, encourages women with unintended pregnancies to continue the pregnancy." Abortion should remain legal—and could be a morally legitimate option—in cases of rape and incest, "a clear threat to the physical life of the woman," or "extreme fetal abnormality," but the church could not necessarily give its approval to abortions that occurred for other reasons. Yet at the same time, there was enough of a residual pro-choice sentiment in the denomination (even if pro-choice advocates were becoming an increasingly beleaguered group) to prevent the denomination from taking a firm stance against elective abortions. The denomination would not endorse laws to restrict abortion before the point of viability, the ELCA said, but neither would it oppose those laws. As long as the law protected access to abortion in extreme cases, the denomination would stand aside from the legal battles and allow its members to follow the dictates of their own consciences on these matters, even as the church as a whole worked to reduce the number of abortions.[24]

None of the mainline Protestant denominations that moved to the right on abortion in the late 1980s and early 1990s joined the Catholic Church or evangelical Protestant denominations in lobbying for restrictive abortion laws. They were still too supportive of abortion access in at least a few exceptional situations to be comfortable endorsing any of the absolutist antiabortion legislation that pro-life activists favored. But beyond that, they were too committed to a generally liberal, pluralistic view of American society to be comfortable with the right-wing politics with which the pro-life movement had become identified. They were still strongly opposed to nuclear arms buildup, a stance that set them apart from the Reagan administration and the Christian Right in the 1980s. The Catholic bishops had for at least a short time combined a strongly antiabortion stance with a similarly strong condemnation of nuclear arms, but mainline Protestants' strong skepticism about state regulation of individual moral behavior and their long-standing view that government restrictions on abortion might threaten religious liberty and church–state separation made them wary of joining the Catholics' campaign for pro-life laws. In 1988, the same year in which the Presbyterian Church (USA) agreed to "restudy" its stance on abortion after hearing from Mother Teresa on the issue, the denomination officially adopted the paper "God Alone Is Lord of the Conscience," which was a defense of religious liberty in a wide variety of contexts, including the right of Native American groups to use illegal drugs in religious rituals.[25] Liberal Protestant memories of their strong opposition to state coercion of individual consciences in the Vietnam War were still fresh enough that many of them shrank back from any suggestion that they should rely on the government to enforce restrictive abortion policies, especially if those abortion policies would offend the consciences of many Jews and some of their fellow liberal Protestants.

For that reason, most did not even endorse the Partial-Birth Abortion Ban that Congress passed in 1996 and that President Bill Clinton then vetoed. The bill banned a form of later-term abortion that made even some moderately pro-choice Americans uncomfortable, which is why the bill passed Congress with the support of a few normally pro-choice Democrats. A Gallup poll taken in 1996 showed that 57 percent of Americans supported a ban on partial-birth abortion with an exception only for saving the life of the pregnant woman.[26] Many mainline Protestant denominational leaders were also uncomfortable with "partial-birth" abortion. In 1997, the Presbyterian Church (USA) passed a resolution saying that the procedure was of "grave moral concern" and should be used only when it was necessary to save a woman's life.[27] The Episcopal Church adopted a resolution that same year warning about the "misuse" of "partial birth abortion."[28] But tellingly, neither resolution expressed an opinion about the Partial-Birth Abortion Ban or any other policy to restrict the procedure. Mainline Protestant denominations were happy to lobby for policy changes on nuclear arms, foreign policy, and social welfare issues, but they did not ask the government to regulate abortion. Instead, their increasingly conservative stances on abortion focused only on personal morality, not government policy.

Indeed, the leading mainline Protestant theologians who expressed opposition to abortion — such as the Methodists William H. Willimon, Stanley Hauerwas, and Richard Hays, all of whom taught at Duke Divinity School — drew a sharp distinction between legal policy and church teaching. In *The Moral Vision of the New Testament* (1996), Hays said that "if the New Testament witness were put into practice, abortion would almost never be seen as necessary within the Christian community." The "cumulative case" of scripture plus church tradition is "weighted heavily against abortion," he argued. Churches should therefore "eschew abortion" even in cases of suspected fetal deformity and "undertake the burden of assisting the parents to raise the handicapped child." But a Christian ethic for the church would not necessarily be appropriate for the legal code of a secular society such as the United States, Hays argued. "We cannot coerce moral consensus in a post-Christian culture," he wrote. "We should recognize the futility of seeking to compel the state to enforce Christian teaching against abortion," because "the convictions that cause us to reject abortion within the church are intelligible only within the symbolic world of scripture."[29]

Hauerwas took a similar stance. In his defense of unborn human life, he repeated many of the arguments that Catholics had been making for decades, such as the argument that countenancing abortion in cases of severe fetal deformity privileges "rationality" as a mark of personhood instead of recognizing severely disabled fetuses as "God's creatures," and that people who argued for abortion in such cases made the mistake of thinking that they could "prevent suffering" by "eliminating the sufferer." But despite his respect for Catholic pro-life arguments, Hauerwas differed from pro-life Catholics in insisting that the church's approach to the abortion issue should focus not on changing the law but on preaching and practicing biblical values of community and care in the church. "Abortion is not a question about the law, but about what kind of people we are to be as the Church and as Christians," he said. When questioners pressed him on what type of abortion law he thought was appropriate, he refused to engage with the premise. "The Church is not nearly at the point where it can concern itself with what kind of abortion law we should have in the United States or even in the state of North Carolina," Hauerwas said. "Instead, we should start thinking about what it means for Christians to be the kind of community that can make a witness to the wider society about these matters."[30]

For all of these mainline Protestant Wesleyan theologians, the difference between biblically shaped Christian ethics and secular American thinking was so strong that it was pointless to try to bring Christian convictions into public law. Christians should therefore be a "called-out community" who would focus on teaching Christian ethics on abortion within the church rather than attempting to impose Christian law on a pluralistic nation. Hauerwas may have adopted this position on a church–state distinction from Anabaptist theology, which influenced his position on several other ethical matters (including his opposition to Christian involvement in war) and which he imbibed partly through his friendship with the Mennonite theologian John Howard Yoder. In keeping with Anabaptists' historic opposition to the church's use of the state to coerce behavior, Mennonites combined moral opposition to abortion with an insistence that the state could not enforce an antiabortion stance in a pluralistic society. In 1980 the General Conference Mennonite Church adopted a resolution that affirmed the high value of fetal life and condemned the individualistic thinking that had led many people to believe that abortion was a matter of a person's individual choice, arguments that Hauerwas later repeated nearly verbatim. Yet at the same time, the

Mennonites' resolution declared, "Though we stress the importance of respect for the life of the fetus and though most of us can support abortion only under the most exceptional of circumstances, we do not believe that this position should be imposed upon the society in general. Because of the diversity of moral conviction in the civil community, we realize that what the law permits is not necessarily Christian moral behavior." That did not mean that the church had nothing to say to policymakers about abortion, but it did mean that neither the General Conference Mennonite Church nor its successor denomination, the Mennonite Church USA, would join the Catholic bishops or some evangelical organizations in lobbying for the Human Life Amendment. Instead, the Mennonites called for "increased welfare payments, adequate and affordable medical care for all, sufficient day care; and to provide other personal and communal support for those one- and two-parent families who feel overwhelmed by the pressure of caring for their children" in order to support women and families, model Christian care for others, offer positive alternatives to abortion, and "witness to society concerning the sanctity of the fetus."[31]

In 2003, the newly constituted Mennonite Church USA reaffirmed most of its predecessor denomination's earlier resolution, but with an even clearer denunciation of both the moral evils of abortion and any use of civil law to enforce the church's stance on the issue. "We oppose abortion because it runs counter to biblical principles," the Mennonite Church USA declared. "Abortion should not be used to interrupt unwanted pregnancies." But "legislation banning all abortions will not stop abortions from happening," said the Mennonites' 2003 resolution. Abortion bans disproportionately hurt women and the poor, while failing to offer real help to the women involved. "Further," the Mennonites' resolution stated, "legislation is using the government to force others to comply with our Christian standards, something our forebears clearly rejected. We believe that the demands of discipleship are to be accepted voluntarily, not imposed legally upon everyone regardless of conviction."[32]

For much of the 1990s and into the early twenty-first century, the Mennonites' approach to the abortion issue seemed to offer a promising pro-life path for mainline Protestants who were morally opposed to abortion but uncomfortable with the idea of using civil law in a pluralistic society to impose Christian moral convictions on those who did not share them. Christians could express their discomfort with abortion and attempt to reduce the abortion rate by caring for women facing crisis pregnancies and encouraging adoptions, while at the same time voting for pro-choice politicians.

BLACK PROTESTANTS

In taking this position, predominantly white mainline Protestant denominations followed the lead of Black Protestants, who had been quick to denounce abortion in the 1970s but who had then distanced themselves from campaigns to make abortion illegal. In the 1970s, African Americans were much more likely than whites to oppose abortion, and even some of the most progressive Black churches therefore combined opposition to abortion with support for social justice causes.

In the 1970s, most African American Protestants who opposed abortion were part of historically Black denominations that were generally theologically conservative (even if they were politically progressive), but even among the relatively small number of African Americans in some of the most theologically liberal, predominantly white denominations, opposition to abortion was stronger than among whites in those same churches. One survey from 1972, for instance, showed that only 9 percent of whites in the most liberal predominantly white denominations (Unitarian, United Church of Christ, Episcopal, Quakers, and United Methodists) opposed abortion in cases of rape or when a pregnancy endangered a woman's health, but 23 percent of Blacks in these same denominations did so. Likewise, Blacks who attended theologically conservative churches were significantly more likely to categorically oppose abortion than whites who were members of theologically conservative denominations. Fifty-three percent of African Americans who were members of a "fundamentalist" church in 1972 opposed abortion even in cases of rape or dangers to a woman's health, for instance, but only 32 percent of white fundamentalist church members did the same.[33] At a time when most white evangelicals, including those in the SBC, were still likely to allow for "therapeutic" abortion in exceptional circumstances, African Americans were early leaders among theologically conservative Protestants in saying that abortion was always wrong, except perhaps in cases when it was necessary to save a woman's life.

African American Christians' moral reservations about abortion in the early 1970s may have reflected the civil rights movement's larger concerns about family planning as a program of white supremacists to reduce the Black population. This was a partial reversal of an earlier stance, because in the mid-twentieth century, some of the most prominent African American ministers had been avid proponents of contraception. Adam Clayton Powell, the pastor of the Abyssinian Baptist Church in Harlem who later became New York's first African American member of the U.S. House of Representatives, publicly spoke out in defense of birth control in the early 1930s. Thirty years later, Martin Luther King Jr. did the same. Contraception was a "profoundly important ingredient" in African Americans' "quest for security and a decent life," he wrote in 1966.[34] Planned Parenthood, which in 1939 had launched the Negro Project to recruit Black ministers to campaign for birth control in Black communities, honored King with its Margaret Sanger Award for his efforts. But in the late 1960s, the rise of Black nationalism in the civil rights movement eroded African American support for birth control, because many Black nationalist organizations, including most prominently the Nation of Islam, denounced birth control as a form of genocide against the Black race. In this climate, even some local chapters of the NAACP—an organization that historically had not been very supportive of the Black nationalist wing of the movement—repeated the charge that family planning clinics were engaged in genocide against Blacks.[35] Sanger's effort to promote birth control in Black communities had in reality been an attempt to eradicate the Black population, they claimed. And Black women were still being forcibly sterilized through government programs. In some cases, they were right. Some politicians were openly suggesting that state-funded birth control programs and legalized abortion for low-income women could be used to reduce welfare rolls. North Carolina did not end its decades-long program of forced sterilization of certain recipients of public assistance until 1973.[36]

Because the campaign to legalize abortion began gaining ground at the exact moment that prominent leaders in the Black community were beginning to label birth control a form of Black genocide, it was not surprising that many African Americans were quick to denounce abortion and that they used the term "genocide" to describe it. Some of the African Americans who described abortion as "genocide" did not differentiate between abortion and contraception, but others did. One of the African American Protestant Christians who conflated at least some birth control methods with abortion and classified all of them as "genocide" was Fannie Lou Hamer, the Mississippi civil rights activist who had had a forced hysterectomy at the hands of a doctor who deceived her about the purpose of her operation. A former sharecropper who had been brutally beaten and jailed for attempting to register to vote, Hamer was legendary in the movement for both her Christian faith and her courage. In her support for civil rights and concerns about the Vietnam War, she was an ally of the political left, but on issues of sex, she was culturally conservative. In a speech at Tougaloo College in Mississippi in 1971, she combined a statement against the Vietnam War and a lament about the murders of African American civil rights leaders with a quick aside about the importance of gender distinctions and the evils of abortion. "The methods used to take human life, such as abortion, the pill, the ring, etc., amount to genocide," Hamer said, using language that was very typical for African Americans of the time who believed that abortion was killing their race. "I believe that legal abortion is legal murder and the use of pills and rings to prevent God's will is a great sin."[37] In 1973, the Progressive National Baptist Convention—the social justice-oriented denomination that Martin Luther King Jr. and other civil rights leaders had helped to create in the early 1960s in a split with the more socially conservative leadership of the National Baptist Convention—passed a resolution declaring that abortion was "genocide" and that pregnancy terminations were acceptable only in cases when a woman's life was in danger.[38]

Yet even though large numbers of African Americans in the early 1970s were opposed to abortion, only a few joined the pro-life movement. In part, that may have been because the pro-life movement was predominantly white and Catholic, while the vast majority of African American

Christians were Protestant. But even as white Protestants began joining the pro-life movement in greater numbers in the late 1970s and early 1980s, most African Americans who opposed abortion did not rush to join pro-life organizations. Indeed, as the movement became increasingly focused on prohibiting abortion through law—and in working with conservative politicians to do so—African American Christians who opposed abortion found themselves alienated from the movement, despite their shared antipathy to abortion. For many African American Christians, addressing the crisis of abortion meant not making abortion illegal—and certainly not punishing anyone involved in the abortion decision—but rather reaching out with social assistance and support to help vulnerable pregnant women while at the same time cherishing all human life. Abortion was wrong because it represented a disregard for the vulnerable and marginalized, so to counteract abortion, Christians should care for the vulnerable and marginalized, they believed.

This was the argument that the Reverend Jesse Jackson made in an article he wrote in 1977 for *National Right to Life News*, "How We Respect Life Is Over-riding Moral Issue." Jackson, who had worked closely with Martin Luther King Jr. at the end of King's career and who was quickly emerging as the nation's most publicly visible civil rights advocate, viewed his pro-life advocacy through the lens of civil rights and especially through the lens of his concerns about poverty. He himself had been born in poverty to an unmarried mother, so for him the issue was "personal," he said. He was also a "minister of the gospel" who was concerned about human life.

Jackson began his article by noting that human life begins at conception, according to biological facts. "Anything growing is living," he wrote. "Therefore human life begins when the sperm and egg join and drop into the fallopian tube and the pulsation of life takes place. From that point, life may be described differently (as an egg, embryo, fetus, baby, child, teenager, adult), but the essence is the same." He supported contraception. "I believe in family planning," he said. He had seen large impoverished families when he was growing up, and he did not think that families needed to have children "by the dozens." But once a child was conceived, it was a human life that deserved to be protected, because life was a "gift from God" that humans did not have the right to "take away."

These arguments were common among opponents of abortion and would have been very familiar to anyone in the pro-life movement. But then Jackson pivoted to concerns that were not necessarily as common among white opponents of abortion, and in doing so presented arguments that resonated with large numbers of Black Christians who opposed abortion at the time. Abortion legalization was a way to avoid social responsibility to the poor, he claimed. "Politicians argue for abortion largely because they do not want to spend the necessary money to feed, clothe and educate more people."

Taking direct aim at the legal reasoning behind *Roe*, Jackson declared that the individualistic version of liberalism on which it was based was flawed. "There are those who argue that the right to privacy is of higher order than the right to life," Jackson stated. "I do not share that view. I believe that life is not private, but rather it is public and universal. If one accepts the position that life is private, and therefore you have the right to do with it as you please, one must also accept the conclusion of that logic. That was the premise of slavery. You could not protest the existence or treatment of slaves on the plantation because that was private and therefore outside of your right to be concerned." In contrast to this exaltation of privacy as an overarching fundamental right, Jackson favored an increase in public concern that would motivate people to welcome the "basic shifts of economic and political power in the world" that would be required to feed the world's hungry and pay the "price of justice."

Abortion, he believed, would not lead to a just world. It would instead lead to further dehumanization and a desensitization to the taking of human life. "What happens to the mind of a person, and the moral fabric of a nation, that accepts the aborting of the life of a baby without a pang of conscience?" he asked. "What kind of a person, and what kind of a society will we have 20 years hence if life can be taken so casually?"[39]

When Jackson wrote this article, there were still plenty of fiscal conservatives who supported abortion rights, and it was therefore easy to believe (as he did) that the abortion rights movement was motivated in part by an opposition to welfare programs and a lack of concern for the poor. The campaign against abortion, he believed, was inseparable from a larger quest for social justice for people of color and those who were in poverty. After all, he pointed out, these campaigns were based on similar concerns. The United States had long denied the full humanity of Blacks, he noted, and it was now denying the full humanity of people in the womb. But as it became increasingly clear that the majority of politicians who wanted to restrict abortion were not very supportive of antipoverty programs, Black Christians who opposed abortion became less supportive of the campaign to enact legal restrictions on abortion, even as they continued to view abortion as immoral.

This was the stance of the African Methodist Episcopal (AME) Church, one of the most politically progressive African American denominations. In 1977, at a time when the United Methodist Church and most other predominantly white mainline Protestant denominations were officially pro-choice, the AME Church differentiated itself from its white counterparts by passing a pro-life resolution that noted that God "endows each human life with a certain sanctity." Because the AME Church believed that the "setting-apart for God's work through His 'sacrificial love' begins from or even before the womb," it said that "abortion, which represents deliberate destruction of that life created by God, is a violation of that sanctity." But if there were similarities between the AME Church's abortion resolution and the antiabortion resolutions passed by a few predominantly white conservative denominations in the 1970s, such as the Christian Reformed Church or the Orthodox Presbyterian Church, there was one critical difference: The AME Church's resolution made no reference to political efforts to make abortion illegal. For predominantly white evangelical denominations that enlisted in the fight against abortion, there was a very quick transition between saying that abortion was the unjustified taking of human life and encouraging Christians to enlist in the campaign to pass antiabortion laws. But the AME Church argued instead that Christians had a duty to "seek first to recognize and prevent the circumstances leading to problem pregnancies." Then, the church said, "we must also surround each parent and child with love and provide them with concrete spiritual, social, economic and educational assistance."[40]

After the beginning of Ronald Reagan's presidency, it became more difficult to associate the right-to-life cause with the campaign to feed the hungry and lift up the impoverished, at least in the political arena. Christian leaders—especially in the Catholic Church—might still try to combine opposition to abortion with a broader concern for the poor and marginalized, but Black Christians did not sense much of this from Republican politicians. In his January 1977 article for the *National Right to Life News*, Jackson had expressed dismay that some politicians who supported government-subsidized abortions for women receiving welfare benefits were unwilling to support school lunch programs. But in the Reagan administration, it was the president himself (an avowed opponent of abortion), along with some of his ostensibly pro-life supporters, who proposed substantial funding cuts for the school lunch program. It was Reagan who frequently complained about welfare programs even as he also decried abortion. Some white pro-life activists did complain about Reagan's position on issues other than abortion, but most of the movement's most prominent leaders—even those who had once been liberal Democrats—argued that Reagan's endorsement of an antiabortion constitutional amendment was sufficient reason for the movement to support him, at least as long as the Democratic Party officially opposed the idea. The National Right to Life Committee and other national pro-life organizations had already announced that they would treat the Human Life Amendment as a political litmus test, endorsing candidates who pledged their support for it and opposing those who did not. When Reagan promised his support for the amendment, the leaders of the National Right to Life Committee—including many who wrote for the *National Right to Life News*, where Jackson had published his article against abortion in 1977—gave Reagan their full support. But Jackson and most other African American ministers did not. "As I see it, there is no room in Reagan's world for us," Jackson told a group of African American civil rights activists in October 1980.[41] In the lead-up to the 1984 presidential race, Jackson entered the Democratic presidential primaries. And in the summer of 1984, he electrified the Democratic National Convention with a speech denouncing the Reagan administration's treatment of the poor.[42]

In the midst of this political activism, Jackson also changed his political position on abortion, but not his personal beliefs on the morality of the matter. He told a *New York Times* reporter in September 1983 that he still believed it was "immoral" for a woman to have an abortion "except under medically extenuating circumstances," but he would not "favor taking away her freedom of choice." Later that year, he also stated that he did not want to cut Medicaid funding for abortion. The *New York Times* noted the shift: "In the past, he has been quoted as equating abortion with murder."[43]

But Jackson's change of position on abortion was not quite as dramatic as some assumed. Unlike his opponents in the race for the Democratic presidential nomination, he refused to simply say that he supported a woman's right to choose. Instead, he insisted on making sure that his audience knew he believed abortion was the wrong choice, even if he now thought women had the right to make it. When asked about his position on abortion at a Democratic presidential primary debate, he said that women who chose abortion "must live [with] the consequences of that choice." "We must never encourage abortion," he added. "More emphasis on sex education," he thought, might reduce the number of abortions.[44] A few weeks later, at another debate among the Democratic presidential candidates, he reiterated his moral reservations about abortion. "I'm not for abortion," he insisted. "I'm for freedom of choice. Even theologically God gives us choice. We must live with the consequences of that choice, whether to go to heaven or hell, but at least we are not robots; we're people that have choice within the law. We have the choice. I would never encourage abortion; I'd not embrace it. I'd put more focus on sex education before the fact, and set discipline before the fact, that people might be responsible and disciplined and matured and make decisions the day before so they will not make decisions the day after. The fact is it is one's choice and it is also one's consequences that must be lived with; that is, it's, for me, it's a matter of fear and trembling, but it's the position I take."[45]

Over the course of the 1980s, this stance quickly became the norm in the progressive African American denominations that had passed antiabortion resolutions in the 1970s. In 1990, when the *Washington Post* asked the senior bishop of the AME Church for his denomination's stance on abortion, the bishop responded that on the question of abortion's morality, most AME Church members believed that "abortion is usually wrong except where a greater wrong would be involved, such as the cases of rape, incest and when the life of the mother is in jeopardy." But he said they also thought that as a policy matter, it should be "a decision of the woman and her family and not of the government."[46]

Among Black evangelicals, a consistent life ethic that included antiabortion laws remained more popular. Tony Evans, a Black Dallas megachurch pastor and author of several books that sold widely among conservative evangelicals of all races, called for legal protections for the unborn and policies to expand health care and protect human dignity.[47] A few embraced a more overt form of Christian conservatism and allied with conservative Republicans. Alveda King, a Christian evangelist who was the niece of Martin Luther King Jr., was a pro-life activist for decades and became a popular speaker on the pro-life circuit while endorsing Republican politicians. King, a postabortive woman who said that she was coerced into her first abortion and felt ongoing guilt about the second, was certainly not the only Black Christian conservative campaigning for abortion restrictions, but she was an outlier.[48] Even Black pro-life activists often placed far more emphasis on ministries to prevent abortion than on passing antiabortion legislation. When the Church of God in Christ, a theologically conservative Black Pentecostal denomination, passed multiple antiabortion resolutions in the early twenty-first century, it didn't say anything about changing the law, but instead focused on creating ministries to offer positive alternatives to abortion. However, it did compare *Roe v. Wade* to *Dred Scott v. Sandford* and *Plessy v. Ferguson*.[49] Black opponents of abortion in the twenty-first century continued to make many of the arguments that their predecessors had made in the 1970s: abortion was bad for the Black community, it was a form of genocide, and, above all, it killed a person created in God's image.

But white liberal Protestants were not taking their cues for abortion policy from Black pro-life advocates, such as Alveda King, Tony Evans, or even the Church of God in Christ. Instead, they were in dialogue with liberal Black Protestant ministers who wanted to keep abortion legal even if they opposed abortion personally. In the 1990s, the denominational positions of Black Protestant churches and predominantly white mainline Protestant churches began to converge, as both groups settled on a position that raised substantial moral questions about abortion even as they agreed on the need to keep it legal. In 1992, the Christian Methodist Episcopal Church adopted a resolution on abortion that, in contrast to Black Protestant denominational resolutions of the 1970s, was almost indistinguishable from abortion resolutions that predominantly white liberal Protestant churches had recently adopted. Like the resolutions recently passed in the general assemblies of the United Methodist Church, Presbyterian Church (USA), and other mainline Protestant denominations, the Christian Methodist Episcopal resolution of 1992 was generally pro-choice, but also expressed ambivalence about the morality of abortion. It suggested that abortion should not be used for "birth control, gender selection, nor for economic purposes." At the same time, it affirmed the pregnant woman's right and responsibility to make the abortion decision herself, with the assurance that she would not be "abandoned by her church."[50]

This emphasis on not "abandoning" women who chose to terminate a pregnancy would find a new emphasis in mainline Protestant denominational statements on abortion in the early twenty-first century. Perhaps not coincidentally, both Black and white women in the church would play a central role in shifting the conversation about abortion from the status of the fetus to a concern for racial and gender equity.

A NEW FRAMEWORK OF REPRODUCTIVE JUSTICE

In 1989, UCC minister Yvonne Delk addressed a theological conference on abortion from her perspective as a pro-choice African American woman whose sisters and ancestors had long been denied the freedom of choice. Not only had they not been able to make reproductive decisions for themselves, but they had also not been able to make the same economic choices or health care choices as whites had. In fact, until only a generation earlier in some places, they had not even been able to choose where to sit on a bus. This was a violation of the principles of Jesus, Delk argued, because choice was central to human dignity. "Choice is the essence of freedom," Delk declared. "It's what African Americans have struggled for. . . . Without choice, women will be objects rather than co-creators with God in the building of a just and humane world."[51]

In the early 1990s, African American women who argued for both racial justice and abortion rights, as Delk had, began calling their campaign a quest for "reproductive justice." Like Delk, they were just as strongly pro-choice as white abortion rights advocates were, but like her, they also recognized that African American women had long been denied the resources and freedom to make this choice, which meant that their campaign could not merely focus on keeping abortion legal but also had to include health care advocacy, economic empowerment, and a fight against racism. But abortion rights were a central part of this package, because without access to abortion, lower-income Black women would remain trapped in poverty. The pro-choice campaign was not merely a campaign for religious freedom, as the Religious Coalition for Abortion Rights (RCAR) had long argued, or even for women's equality but for racial and economic justice. When that shift in thinking occurred, it helped to galvanize liberal Protestant support for abortion rights to a greater degree than ever before.

The effort to ground the pro-choice campaign in a larger quest for racial and economic justice was not entirely new, of course. Even in the late 1960s and early 1970s, liberal Protestant advocates of abortion rights had argued that restrictive abortion laws hurt poor women far more than wealthier women, which meant that abortion restrictions exacerbated the divide between rich and poor. In the late 1970s and early 1980s, the UCC and RCAR opposed the Hyde Amendment on the grounds that it deprived poor women of the freedom of choice that middle-class women enjoyed. Racial and economic justice also featured prominently in the first major book-length defense of abortion rights written by a prominent academic Christian theologian, Union Theological Seminary professor Beverly Wildung Harrison's *Our Right to Choose: Toward a New Ethic of Abortion*, published in 1983. Harrison, a feminist theologian affiliated with the Presbyterian Church (USA), argued that abortion rights were first and foremost women's rights, but she also argued that they intersected with issues of equity for racial minorities and the poor.[52]

But for the most part, liberal Protestants—including those who were pro-choice—did not view abortion access as a social justice issue in the same category with poverty relief or civil rights for African Americans. In 1984, Illinois state RCAR coordinator Barbara Moore reported that for many progressive religious leaders in her state, "the hunger issue is very important, that there is a lot of concern about Central America and nuclear disarmament. But abortion rights—a lot of people's feelings are that it's taken care of. It's really difficult to find people who are activist types, who are not already committed to other issues."[53] The Hyde Amendment had already been in effect for eight years at that point, but many pro-choice liberal Protestant ministers did not think that it was worth the effort to fight it. Moore noted that many of them also knew a substantial number of their own congregants opposed abortion, which meant they knew the issue would be divisive. As long as abortion remained legal, it was safer to focus on other social justice matters and say very little about abortion.

For much of the 1990s and early twenty-first century, a politically left-leaning coalition of mainline Protestants, progressive evangelicals, and Catholic Democrats consistently voted for pro-choice liberal candidates while at the same time expressing some moral reservations about abortion and advocating economic and health care policies that they claimed would reduce the abortion rate. This was the stance that *Sojourners* magazine adopted, and it closely echoed the denominational pronouncements on abortion that several mainline Protestant denominations had issued in the late 1980s and 90s. And it closely echoed the position that Mario Cuomo had adopted on abortion in 1984, which became near-universal among all but a handful of Catholic Democratic politicians by the beginning of the twenty-first century.

Even the Democratic Party, while remaining firmly pro-choice, also expressed some degree of moral ambiguity about abortion and promised measures to reduce the abortion rate. "Our goal is to make abortion less necessary and more rare, not more difficult and more dangerous," the Democratic Party platform of 2000 proclaimed, in a close echo of President Bill Clinton's promise eight years earlier to make abortion "safe, legal, and rare." "The abortion rate is dropping. Now we must continue to support efforts to reduce unintended pregnancies, and we call on all Americans to take personal responsibility to meet this important goal." In a recognition of the morally contested nature of abortion, the Democratic Party platform also added, "We respect the individual conscience of each American on this difficult issue, and we welcome all our members to participate at every level of our party."[54] In most respects, this platform could have been the position statement of any of a number of mainline Protestant denominations that had combined an expression of moral reservations on abortion with a commitment to keeping abortion legal, while also recognizing the diversity of positions among their own members on the issue.

As long as a substantial percentage of mainline Protestants saw abortion as a morally problematic choice, it was going to be difficult for mainline Protestant denominations to frame abortion rights as a positive good that people could rally around. Some pro-choice mainline Protestants admitted as much, but for decades they didn't seem to mind. "Mainline Protestants' nuanced position on abortion may not bring people to the barricades, but it points to a coherent, responsible policy," the *Christian Century* editorialized in December 2012. "It is possible to move toward a society in which abortion is safe, legal and rare."[55] But shortly after the *Christian Century* made this statement, several things happened in a short period of time to shift mainline Protestants and progressive evangelicals' view of abortion from a morally dubious action to a fundamental social justice issue.

One of those was a series of denominational splits over sexuality and same-sex marriage. In the late 1980s and 1990s, the mainline Protestant advocates of stronger antiabortion resolutions were almost invariably conservatives on issues of sex, and their campaign periodicals, and also the denominational resolutions they sponsored, frequently coupled denunciations of abortion with affirmations of the traditional Christian doctrine that sex outside of marriage was forbidden. Their reasons for opposing abortion went far beyond concerns about premarital or extramarital sex, but it was hard to deny the close connection between abortion and out-of-wedlock pregnancy at a time when more than 80 percent of women seeking abortions were unmarried. But their insistence on a conservative Christian sexual ethic went beyond the merely pragmatic goal of reducing the abortion rate. Instead, by the late 1980s and early 1990s, opposition to abortion had become inseparably linked in Protestant denominations with a strong insistence on biblical authority and theological conservatism across a whole range of issues, which is why pro-life advocates among mainline Protestants were often engaged in a much more sweeping effort to reclaim their denominations for biblical conservatism. In this campaign to steer their denominations in a more theologically conservative direction, they often felt like a beleaguered minority, because they never had enough votes on their side at denominational meetings to do more than add modest caveats to their denominations' generally pro-choice resolutions. Nevertheless, for a while they were willing to stay in their denominations and continue their fight as long as they thought they could find a sufficient quorum of likeminded conservatives. That changed when their denominations began ordaining gay clergy and endorsing same-sex marriage.

In 2003, the Episcopal Church ordained its first openly gay bishop. In 2009, the Episcopal Church's General Assembly passed resolutions affirming the full inclusion of same-sex couples in the life of the church and began advocating for transgender rights by endorsing laws that banned discrimination based on gender identity. The conservative side of the debate on issues of sexuality had clearly lost, and some responded by leaving the denomination. In 2009, conservatives within the Episcopal Church formed the breakaway Anglican Church in North America, an action that led to several years of legal battles over church property. By 2024, the Anglican Church in North America had 125,000 members.[56]

Presbyterians, Methodists, and Lutherans also experienced similar splits over sexuality in the second decade of the twenty-first century. In 2010, the Presbyterian Church (USA) voted to repeal its "fidelity and chastity" clause that had served as an implicit prohibition of same-sex sexual relationships for clergy. When a majority of the presbyteries ratified this repeal in 2011, the Presbyterian Church (USA) began ordaining openly gay clergy who were in same-sex relationships. The following year, dozens of congregations who objected to this change left the Presbyterian Church (USA) and formed a new denomination, ECO: A Covenant Order of Evangelical Presbyterians.[57] Something very similar happened in the Evangelical Lutheran Church in America (ELCA) shortly after it adopted the report "A Social Report on Human Sexuality: Gift and Trust" in 2009. The report, while acknowledging a conservative counterperspective among some members of the ELCA and affirming the high and unique value of lifelong, monogamous marriage, suggested the possibility of treating committed same-sex relationships, along with other monogamous relationships outside marriage, as potentially legitimate sexual relationships. The next year, in 2010, conservatives left the ELCA to form the North American Lutheran Church, which by the early 2020s had more than 140,000 members.[58] In the United Methodist Church, conservatives and liberals agreed in 2019 to a plan of separation after years of debating LGBTQ+ issues. More than 7,000 congregations left the United Methodist Church between 2019 and 2023, with about half of them joining the newly formed conservative Global Methodist Church and many of the others joining smaller conservative Wesleyan denominations or becoming independent churches.[59]

In each of the denominations that experienced a split over sexuality, the more liberal group remained larger than the conservative splinter group, yet nevertheless experienced steep membership declines. Between 2013 and 2022, the Episcopal Church's membership declined by 21 percent. The Presbyterian Church (USA) lost nearly 30 percent of its members between 2016 and 2022. The United Methodist Church lost nearly 25 percent of its congregations between 2019 and 2023.[60]

The result was a much smaller—and arguably less politically or socially influential—liberal Protestantism. By 2024, the 5.5 million-member United Methodist Church was only half as large as it had been at the beginning of the 1970s, when its total membership of 11 million had been only slightly smaller than the 13 million Southern Baptist Convention, the nation's largest Protestant denomination at the time.[61] Indeed, by 2024, the total *combined* membership of the United Methodist Church, the Episcopal Church, the Presbyterian Church (USA), and the Evangelical Lutheran Church in America did not even equal the number of members of the SBC, which, incidentally, was experiencing its own struggle to retain members. Or, to put it another way, the total combined membership of all of the old mainline Protestant denominations that advocated for abortion rights and gay rights—that is, the Episcopal Church, the United Church of Christ, the United Methodist Church , the Presbyterian Church (USA), the Evangelical Lutheran Church in America, and the Disciples of Christ—was less than 5 percent of the U.S. population, whereas evangelicals made up about 20 percent of the population and Catholics another 20 percent.

But if the loss of the conservatives left the liberal Protestant denominations smaller, it also left them more homogenously liberal and more unified around both LGBTQ+ rights and abortion rights. By supporting gay rights, liberal Protestants made it clear that they valued equality of marginalized groups more than traditional Christian theological views of sex. They endorsed a progressive interpretation of scripture that was at odds with the biblical hermeneutic that conservatives in their tradition endorsed. They were thus open to the type of abortion rights argument that Presbyterian Church (USA) minister and religious studies professor Rebecca Todd Peters presented in *Trust Women: A Progressive Argument for Reproductive Justice* (2018), which argued that the Christian antiabortion position reflected a "deeply embedded" misogynist tradition in Christian history and theology. It was time, Peters argued, for Christians to abandon the idea that there was something sinful or shameful about abortion, an idea that had informed not only the Christian pro-life movement but even the pro-choice resolutions of liberal Protestant denominations ever since the 1960s. Even among liberal Protestants, pro-choice resolutions had expressed moral reservations about abortion and had discouraged the "casual" use of abortion as a form of birth control. But it was now time to "trust women," Peters said—not merely give women permission to make their own moral choices, but genuinely trust them to make the right moral choices. It was also time to empower them to make those choices by ensuring that they had access to a full range of reproductive services, because abortion care was both health care and part of a larger health care package.[62]

Peters took the same position toward fetal life that most mainline Protestants who supported abortion rights had held since the 1960s—the fetus had value as a potential human being but was not yet an actual human being. For decades, liberal Protestants who held that position had passed denominational resolutions that advocated making abortion legally available while at the same time cautioning against adopting too casual an attitude toward it. But Peters, a feminist Christian ethicist, said that women did not need those resolutions and the patriarchal attitudes behind them; they instinctively knew the value of the unborn human life they were carrying, and Christians should trust them to make the right decisions on behalf of that life. "The bulk of social-scientific research demonstrates that the vast majority of women who have abortions make the decision in light of their capacity to be a good mother to a *potential* child. . . . They recognize the significant moral and material obligations of having a child. At the same time, because the prenate is not yet a child and does not hold equivalent moral status to a person, and because the decision to have a baby and to become a mother is a personal and private decision, the question of whether to continue a pregnancy can and should only be made by pregnant women with the support of their families and communities."[63]

Peters rejected the conservative Christian argument that sex should be reserved exclusively for marriage, that the Bible presented a consistent sexual ethic, or that biblical teaching about sex was necessarily an authoritative guide for the present rather than a reflection of ancient cultural ideas that needed to be modified in light of feminist principles. General ethical guidelines grounded in principles of love and respect rather than precise stipulations guided her approach. And in the end, the ultimate moral authority was not church teaching or a set of Bible verses but rather personal intuition, guided by prayer and community support. These ideas were not entirely new. Liberal Protestants of the 1960s had made many of the same arguments. And in 1983, the Presbyterian Church (USA) minister and seminary professor Beverly Wildung Harrison had presented a feminist argument for abortion rights that closely presaged Peters's position. But in the 1980s, when Harrison wrote, neither feminists nor other theological liberals had full control over the Presbyterian Church (USA) or most other mainline Protestant denominations. As a result, denominational resolutions on issues of sexuality and reproduction were almost invariably a product of compromise between different factions in the denomination. From 1996 until 2010, the Presbyterian Church (USA) continued to require its clergy to reserve sex for (heterosexual) marriage, despite the presence of more theologically liberal, feminist clergy such as Peters who did not support that stance. By 2018, the situation was different. Liberal Protestant denominations, though now substantially smaller than they had been a generation earlier, were more thoroughly feminist, less attached to traditional Christian theologies of sexuality and reproduction, and far more open to a feminist abortion rights argument.

They were also eager to exchange their traditional middle-class-centered pro-choice rhetoric for a reproductive justice framework that originated from African American supporters of abortion rights and that centered on justice for poor women. In the late twentieth century, pro-choice liberal Protestants had usually spoken of abortion rights as a matter of conscience, but in the second decade of the twenty-first century they began following the lead of African American reproductive justice advocates in speaking of abortion access as health care. Supporting women's reproductive choice was necessary not only to protect their dignity as moral decision-makers who had a right and responsibility to follow the dictates of their own conscience but also because reproductive health care was an essential part of a comprehensive health care package that was necessary to allow all people to flourish as human beings. Since people who were living in poverty—and especially Black women living in poverty in socially conservative states—were likely to lack comprehensive reproductive health care, the campaign for equal access to this type of health care was a matter of racial and socioeconomic justice. When abortion rights were reframed as a health care equity issue, the cause seemed far more Christian than it had before. After all, Jesus came to heal the sick and bring justice and relief for the poor, he declared in Luke 4. For those who followed a Savior who went out of his way to reach out to socially marginalized women and care for the poor and the ailing, it made sense that the cause of reproductive justice and abortion care was the work of Jesus. And as liberal churches gave greater prominence to issues of racial justice in the wake of the Black Lives Matter movement of the 2010s and 2020s, it made sense that if reproductive justice was framed as a way to fight structural racism, it would attract a great deal more liberal Christian support.

If new paradigms on race pushed liberal Protestants to the left on the abortion question, so did a change in the place of women in liberal Protestant denominational leadership. In the late 1970s, most mainline Protestant denominations were willing to ordain women, but nevertheless, because women were less than 3 percent of the clergy in mainline Protestant denominations, abortion resolutions in these denominations were written mainly by men. And in the late 1980s and early 1990s, when mainline Protestant denominations were moderating their pro-choice resolutions and moving closer to the political center on the abortion question, women still made up less than 15 percent of mainline Protestant clergy. But by 2017, 32 percent of all mainline Protestant clergy were women, which meant that women were now a large enough force in the leadership of these denominations to exercise a substantial influence on how abortion resolutions were framed.[64] Mainline Protestant male church leaders and female church leaders did not usually disagree on abortion per se; both were generally supportive of abortion rights. But some mainline Protestant female clergy who were pro-choice were more likely than their male colleagues to object to language in the denominational resolutions that might imply that abortion was a morally problematic or shameful choice for women. Like Rebecca Todd Peters, they wanted to affirm women's power of moral decision-making without any suggestion that the moral choices they made could be sinful or morally questionable.

In the 2010s and early 2020s, liberal Protestant denominations therefore passed the most strongly pro-choice abortion rights resolutions they had ever adopted. In 2012, the General Assembly of the Presbyterian Church (USA) approved the resolution "On Providing Just Access to Reproductive Health Care," which called "full access to health care" a "basic human right," and said that this included "full access to reproductive health care for both women and men in both private and public health plans."[65] The Episcopal Church did the same in 2018. "Women's reproductive health and reproductive health procedures" should "be treated as all other medical procedures," said the Episcopal Church. "Equitable access to women's health care, including women's reproductive health care, is an integral part of a woman's struggle to assert her dignity and worth as a human being."[66]

Despite these denominational resolutions, it's not clear that the percentage of mainline Protestants who were pro-choice changed much during this period. A PRRI poll showed that the percentage of white mainline Protestants who said that abortion should be legal in all or most cases increased by only 3 percentage points between 2010 and 2023—that is, from 65 percent in 2010 to 68 percent in 2023.[67] White mainline Protestants had been generally supportive of abortion rights for a long time, and they didn't necessarily become substantially more so in the 2010s and early 2020s, regardless of what their denominational resolutions indicated. And, ironically, those who were most likely to oppose abortion rights were the ones who attended church most frequently and who practiced other acts of religious devotion most regularly, even though their pastors were highly likely to support abortion rights. The new pro-choice denominational resolutions didn't change that. What did change, however, was liberal Protestant denominations' commitment to the cause. Before the 2010s, liberal Protestant denominational general assemblies had often tried to balance their pro-choice commitments with cautious admonitions against the casual use of abortion or with acknowledgments of the diversity of views on the issue within the denomination, but after the 2010s, they were much more direct about endorsing abortion access as a fundamental human right.

The new mainline Protestant focus on abortion as health care coincided with a substantial increase in the percentage of Black Protestants who supported abortion legalization. For decades, Black Protestants had had strong moral reservations about abortion. From 2010 to 2019, only a slight majority (about 56 percent) of Black Protestants said that abortion should be legal in all or most cases. But in 2019, as a wave of Republican states passed restrictive abortion laws, and as advocates of abortion rights pivoted toward a reproductive justice framework, Black Protestant support for the removal of legal restrictions on abortion started to increase dramatically, and this trend continued after *Dobbs*. By 2023, 72 percent of Black Protestants supported making abortion legal in all or most cases. For the first time in U.S. history, Black Protestants—who in the 1970s were even more strongly opposed to legal abortion than white Catholics or white evangelicals—were the Christian group most strongly supportive of legal abortion.[68] And when they spoke about abortion, they did so using the language of reproductive justice and abortion as vitally needed health care. White mainline Protestant clergy followed their lead.

At the same time, most of the newly formed conservative breakaway mainline Protestant denominations adopted conservative positions not only on sexuality but also on abortion. The North American Lutheran Church quickly became a strong supporter of the pro-life cause, issuing theological statements such as "'The Lord Is with You': A Word of Counsel to the Church: The Sanctity of Nascent Life" (2012).[69] The Anglican Church in North America adopted a similar stance. Its founding articles included the statement, "God, and not man, is the creator of human life. The unjustified taking of life is sinful. Therefore, all members and clergy are called to promote and respect the sanctity of every human life from conception to natural death." In a sign of how strongly committed to the pro-life cause the Anglican Church in North America was, more than a third of the denomination's bishops—including the denomination's titular head, Archbishop Robert Duncan—participated in the 2013 March for Life in Washington, DC.[70] The Global Methodist Church likewise adopted a conservative statement on abortion: "The sacredness of all life compels us to resist the practice of abortion except in the cases of tragic conflicts of life against life when the wellbeing of the mother and the child are at stake."[71] And although ECO did not adopt a formal position on abortion, the Evangelical Presbyterian Church, which broke away from the Presbyterian Church (USA) before ECO did, doubled down on its pro-life stance, releasing a position paper on abortion in February

2019 that declared that "the Evangelical Presbyterian Church continues to strongly and unequivocally affirm the dignity and value of every human life — born and unborn." "The Bible does not distinguish between prenatal and postnatal life," the Evangelical Presbyterian Church said. "It attributes human personhood to the unborn child. This extends to the unborn child ex utero as no less a human being than the child in the mother's womb. . . . The Evangelical Presbyterian Church grieves over the murder of more than 61 million unborn children who were made in the image of God. We also stand in strong opposition to the legal and political decisions that have led to this tragedy."[72]

PROGRESSIVE EVANGELICALS JOIN THE REPRODUCTIVE JUSTICE COALITION

As the new breakaway denominations that split from mainline Protestant church bodies mobilized against abortion, another group of longtime abortion opponents converted to the pro-choice side: progressive evangelicals. For decades, progressive evangelicals such as those associated with Jim Wallis's *Sojourners* magazine and Ron Sider's Evangelicals for Social Action had promoted the consistent life ethic that they had acquired from left-leaning Catholics. Though they had long voted for pro-choice Democrats, they did so on pro-life grounds. Because they believed that fighting poverty was the best way to reduce abortion rates, they argued that Democrats' progressive positions on economics and health care made it more likely that abortion rates would decline when a Democrat was in the White House. "On abortion, I will choose candidates who have the best chance to pursue the practical and proven policies which could dramatically reduce the number of abortions in America and therefore save precious unborn lives, rather than those who simply repeat the polarized legal debates and 'pro-choice' and 'pro-life' mantras from either side," Wallis wrote in 2008.[73]

Unlike mainline Protestants, such as Richard Hays, or pro-choice Catholics, such as Mario Cuomo, who claimed that their personal opposition to abortion should not be translated into secular law in a pluralistic society, evangelicals on the left commonly said that their ideal candidate would be a progressive Democrat who shared their consistent life ethic and believed in protecting the unborn in public law. They criticized President Clinton for vetoing the Partial-Birth Abortion Ban Act. "One cannot escape the clarity that it is indeed a human life destroyed in this procedure. From the perspective of a consistent life ethic, Clinton's veto cannot be condoned," *Sojourners* staff writer Julie Polter wrote in 1996.[74] When the Democratic Party strengthened its pro-choice platform in 2004, Jim Wallis sometimes chided the Democrats for their strategic foolishness in not extending more of an olive branch to politically progressive pro-life Christians who wanted to vote for them but found it difficult to do so in good conscience because of the party's staunch support for legal abortion. And when Ron Sider endorsed Hillary Clinton for president in 2016, he wrote, "She and the Democratic platform are wrong on abortion—period," even though he still considered her a much better choice than Donald Trump.[75]

But sometime during Trump's term in office, *Sojourners* and its progressive Christian coalition began shifting away from their traditional pro-life views. The magazine began insisting that abortion must remain legal, even if abortion was still a morally problematic choice and even if the reduction of abortion rates was still a worthy goal. "Reproductive health care," one *Sojourners* article proclaimed in 2020, was a "human right," and access to the full range of reproductive health care services (including abortion) needed to be expanded.[76] At the same time, the magazine also began publishing articles by people who said they were abandoning the word "evangelical," which had become too closely associated with the political right and with Trump supporters. With the abandonment of a moral opposition to abortion—and an embrace of the mainline Protestant position that abortion was health care and a human right—progressive Christians who had once viewed themselves as part of the evangelical coalition severed the last vestigial tie they had to contemporary evangelicalism. And though there were still some Catholics who held to a moderately politically liberal consistent life ethic and might try to combine pro-life advocacy with Democratic voting, even these were becoming few in number. By the end of the 2010s, Christians who were political progressives were more likely than ever to be supporters of reproductive justice, while those who leaned conservative were more likely than ever to be pro-life.

This may have had something to do with party identification. As Democrats became increasingly monolithically pro-choice in 2016 and afterward, it became more difficult than ever for Christians who had long voted Democratic and who strongly opposed Trump to support a cause that was now publicly identified almost exclusively with Trump's party. It was probably no coincidence that both progressive evangelicals and African American Christians—two groups of religious Democrats that had long included sizable numbers of abortion opponents—began moving sharply away from their earlier pro-life convictions during the Trump presidency. But in addition, the increasing acceptance of same-sex marriage among both progressive evangelicals and African American Protestants—two groups that had also been much slower than liberal white Protestants to support this cause—made it more likely that they would shift on abortion too. Most likely, a confluence of mutually reinforcing factors rather than one single cause accounted for the rapid shift of both progressive evangelicals and African American Protestants into the reproductive justice advocacy camp. In addition to Trump's election and the identification of the pro-life cause with a candidate whom progressive Christians viewed as racist and misogynistic, the shift of the pro-choice campaign toward a reproductive justice framework made it much easier for erstwhile consistent life ethic advocates who cared about racial equality and poverty relief to embrace the cause. By the early 2020s, it was difficult to find much commitment to the pro-life cause among progressive evangelicals, mainline Protestants, Black Protestants, or even politically liberal Catholics. Yet white conservative evangelicals, Hispanic evangelicals, conservative Catholics, and a large number of African Americans who attended multiracial evangelical churches identified more strongly than ever with the pro-life cause.

Conservative Christians' increasing commitment to the pro-life campaign was not merely a product of their increasing affinity for the Republican Party. In fact, from the 1990s through the Trump presidency and beyond, Republican Party leaders tried hard to moderate their party's stance on the issue. As his party's presidential nominee in 1996, Bob Dole tried unsuccessfully to add a statement to the Republican Party platform acknowledging the diversity of views within the party on the issue, but activists from the Christian Right and the pro-life movement prevented him from doing this. In 2000, George W. Bush downplayed his opposition to abortion on the campaign trail, saying that "good people can disagree" about the issue.[77] In 2008, Republican presidential nominee John McCain wanted to pick pro-choice senator Joe Lieberman (I-CT) as his running mate, but his advisors convinced him that this would alienate pro-life and Christian Right voters. In 2012, the Republican Party nominated a presidential candidate, Mitt Romney, who had formerly won elected office on a pro-choice platform, and in 2016 the party nominated the formerly pro-choice Trump as its standard-bearer. Although Trump ended up appointing three Supreme Court justices whose votes were critical for overturning *Roe v. Wade*, he gave so few signals on the campaign trail that he was committed to the pro-life cause that several prominent Christian Right leaders publicly questioned whether he would do anything to restrict abortion. Some pro-choice activists accused Catholic leaders or other pro-life Christians of emphasizing the abortion issue because they wanted to elect Republicans, but actually, the reverse was probably true: Pro-life activists and conservative Christians were the ones pushing the Republican Party to do something about abortion because they cared about the issue, while many Republican Party leaders would have preferred to downplay abortion and frame their campaigns around something less politically polarizing.

If conservative Christians' increasing commitment to the fight against abortion in the early twenty-first century was not a product of their partisan loyalty, what was its cause? The answer is probably an increasing sense that many conservative Christians had that they were losing the fight against a secular and sexually permissive culture.[78] This sense of fear was a central reason why conservative evangelicals had enlisted in the pro-life campaign in the late 1970s, and it remained a key motivating factor in the movement throughout the late twentieth century, with the most radical pro-life activists—such as those in Operation Rescue who were willing to go to jail for their acts of civil disobedience—most likely to express a fear of secularization and a vehement opposition to cultural liberalism. The increasing cultural acceptance of same-sex marriage in the early twenty-first century, combined with the Obama administration's mandate that its health care plan include coverage for contraceptives that many pro-life activists considered abortifacients, increased their fear that the culture was secularizing and that the federal government was against them. Many of them believed that liberals in the federal government would be all too willing to deprive them of their religious liberty to dissent if they tried to stand in the way of LGBTQ+ rights mandates or refused to comply with health care directives that included abortion. The pro-life cause became an anchor for them in the midst of their opposition to a secular, liberal culture. They doubled down on their attempts to pass abortion restrictions. To their delight, they found that many conservative state legislatures were receptive to their cause. Between 2011 and 2013, pro-life activists succeeded in enacting seventy new restrictions on abortion in twenty-two states; they passed more restrictions in this two-year period than they had in the entire previous decade.[79] The political momentum gave them hope that they could finally win the battle against abortion—maybe even by rescinding *Roe v. Wade*.

But the reversal of *Roe v. Wade* did not lead to the reduction in abortion rates that they had hoped. Nor did it lead the country any closer to a national pro-life consensus, as they had anticipated. Instead, the Supreme Court's decision in 2022 polarized the country, just as *Roe* itself had nearly a half century earlier. This time, though, the battle lines were not drawn in precisely the same places they were in the early 1970s. The division among Christians was now between progressives who endorsed both sexual equality and the Democratic Party and conservatives who believed in a transcendent, unchanging moral standard and a fixed code of sexual ethics. Conservative Catholics and conservative evangelicals were firmly on one side of that division, while most liberal Protestants, Black Protestants, progressive evangelicals, and theologically liberal Catholics were on the other. And this time, the debate was no longer primarily over religious liberty, as it had been for pro-choice Christians in an earlier generation. Instead, it was a contest over the future identity of both the United States and the meaning of Christianity.

CHAPTER 7

THE CONSERVATIVE CHRISTIAN COALITION THAT OVERTURNED *ROE*

In 1994, some of the most prominent evangelicals and Catholics in the United States issued the most ecumenical document that the two religious groups had ever agreed upon: "Evangelicals and Catholics Together." For most of the previous two hundred years, evangelicals and Catholics had been bitter enemies. In 1960, prominent Southern Baptist and evangelical pastors had waged a campaign to save the country from the prospect of a Catholic president. Even in the late 1960s, when the Catholic Church began engaging in dialogue with Protestant denominations, the hostility from evangelicals was still such a recent memory that Catholic bishops conducted nearly all of their ecumenical conversations with mainline Protestant denominational leaders rather than with evangelicals. But that changed dramatically in 1994, when leading evangelical culture warriors such as Charles Colson and Pat Robertson, along with a large number of evangelical seminary presidents, academics, and denominational leaders—including the Southern Baptist Convention's Christian Life Commission president, Richard Land—signed a document affirming

Catholics as fellow Christians who shared the essential tenets of the faith and who were part of the one church that Jesus founded. Equally prominent Catholics also signed. Cardinal John O'Connor, Catholic apologist Peter Kreeft, Harvard law professor Mary Ann Glendon, and conservative commentator George Weigel were only a few of the prominent Catholic clergy and lay cultural leaders who endorsed the document affirming that evangelicals and Catholics could work together as fellow Christians. Perhaps it was fitting that the signatories published the statement in a magazine that was edited by a Catholic priest who had once been a Protestant minister himself. *First Things*, the magazine that the Lutheran-turned-Catholic Fr. Richard John Neuhaus edited, was rapidly becoming the leading voice for a Catholic-centered, ecumenically minded, cultural conservatism centered on defense of the right to life for the unborn and for all humans from conception to natural death. Indeed, if there was one cause that brought these particular Catholics and evangelicals together, it was the campaign against abortion.

The signatories of "Evangelicals and Catholics Together" recognized this themselves. "The pattern of convergence and cooperation between Evangelicals and Catholics is, in large part, a result of common effort to protect human life," the statement said. The signatories therefore pledged to "multiply every effort" to "secure the legal protection of the unborn," because abortion was "the leading edge of an encroaching culture of death."[1]

For the next three decades and beyond, evangelicals and conservative Catholics formed a united front in the pro-life cause, with both groups viewing the political fight against abortion as the foundation for a broader resistance against a secular culture that they believed was vehemently opposed to life and religious liberty. The common ground that they forged in "Evangelicals and Catholics Together" enabled the formation of a political coalition that would ultimately succeed in overturning *Roe v. Wade*. But by the time of that legal victory, the evangelical and Catholic pro-life campaign had become so closely identified with a conservative Christian nationalist platform that it had almost no appeal to those outside of that conservative coalition. As a result, *Dobbs v. Jackson Women's Health Organization* (2022), the Supreme Court triumph that evangelicals and Catholics had long sought, appeared likely to become only a pyrrhic victory, or, at best, a step toward further polarization on abortion rather than a resolution of the conflict.

CATHOLIC PRO-LIFE THEOLOGY

For Catholics who attended Mass regularly and sought to follow church teaching, the trends that had begun in the 1970s and 1980s toward making abortion a high political priority increased in the 1990s and 2000s. In 1989, the National Conference of Catholics Bishops (NCCB) declared that "at this particular time, abortion has become the fundamental human rights issue for all men and women of good will," a statement that clarified that abortion had indeed become the foremost political concern for the bishops, not merely one concern among several. The bishops also made clear that this had implications for ballot choices. "No Catholic can responsibly take a 'pro-choice' stand when the 'choice' in question involves the taking of innocent human life," the bishops said.[2]

The bishops' boldness in categorically saying that a pro-choice political stance was incompatible with Catholicism was not entirely new; even politically progressive bishops in the 1970s had said similar things. But many of the progressive bishops in the 1970s and early 1980s had attempted to ground the pro-life stance in a larger "seamless garment" consistent life ethic, whereas bishops in the late 1980s and afterward were more likely to treat the "sanctity of life" as the single highest political priority. They wanted to make abortion the central focus of all "sanctity of life" teaching on the grounds that legal abortion was the single greatest threat to human life in the contemporary United States.

This was partly a reflection of Pope John Paul II's priorities. Although John Paul II believed in all of the issues that formed part of the seamless garment, he treated abortion as a singularly important issue that superseded all others, and he wrote far more on abortion than any previous pope had. Not only did he give regular homilies on the issue, but he also produced the encyclical *Evangelium Vitae* (1995), which claimed to "reaffirm with the authority of the Successor of Peter the value of human life and its inviolability." Over the course of dozens of pages, the encyclical laid out the case for the preservation of unborn life from the Bible, church history, genetic science, and political philosophy. Although several other twentieth-century popes had written on abortion, none did so at such great length. John Paul II wrote more on abortion than any of his predecessors did partly because he saw abortion as a uniquely important challenge in the late twentieth century and partly because he wanted to lay to rest any doubts that some liberal Catholics had about whether the church's teaching on abortion was infallible. The pope suggested it was. Although he did not invoke the claim to speak *ex cathedra* in defining the doctrine, he came as close as he otherwise could to defining the church's prohibition on abortion as an infallible doctrine when he said that the teaching was "unchanged and unchangeable." The church had always taught this, he said, but to make the matter even clearer, he invoked his papal authority in saying it again:

> By the authority which Christ conferred upon Peter and his Successors, in communion with the Bishops—who on various occasions have condemned abortion and who in the aforementioned consultation, albeit dispersed throughout the world, have shown unanimous agreement concerning this doctrine—I declare that direct abortion, that is, abortion willed as an end or as a means, always constitutes a grave moral disorder, since it is the deliberate killing of an innocent human being. This doctrine is based upon the natural law and upon the written Word of God, is transmitted by the Church's Tradition and taught by the ordinary and universal Magisterium. No circumstance, no purpose, no law whatsoever can ever make licit an act which is intrinsically illicit, since it is contrary to the Law of God which is written in every human heart, knowable by reason itself, and proclaimed by the Church.[3]

The *Catechism of the Catholic Church*, published two years after the pope's pronouncement, emphasized the absolute permanence of this injunction against abortion. The church had "affirmed the moral evil of every procured abortion" since the first century, stated the 1997 edition of the *Catechism*. "This teaching has not changed and remains unchangeable," which was a line copied almost verbatim from *Evangelium Vitae*.[4]

But abortion, John Paul II said in his encyclical, was not merely an individual sin but rather a structural evil of a secular society that had rejected God and, as a result, had forgotten the value of human life. The remedy for this structural evil therefore could not be merely individual; it had to involve political and societal remedies too. The pope wrote:

> Responsibility [for abortion] likewise falls on the legislators who have promoted and approved abortion laws, and, to the extent that they have a say in the matter, on the administrators of the health-care centers where abortions are performed. A general and no less serious responsibility lies with those who have encouraged the spread of an attitude of sexual permissiveness and a lack of esteem for motherhood, and with those who should have ensured—but did not—effective family and social policies in support of families, especially larger families and those with particular financial and educational needs. Finally, one cannot overlook the network of complicity which reaches out to include international institutions, foundations and associations which systematically campaign for the legalization and spread of abortion in the world. In this sense abortion goes beyond the responsibility of individuals and beyond the harm done to them, and takes on a distinctly social dimension. It is a most serious wound inflicted on society and its culture by the very people who ought to be society's promoters and defenders. As I wrote in my Letter to Families, "we are facing an immense threat to life: not only to the life of individuals but also to that of civilization itself." We are facing what can be called a "structure of sin" which opposes human life not yet born.[5]

In framing the fight against abortion as a battle against secular liberalism in political and social structures, John Paul II positioned the church for a political fight for the preservation or recovery of Christian principles.

Most of the bishops he appointed in the United States shared that vision, which meant that their political views often differed from the bishops who had presided over the American church in the late 1960s and 1970s, and, to an even greater extent, from the majority of priests ordained in that period. In the years before John Paul II's papacy—and especially from 1964 to 1978 in the wake of Vatican II and the social changes in the church and society—a large percentage of the men who had joined the priesthood were progressives in both theology and politics.[6] Rather than seeing politics as a battleground between Christian truth and secularism, they believed that Christians needed to respect pluralism in a democratic society and focus on promoting principles of peace and equality that they believed reflected Jesus's concern for the marginalized. To some of them, the church's less popular teachings on sexuality—especially its categorical opposition to artificial contraception—were an embarrassment. But in appointing bishops, John Paul II passed over most of the progressives and made a concerted effort to appoint theological traditionalists who aligned with his views on theology, social ethics, and sexual conservatism. It was thus not surprising that by the mid-to-late 1980s, American bishops were already leaning to the right in their political framing of the abortion issue. Following Cardinal John O'Connor's lead, they were less likely to turn a blind eye when Catholic politicians took a pro-choice stance. By the early twenty-first century, an increasing number of them were willing to take the drastic step of denying Communion to pro-choice Catholic politicians or possibly even to private citizens who voted for pro-choice candidates.

CATHOLIC PRO-CHOICE POLITICIANS
AND COMMUNION CONTROVERSIES

Both excommunication and denial of Communion were extreme penalties in Catholicism that, nevertheless, the church had long said were appropriate for those who engaged directly in the sin of abortion. The 1917 canon law on abortion said that anyone who had an abortion or who was an accomplice in one incurred automatic excommunication. The revision of canon law issued in 1983 reiterated this sentence. But canon law did not say that those who voted for abortion legalization (but did not have abortions themselves) would be automatically excommunicated. Both bishops and popes had long said that Catholics had a duty to seek the protection of the unborn in civil law, but did that necessarily mean that those who did not follow this teaching would lose the privilege of Communion? For years, most bishops said no. When one Ohio pro-life activist asked Archbishop Joseph Bernardin in 1975 why he and other bishops did not deny Communion to pro-choice Catholic politicians, Bernardin explained that there were no "quick and easy solutions" to convincing Catholics to follow church doctrine on the issue, and that using the coercion of Communion denial would accomplish less than patient teaching. "The Church's position on abortion is certainly clear," he said. "The problem is not in making that position known; it is in convincing people of the validity of the position and motivating them to do something about it." When dealing with the political applications of the church's teaching, he preferred to use the power of teaching rather than the coercion of ecclesiastical penalties.[7]

But by the late 1980s, a few bishops were ready to deny Communion to Catholic politicians who supported abortion rights. In 1989, San Diego bishop Leo Maher declared that Democratic state assemblywoman Lucy Killea could no longer receive Communion after she ran several campaign ads emphasizing her support for abortion rights. Pro-life activists in California were delighted. "For far too long, those of us who do daily battle have watched the most militant oppressors vote for the slaughter and then put on the cloak of respectability when they label themselves as 'Catholic,'" said Jeannette Dreisbach, legislative director of the California Pro-Life Medical Association. She and others were grateful for Maher's "moral leadership in the battle to stop the holocaust against innocent preborn babies."[8]

Governor Mario Cuomo (D-NY), predictably, condemned Maher's action as inconsistent, asking if he would also deny Communion to Catholic politicians who supported the death penalty or contraception. Maher's diocesan office explained that the bishop viewed abortion as a much more imminent threat to human life than the other issues Cuomo mentioned, but this was not Cuomo's view. Nor was it the view of most other

Catholic Democrats. As the Democratic Party continued to move to the left on abortion, while the bishops moved to the right, confrontations between the nation's bishops and pro-choice Catholic politicians (most of whom were Democrats) became more frequent. As some of the bishops appointed by John Paul II moved into positions of influence, they made it clear to Democratic pro-choice Catholic politicians that their refusal to protect unborn human life in public law was a serious problem that the church could no longer ignore.

"We urge those Catholic officials who choose to depart from Church teaching on the inviolability of human life in their public life to consider the consequences for their own spiritual well-being, as well as the scandal they risk by leading others into serious sin," the bishops said in 1998, in a statement written by Cardinal Bernard Law, archbishop of Boston, who was one of the country's most powerful prelates until his sudden fall from grace in 2002 because of his own scandal of covering up clerical sex abuse in his diocese. "No appeal to policy, procedure, majority will or pluralism ever excuses a public official from defending life to the greatest extent possible."[9]

When the Democratic Party nominated a pro-choice Catholic, Senator John Kerry of Massachusetts, as its presidential candidate in 2004, several bishops decided they had to publicly call him to repentance. Kerry frequently mentioned his experience as an altar boy as an example of his deep Catholic roots, and he continued to attend Mass while on the campaign trail. He was a "believing and practicing Catholic," he said. But like most Catholic Democratic politicians at the time, his Catholic belief and practice did not extend to the abortion issue in public life, as the bishops insisted it should. He had a 100 percent pro-choice voting record, according to NARAL. Like other Catholic pro-choice politicians, including Mario Cuomo and Geraldine Ferraro, he insisted that he was "personally" opposed to abortion and that he believed that "life does begin at conception." But, like other Catholic pro-choice politicians, he said that he could not impose this belief on those outside his faith because of the "separation of church and state."[10]

Catholic bishops had repeatedly argued against this stance in the past, saying that it represented a misunderstanding of church–state separation and a confusion between moral principles, such as the right to life, that were an appropriate matter for legislation, and religious dogma that was not. This time, though, some bishops decided to do more than merely state their disagreements with Kerry. When they had last dealt with the issue of a pro-choice Catholic candidate on a national ticket, Ferraro in 1984, the pope had not yet issued *Evangelium Vitae*, and there were still some liberal Catholic theologians who were making the argument that the church's statements on abortion were not a matter of church dogma and that dissent from those statements was not an excommunicable offense. But after John Paul II's encyclical *Evangelium Vitae* (1995), it became harder to make that argument. The church's teaching on abortion was clear, unequivocal, and nonnegotiable, so Catholics who dissented from that teaching were out of harmony with the church. Given that, some suggested that when a Catholic politician argued for abortion rights, extreme measures of church discipline might be warranted.

In February 2004, Archbishop Raymond Burke of St. Louis announced that Kerry was not welcome to take Communion in that archdiocese because of his pro-choice platform.[11] Most bishops were reluctant to take that stance, not because they thought that it was acceptable for a Catholic politician to support abortion rights but because they believed that forcibly denying the Eucharist to a parishioner was such an extreme penalty that it might not be an appropriate act of church discipline even for a grave error such as voting to keep abortion legal. Cardinal Sean O'Malley, archbishop of Boston (where Kerry lived), said that he would not forcibly deny Communion to a pro-choice politician who came forward to receive it, but that politicians who supported abortion rights or any other policy that directly contradicted church teaching should abstain from Communion on their own. Kerry didn't follow this admonition. Reporters who followed Kerry to church on Easter Sunday in 2004 witnessed him taking Communion at the Paulist Center, near his home in Beacon Hill.[12]

A few weeks later, though, when the archbishop of Newark, John Myers, joined O'Malley in asking Catholic politicians who supported abortion rights to voluntarily abstain from Communion, the pro-choice Catholic Democratic governor of New Jersey, James McGreevey, said that he would choose to abstain. This was probably not exactly what the archbishop had hoped; he would have preferred that McGreevey bring his policies into line with the church. But at least the governor seemed to recognize the nonnegotiability of the bishops' stance. "With abortion, there can be no legitimate diversity of opinion," the Newark archbishop declared. "The direct killing of the innocent is always a grave injustice." "There is no right more fundamental," he stated, "than the right to be born and reared with all the dignity the human person deserves."[13]

The controversy reached new heights when the bishop of Colorado Springs became the first in the nation to say that he would deny Communion not only to pro-choice politicians but also to any voters who supported pro-choice candidates. "Anyone who professes the Catholic faith with his lips while at the same time publicly supporting legislation or candidates that defy God's law makes a mockery of that faith and belies his identity as a Catholic," the bishop wrote. He insisted that his action was not a "political statement" but rather an application of "church teaching." Other bishops pushed back against this view. "I do not favor a confrontation at the altar rail with the sacred body of the Lord Jesus in my hand," said Cardinal Theodore McCarrick, archbishop of Washington, DC. Cardinal Roger Mahony, archbishop of Los Angeles, also objected, saying that even if other bishops refused to admit pro-choice politicians to Communion, John Kerry was welcome to take Communion in his diocese.[14]

The bishops held an emergency meeting in June 2004 to discuss the matter of Communion for pro-choice Catholic politicians. Despite their differences on the matter, the bishops were united in affirming that "the killing of an unborn child is always intrinsically evil and can never be justified." They were also united in believing that they had a responsibility to "counsel Catholic public officials that their acting consistently to support abortion on demand risks making them cooperators in evil in a public manner." "We will persist in this duty to counsel, in the hope that the scandal of their cooperating in evil can be resolved by the proper formation of their consciences," the bishops said. But on the matter of whether a Catholic pro-choice politician should be denied Communion, the bishops did not reach consensus. Each bishop had the authority to decide this matter at the local level for his own diocese, they said.[15]

Faced with this division in practice, the bishops sought guidance from the Vatican. Cardinal Joseph Ratzinger (who was then serving at the Vatican as prefect for the Congregation of the Doctrine of the Faith, and became Pope Benedict XVI in 2005) sent a letter to Cardinal McCarrick in early July 2004 clarifying that there were some sins that could disqualify a person from Communion, and that support for abortion rights might be one of them. "There may be a legitimate diversity of opinion even among Catholics about waging war and applying the death penalty, but not however with regard to abortion and euthanasia," Ratzinger wrote. The common pro-choice Catholic argument that Mario Cuomo and others had been making since the 1980s that questioned why bishops would deny Communion to supporters of abortion rights but not to supporters of nuclear arms buildup or capital punishment was therefore invalid, Ratzinger's memo implied; abortion was a higher-order issue that the church had made official teaching in a way that it had not done with other issues of political controversy. For that reason, Ratzinger said, "if a Catholic were to be at odds with the Holy Father on the application of capital punishment or on the decision to wage war, he would not for that reason be considered unworthy to present himself to receive Holy Communion." But when it came to the "grave sin of abortion or euthanasia," any "formal cooperation" with the sin could disqualify a person from taking Communion. "When a person's formal cooperation becomes manifest," such as "in the case of a Catholic politician . . . consistently campaigning and voting for permissive abortion and euthanasia laws," "his Pastor should meet with him, instructing him about the Church's teaching, informing him that he is not to present himself for Holy Communion until he brings to an end the objective situation of sin, and warning him that he will otherwise be denied the Eucharist," Ratzinger stated.

But if these measures did not work and "the person in question, with obstinate persistence, still presents himself to receive the Holy Eucharist, 'the minister of Holy Communion must refuse to distribute it,'"

Ratzinger said. Cardinal O'Malley and Archbishop Myers were therefore correct in requesting that politicians in their dioceses who supported abortion rights voluntarily abstain from Communion. But attempts to deny Communion to all voters who supported pro-choice candidates went too far. Those who supported pro-choice candidates *because* of their support for abortion rights were guilty of "material cooperation" in abortion and should voluntarily abstain from Communion, Ratzinger wrote, but if a Catholic "does not share a candidate's stand in favour of abortion and/or euthanasia, but votes for that candidate for other reasons, it is considered remote material cooperation, which can be permitted in the presence of proportionate reasons."[16] The Catholic Church, in other words, was not telling people how to vote in a presidential election, so bishops should not deny Communion to voters merely because they cast their ballots for pro-choice candidates. But if the church did not categorically rule out voting for pro-choice candidates for "proportionate reasons," it drew a firm line against any support for abortion legalization, which seemed to suggest that politicians who supported abortion rights could no longer plausibly claim that their pro-choice stances could be harmonized with Catholic teaching, or, at least, with the Vatican's official understanding of that teaching. Ratzinger's memo seemed to offer support for the bishops who encouraged Kerry and other Catholic supporters of abortion rights to voluntarily refrain from taking Communion.

Kerry's narrow defeat in the election laid the issue to rest for a while, but as the bishops prepared for the 2008 presidential election, they signaled that they intended to follow the dictates of the letter that Cardinal Ratzinger (now Benedict XVI) had sent them in 2004. In 2007, the United States Conference of Catholic Bishops (USCCB), the successor organization of the old NCCB, declared in "Forming Consciences for Faithful Citizenship" that "a Catholic cannot vote for a candidate who takes a position in favor of an intrinsic evil, such as abortion or racism, if the voter's intent is to support that position. In such cases a Catholic would be guilty of formal cooperation in grave evil." Catholic social teaching on other issues besides abortion was also important, the bishops said, but human life issues such as abortion headed the list; abortion was not just "one issue among many." Though stopping just short of saying that a Catholic could not vote for a pro-choice candidate (the bishops allowed that for "grave moral reasons," a Catholic could theoretically do so in exceptional circumstances), the Catholic bishops effectively made it impossible for any Catholic politician to remain in good standing with the church while championing the pro-choice cause, and they cast grave doubt about whether Catholic voters should support candidates who advocated keeping abortion legal. Cardinal O'Malley of Boston said in 2007 that the support of Catholics in Massachusetts for pro-choice Democratic candidates "borders on scandal."[17]

Yet in practice, this was hard to enforce. When Senator Barack Obama (D-IL), the Democratic presidential nominee, selected a pro-choice Catholic, Senator Joe Biden (D-DE), as his running mate, some Catholic bishops grumbled, but for the most part, their reactions were noticeably quieter than they had been to Kerry's candidacy in 2004. The bishop of Scranton, Pennsylvania, where Biden had grown up, said that the pro-choice senator was not welcome to take Communion in his diocese, but few other bishops said the same.[18] Perhaps that was because Biden had a more moderate record on abortion than Kerry or Ferraro. He had voted for the Partial-Birth Abortion Ban Act and was a longtime supporter of the Hyde Amendment. He was also part of a campaign that was working harder than some previous Democratic campaigns to make pro-life Democrats feel welcome in the party. The 2008 Democratic National Convention gave a primetime speaking slot to Senator Bob Casey Jr. of Pennsylvania, who identified as a pro-life Democrat. Casey's father, Pennsylvania governor Bob Casey Sr., was famously denied a speaking opportunity at the 1992 Democratic National Convention because of his opposition to Bill Clinton's candidacy over abortion, so the selection of Casey Jr. to deliver an address at the 2008 convention was a deliberate olive branch from Obama that signaled his desire to reach out to politically moderate evangelicals and Catholics. Obama knew that even if they might differ with the party's official stance on abortion, they likely supported the Democrats' position on universal health care or concern for the environment.

RELIGIOUS LIBERTY AND THE PRO-LIFE ISSUE

Regardless of the truce that might have existed between pro-life Catholics and Obama before he entered the White House, the confrontations between the bishops and Democratic politicians quickly became more heated after Obama's election, partly because Obama underestimated what he would need to do to placate pro-life Catholics. Pro-choice Democrats in Congress (along with the president) assumed that they could pass the president's health care plan and appease the small number of pro-life Democrats whose support they needed to secure the bill's passage merely by extending the language of the Hyde Amendment to the Affordable Care Act—that is, by guaranteeing that federal funds would not be used to cover abortions under Obamacare. But when Representative Bart Stupak, a pro-life Democrat from Michigan, offered an amendment to go further by also prohibiting private insurance plans purchased through Obamacare from covering abortion, the nation's Catholic bishops began lobbying for the Stupak amendment, threatening to pull their support for Obama's health care plan if the plan covered abortions in any form. They encouraged priests to discuss the matter in church and pray for the amendment's passage. The pressure worked. Although pro-lifers were a small minority in the party, they had just enough power in Congress to force the pro-choice party leadership to accept the Stupak amendment, despite their reservations. Obamacare would not cover abortions, even through private insurance plans.[19]

But that was not the end of the bishops' concerns about Obamacare. Obama promised that his health care plan would not cover abortifacients, but his definition of abortifacient—which reflected the official medical definition—was not the same as the Catholic Church's. Catholic ethicists and church leaders understood pregnancy to begin the moment in which an egg was fertilized and became a zygote, with a unique chromosomal identity. This is how the bishops and pro-life activists had always spoken of the beginning of human life. It is how the Vatican described conception in *Donum Vitae* in 1987 and how John Paul II did so in his encyclical *Evangelium Vitae* in 1995: "From the time that the ovum is fertilized, a life is begun which is neither that of the father nor the mother; it is rather the life of a new human being with his own growth."[20] But this is not how the medical community defined the beginning of pregnancy; according to medical definitions, abortions could occur only after a fertilized egg was implanted in the uterus, not merely after fertilization. The Guttmacher Institute wrote in 2005, "Federal policy has long been both consistent and in accord with the scientists: Drugs and devices that act before implantation prevent, rather than terminate, pregnancy."[21] Thus, according to the Food and Drug Administration, medications such as Ella (the "morning-after pill") and Plan B, which blocked implantation of fertilized eggs, were not abortifacients; they were "emergency contraception." But according to most pro-life activists and the Catholic bishops, they were abortion-inducing drugs, because they destroyed fertilized eggs that had unique chromosomal identities and were therefore (in their understanding) divinely created human persons.

Although the Obama administration had given into pro-life Catholic demands earlier, it stood firm on Ella and Plan B: Employers had to pay for health care coverage that included emergency contraception, regardless of their conscientious objections to it. This alarmed not only conservative Catholics but also some conservative evangelicals. Although most evangelicals (unlike some conservative Catholics) accepted forms of contraception that did not destroy fertilized eggs, they shared the Catholic bishops' view that Ella and Plan B were not merely contraceptives but were abortifacients. The evangelical owners of Hobby Lobby refused to provide insurance plans for their employees that covered these drugs, claiming that it violated the company owners' religious freedom. The Obama administration took the Hobby Lobby owners to court in an attempt to force them to purchase this coverage. In a 5–4 decision, the Supreme Court sided with Hobby Lobby. *Burwell v. Hobby Lobby Stores, Inc.* (2014), in which Samuel Alito wrote the majority opinion, said that if a corporation's owners had religious objections to the contraceptive coverage mandated by Obamacare, they did not have to provide it.[22] Many pro-life Catholics and evangelicals were jubilant. But it had been a close call. Justice Ruth Bader Ginsburg wrote a strong dissent. If she had had just one more justice on her side, her dissenting opinion would have become the majority, and employers would not have had the right to act on their convictions by refusing to pay for contraceptives they considered abortifacients.

The standoff with the Obama administration made the bishops and other conservative Catholics (and many evangelicals) more fearful than they had been in forty years about the possible loss of their religious liberty in the area of abortion rights. For a brief moment in 1973, immediately after *Roe v. Wade*, Catholic bishops had worried that the government might require Catholic hospitals to offer abortions or force Catholic doctors and nurses to assist in abortion procedures. But bipartisan legislation created by Senator Frank Church, a pro-choice Democrat from Idaho, allayed their fears. The Church Amendments of 1973 prohibited the government from requiring recipients of federal funds for medical procedures to offer abortions. The Hyde Amendment, which was passed three years later with strong support from members of both parties, restricted Medicaid funding of abortions. From the mid-1970s until the beginning of the Obama administration, therefore, Catholic bishops did not worry too much about whether the federal government would force Catholics (or others) to violate their conscience by funding or providing abortions. Now they began to worry. From this point on, the cause of religious liberty was almost inseparable from the pro-life campaign.[23]

Pro-life conservative Catholics thought they had good reason to believe that both the courts and Democratic politicians were arrayed against them in the final years of the Obama administration. In 2015, the Democratic-controlled legislature of California passed the Reproductive FACT Act, which required licensed medical facilities offering pregnancy services—including pro-life crisis pregnancy centers that met the criteria for a licensed medical facility in the state—to post public notices at their facility advising patients that California offered free or low-cost abortion services. Several crisis pregnancy centers sued the state, arguing that this requirement violated their rights of conscience and free speech. "No one would require Alcoholics Anonymous to promote liquor stores," said the president of the National Institute of Family and Life Advocates. "Pro-life clinics deserve the same respect." But many progressives disagreed.

Pro-life clinics eventually won their case when the Supreme Court ruled in their favor in 2018 (*NIFLA v. Becerra*), but it was a 5–4 decision, with all of the Court's liberal justices siding with the state of California instead of the crisis pregnancy centers.[24]

In 2015 or 2016, there was no way to predict that Court victory, since the narrowly decided ruling was dependent on a Trump nominee who was not yet on the Court. In the months leading up to the 2016 election, the Court appeared to be tacking to the left on issues of reproduction and sexuality. In 2016, the Supreme Court ruled in *Whole Woman's Health v. Hellerstedt* that restrictive abortion laws that created an "undue burden" for people seeking abortion were unconstitutional. When coupled with the Court's decision the previous year in *Obergefell v. Hodges* (2015) that required states to legally recognize same-sex marriages, it seemed clear to many conservative Catholics that the Supreme Court was opposed to their values and that it would pose a further threat to their religious liberty if another Democratic president was elected who would nominate more progressive justices. The Democratic platform of 2016 signaled as much by featuring a lengthy section on LGBTQ+ rights that included the line, "We support a progressive vision of religious freedom that respects pluralism and rejects the misuse of religion to discriminate." Many conservative Catholics and evangelicals had no doubt that Democratic-nominated justices would use this principle to force them to do things that their consciences prohibited. For decades, Catholics for Choice and many liberal Protestant advocates of abortion rights had talked about the primacy of freedom of conscience, but now it appeared to pro-life Catholics that it was pro-choice progressives who were least concerned about conscience rights. The Democratic Party platform of 2016 also included a promise to repeal the Hyde Amendment and begin nationally funding elective abortion through Medicaid once again. Never before had a Democratic Party platform called for a repeal of the Hyde Amendment, but the 2016 platform was the most overtly pro-choice platform that the party had ever adopted.[25]

That is why some of the nation's bishops were reluctant to follow Pope Francis's lead in finding common ground with progressives by emphasizing the entirety of the consistent life ethic instead of focusing narrowly on abortion. The consistent life ethic had characterized the U.S. church hierarchy's framing of the abortion issue in the late 1970s and early 1980s, but for most of the bishops in the 1990s and afterward, abortion seemed to be a much more important issue than any of the other components of the consistent life ethic. That was not Pope Francis's view. When Francis became pope in 2013, he insisted that he and the church would always oppose abortion — which he called a "crime, an absolute evil" — but it was essential for the church to frame this pro-life advocacy as part of a larger concern for all human life and to avoid the alliances with the political right that had characterized much of conservative Catholicism in the United States. "This defence of unborn life is closely linked to the defence of each and every other human right," Francis wrote in his first encyclical, *Evangelii Gaudium* (2013). "It involves the conviction that a human being is always sacred and inviolable, in any situation and at every stage of development. Human beings are ends in themselves and never a means of resolving other problems. Once this conviction disappears, so do solid and lasting foundations for the defence of human rights."[26]

This was hardly a new message, of course; pro-life Catholics had been making this argument for decades. But Francis was concerned that some conservative Catholics who championed the rights of the unborn had not devoted sufficient effort to the "defence of [other] human rights" (*Evangelii Gaudium*) that he thought should accompany concern for the life of the unborn. He issued an encyclical on environmental stewardship and climate change, strengthened the church's opposition to the death penalty, and made opposition to wars around the globe a central part of his papacy. In each case, he saw his progressive political advocacy as a natural corollary to his defense of unborn human life. "Since everything is interrelated, concern for the protection of nature is also incompatible with the justification of abortion," he wrote in *Laudato Si'* (2015), his encyclical on environmental stewardship. "How can we genuinely teach the importance of concern for other vulnerable beings, however troublesome or inconvenient they may be, if we fail to protect a human embryo, even when its presence is uncomfortable and creates difficulties? 'If personal and social sensitivity towards the acceptance of the new life is lost, then other forms of acceptance that are valuable for society also wither away.'"[27]

Francis was also deeply concerned about the rights of immigrants, which is why he issued a public rebuke of Donald Trump. "A person who thinks only about building walls, wherever they may be, and not building bridges, is not Christian," he said in early 2016, in an unusual insertion of papal opinion into the U.S. election process.[28]

At least some of the U.S. bishops whom Francis appointed were a little more likely than some of their older counterparts to champion the consistent life ethic and avoid the single-issue politics that had come to characterize much of the country's episcopacy during the previous two or three decades. Likewise, the bishops whom he made cardinals included outspoken supporters of gun control and strong advocates of a compassionate stand toward immigrants and refugees. But in a church where bishops usually serve for more than a decade, the Francis-appointed bishops were only a small minority in the church in 2016. Indeed, not until 2024 would the number of Francis-appointed bishops reach even 50 percent of the total number of actively serving bishops; many of the bishops appointed by John Paul II or Benedict XVI were still serving in their positions well into the 2020s.[29]

But even with Pope Francis's interest in appointing consistent life advocates rather than single-issue conservative ideologues to high positions in the U.S. church, the Francis-appointed bishops found a great deal of common ground with their older conservative peers in the episcopate. Indeed, any disagreements they had were more on matters of emphasis than on policy per se. Even the staunchest conservatives among the bishops affirmed the human dignity of undocumented immigrants. One of the church's most strongly conservative antiabortion bishops—Archbishop Charles Chaput of Philadelphia, who had suggested in 2004 that it might be a sin for Catholics to vote for John Kerry because of his pro-choice views—wrote in 2013 about the Christian imperative to treat undocumented immigrants with compassion and dignity: "The Catholic commitment to the dignity of the immigrant comes from exactly the same roots as our commitment to the dignity of the unborn child."[30] Nor did any of the more progressive bishops appointed by Francis suggest that the church should back away in any way from its defense of unborn human life. Abortion was a settled issue for the Catholic Church, and even the most progressive bishops were strongly committed to the right to life for the unborn. That was certainly true of Bishop Robert McElroy of San Diego, widely regarded as one of the leading members of the progressive wing of the Catholic episcopacy in the United States, and a prelate whom Pope Francis would later reward with a cardinal's hat. During the bishops' controversy over Kerry a decade earlier, McElroy had spoken out against denying Communion to pro-choice Catholic politicians. In the lead-up to the 2016 election, he urged his fellow bishops to give more attention to climate change and antipoverty initiatives in their political pronouncements instead of focusing so narrowly on the single issue of abortion. But despite his progressivism, McElroy's views on the morality of abortion were thoroughly orthodox. Abortion was "intrinsically evil," he said, and it was therefore "an imperative of conscience for Catholic disciples to seek legal protections for the unborn." But he added that the church could not dictate exactly how individual voters and politicians should apply these imperatives to specific situations, and it would weigh competing priorities in a world of imperfect political choices, because "like the issues of fighting poverty and addressing climate change, the issue of abortion in law and public policy is a realm where prudential judgment is essential and determinative."[31]

Fighting poverty was, in fact, a way to reduce the incidence of abortion, some bishops claimed; the two causes were mutually reinforcing, not mutually exclusive. Given that abortion was disproportionately concentrated among the poor, the single best way to reduce abortion rates was to "fight poverty," said Richard Doerflinger, the deputy director of the USCCB's Secretariat for Pro-Life Activities.[32] The realization that the party that might do the most to reduce abortion rates was not necessarily the party that would do the most to overturn *Roe v. Wade* or restrict abortion through law made pro-life Catholics' political choice all the more difficult, and made it challenging for the bishops to agree on how to frame their political guidance to the faithful. Even though the bishops avoided directly endorsing specific candidates or parties, they also knew that the public would inevitably interpret the way in which they prioritized issues—such as whether they emphasized the right to life more than the moral imperative of fighting poverty, or vice versa—as an implied endorsement of one side or the other.

When faced with the choice between Donald Trump (whose stances and public rhetoric on immigration and climate change were diametrically opposed to the teachings of Pope Francis) and the 2016 Democratic Party platform (which was the most strongly pro-choice, pro-LGBTQ+ rights platform that the party had ever adopted up to that point), the bishops debated with each other whether it was best to highlight abortion and marriage issues in their discussions of the upcoming election or whether they should instead make a greater effort to discuss climate change and other concerns that reflected Pope Francis's new priorities. Both the Republican and Democratic platforms were far from ideal, the bishops could agree. Even McElroy, one of the most outspoken progressives in the USCCB, would eventually express great concern about the Democratic Party's abandonment of its previous moderate language on abortion and its willingness to "simply block out the human identity and rights of unborn children."[33] And on immigration, the bishops also agreed that the Trump-era Republican Party was badly misguided. "We will work to promote humane policies that protect refugees and immigrants' inherent dignity, keep families together, and honor and respect the laws of this nation," the USCCB said in November 2016. "Serving and welcoming people fleeing violence and conflict in various regions of the world is part of our identity as Catholics."[34] But despite their concerns about the Republicans' policies on immigration, the conservative approach of emphasizing abortion over other issues won out among the bishops in the end. The updated edition of "Forming Consciences for Faithful Citizenship" that the USCCB issued for the 2016 election was very similar in approach to the bishops' guides to the 2008 and 2012 elections; like the earlier guides, it highlighted abortion and marriage as foundational concerns. Although a handful of bishops called for a thorough revision to emphasize antipoverty efforts as a moral imperative alongside fighting abortion, the USCCB adopted the conservative version of the document by a vote of 210 to 21.[35]

This vote was only one indication of a larger, decades-long culturally conservative shift among bishops in the United States that had resulted in making the abortion issue the foundation for a socially conservative campaign for moral absolutes and opposition to secularism. A 2016 survey of Catholic bishops — the vast majority of whom had been appointed by either John Paul II or Benedict XVI — revealed that they were overwhelmingly conservative in their theological views, with about one-third falling into the category of hardline ideological culture warriors. For all of them, abortion was *the* central issue of political concern. One hundred percent of the bishops said they had written a pastoral letter, a column in a Catholic newspaper, or post in some other public forum about the "sanctity of life," with 82 percent saying that they wrote about this topic "often" or "on a regular basis." No other issue received nearly as much attention from the bishops.[36]

In 2017, the bishops signaled their continued interest in making a single-minded focus on abortion the centerpiece of their political efforts when they selected Archbishop Joseph Naumann instead of Cardinal Blase Cupich to lead the USCCB's Committee on Pro-Life Activities. Both Naumann and Cupich, of course, opposed abortion, but Cupich, who had received his appointment as cardinal from Pope Francis, was a devotee of the consistent life ethic and an enthusiastic admirer of Cardinal Joseph Bernardin's approach, while Naumann favored making abortion a single issue of focus, just as Cardinal John O'Connor had. Unlike some of the consistent life ethic advocates who were willing to find common ground with pro-choice politicians who shared their concerns about gun violence or climate change, Naumann insisted that since abortion was an "intrinsic evil" that was of higher "moral priority" than other issues, Catholic politicians who supported abortion rights should abstain from Communion. In previous committee elections, the bishop who wore a cardinal's hat had almost always prevailed over the candidate who did not, but in this case, Cardinal Timothy Dolan, archbishop of New York, endorsed Naumann. The bishops followed Dolan's lead. Even though the pro-life committee had been led by a cardinal for the previous thirty years, the bishops elected Archbishop Naumann over Cardinal Cupich by a vote of 96 to 82. Both Catholic and secular news media interpreted the vote as a sign that the bishops were not on board with Pope Francis's attempts to revive the consistent life ethic; they wanted a hardline culture war campaign against abortion.[37]

In November 2019, the USCCB issued a letter to the faithful declaring that although there were many important issues of moral significance in the 2020 presidential election, "the threat of abortion remains our preeminent priority because it directly attacks life itself, because it takes place within the sanctuary of the family, and because of the number of lives destroyed."[38] Two weeks after Biden's election, the president of the USCCB, Los Angeles archbishop José Gomez, said he anticipated that the bishops and Biden could find common ground on much of Catholic social teaching, but the president-elect's opposition to the Hyde Amendment and his commitment to *Roe v. Wade* were "against some fundamental values we hold dear as Catholics." "Both of these policies undermine our preeminent priority of the elimination of abortion," Gomez said.[39]

The bishops then opened a monthslong study into whether pro-choice Catholic politicians such as Biden could be denied Communion, an issue that they did not think had been laid to rest by the directives they had received from the Vatican in 2004. Biden posed a particular problem for them, because he frequently attended Mass and routinely invoked his love for the Catholic faith. But he was also a liberal pro-choice Catholic in the mold of Mario Cuomo. Like many other churchgoing liberal Catholics of his generation of Democratic politicians, Biden insisted that he could square his personal faith-based moral opposition to abortion with a firm commitment to keeping abortion legally available. Catholic bishops had insisted for decades that this position represented an incorrect understanding of the church's moral teaching, and now some of them were ready to take disciplinary action against politicians who persisted in defying the church on this matter.

Some conservative Catholics believed that the denial of Communion to those who supported abortion rights was simply an enforcement of existing church doctrine, but more liberal Catholic theologians saw it as a change in the nature of a "Catholic" understanding of the church. Massimo Faggioli, a theology professor at Villanova University, said that such a move would lead to "a full-blown 'evangelicalization' of U.S. Catholicism—'evangelicalization' in the sense of U.S. conservative white evangelicals, and the loss of a Catholic sense of the church."[40] The question for them was not necessarily whether the bishops were right in their understanding of Catholic doctrine on abortion and the implications of that teaching in political life. The question was rather whether they were right to turn the Eucharist into a political gatekeeper. The church had long denied the sacraments to those who refused to repent of grave sins, including abortion. But never before had the church's disciplinary penalties had such clear potential partisan implications in national politics. If the church began routinely denying Communion to politicians who endorsed the Democratic Party platform on abortion, as some bishops wanted, it would align the church against a major political party, and it would then be impossible to separate the church from political partisanship. This worried some Catholics, even some who were pro-life.

In the end, Pope Francis, in keeping with his desire to expand the availability of the sacraments as much as possible, signaled his strong preference that pro-choice Catholic politicians not be forcibly denied the Eucharist. When it became apparent that Francis would almost certainly use his papal power to veto the bishops' declaration if they insisted on issuing a hardline policy excluding pro-choice politicians from Communion, the bishops instead issued a much more moderate document. Instead of discussing whether political support for abortion rights disqualified a person from Communion, the bishops' declaration "The Mystery of the Eucharist in the Life of the Church" instead reiterated the seriousness of Communion, the value of the unborn, and the need for Catholics to examine their consciences before partaking, directives that few theologically informed Catholics could object to and which the *National Catholic Reporter* characterized as "milquetoast" in comparison to what some conservatives in the church had anticipated.[41] Biden would continue taking Communion, even as he remained committed to protecting abortion rights. But though some of the conservative bishops may have backed down from their efforts to use the Mass to enforce orthodoxy on abortion, the church's clergy remained overwhelmingly conservative. Indeed, by 2024, the youngest cohort of priests was more conservative in both theology and politics than any cohort ordained in the previous half century. As strong culture warriors, they believed that fighting against secularism and a liberalized sexual ethic was central to the church's mission, and they viewed the pro-life cause as the linchpin of their campaign.[42]

A majority of Catholics who frequently attended Mass agreed with the clergy on this matter. Sixty-eight percent of Catholics who attended Mass at least once a week wanted to make abortion mostly or entirely illegal, according to a 2022 Pew survey. But by 2022, these weekly churchgoers were a minority among the country's Catholics, because only one-third of Catholics attended Mass weekly, while 50 percent never or "seldom" attended. And among those who did not attend church very often, supporters of abortion rights outnumbered pro-lifers by 2 to 1.[43]

The fact that between half and two-thirds of self-identified Catholics didn't go to church very often—and, in most cases, didn't feel bound by church teaching on abortion or any other issue—meant that public opinion surveys consistently showed that the majority of Catholics were pro-choice and voted accordingly. In the 1950s, three-quarters of Catholics went to church every week, and two-thirds had complied with church teaching on contraception, despite its unpopularity.[44] In the early twenty-first century, there were still Catholics who went to church every week and treated church teaching on issues of sexuality and reproduction as authoritative. But this group now constituted only a minority of Catholics. There was now a pronounced bifurcation between frequent churchgoers and less frequent churchgoers on abortion, partly because the two groups had adopted very different frameworks and sources of moral authority for looking at the issue.

This gap also extended to Hispanics. A 2022 Pew survey found no real difference between the abortion views of Hispanic and white non-Hispanics. First-generation Latino immigrants and those who attended church frequently were highly likely to oppose abortion, but since only 22 percent of Hispanic Catholics attended church once a week, it was not too surprising that the majority of Hispanics—especially young Gen-Zers—adopted the pro-choice views of their peers. But among evangelical Hispanics (most of whom were Pentecostals or charismatics), opposition to abortion was strong, just as it was among non-Hispanic white evangelicals. Abortion views among Hispanics thus closely paralleled those of white non-Hispanics: Devout Catholics who regularly attended church found common ground with evangelicals, while those who attended church infrequently adopted pro-choice views that were indistinguishable from those of religiously non-affiliated Americans.[45]

EVANGELICALS' CONTINUED PRO-LIFE COMMITMENT

Like conservative Catholics, most conservative evangelicals maintained and even deepened the antiabortion convictions that they had solidified in the 1980s. Because the pro-life cause for most evangelicals outside of progressive circles had always been closely linked to their desire to rescue the country from secularization and the sexual revolution, their commitment to pro-life activism became even stronger as they perceived that they were losing the battle against gay rights, same-sex marriage, and the preservation of Christian values in public life. The Southern Baptist Convention (SBC), in particular, used its political power as the nation's largest Protestant denomination to lobby for the Partial-Birth Abortion Ban Act in the 1990s and early 2000s, and to push for restrictions on embryonic stem cell research during President George W. Bush's first term in office. The SBC passed a resolution rebuking President Bill Clinton for his support for abortion rights and lauded George W. Bush for his pro-life stance. And it included a statement on behalf of the rights of the unborn from the moment of conception in the *2000 Baptist Faith and Message* (*BFM*), the closest thing the denomination had to a creed. "We should speak on behalf of the unborn and contend for the sanctity of all human life from conception to natural death," the *BFM* said.[46]

In 2003, Southern Baptists marked the thirtieth anniversary of *Roe v. Wade* by publicly apologizing for their denomination's support for a moderate position on abortion in the early 1970s. The denomination had never been fully pro-choice, but Southern Baptists of the early twenty-first century considered the therapeutic abortion laws that the SBC endorsed in the 1970s bad enough. If the fight against abortion was a battle for the nation's soul, the SBC's moderation on the issue in the 1970s put the denomination on the wrong side of the most important moral issue the country faced. "We lament and renounce statements and actions by previous Conventions and previous denominational leadership that offered support to the abortion culture," the SBC resolution said. "We humbly confess that the initial blindness of many in our Convention to the enormity of Roe v. Wade should serve as a warning to contemporary Southern Baptists of the subtlety of the spirit of the age in obscuring a biblical worldview. . . . We urge our Southern Baptist churches to remain vigilant in the protection of human life by preaching the whole counsel of God on matters of human sexuality and the sanctity of life." This resolution made clear that Southern Baptists of the early twenty-first century perceived the abortion issue as the foundation for a larger culture war that was inextricably connected to matters of "human sexuality" and "the sanctity of life."[47] They were aghast that some of their predecessors of the 1970s, who shared their concerns about homosexuality and pornography, had nevertheless failed to discern the full evil of abortion, which they thought was inseparable from those other cultural sins.

Evangelicals' concern about abortion was never far removed from their political program, but it also took an increasingly personal turn after the 1980s, as evangelicals created pro-life crisis pregnancy centers (CPCs) to encourage pregnant women who were considering abortion to give their unborn children the gift of life instead. By the early 2020s, more than 2,500 CPCs were operating in the United States, and most of them were faith-based. Although Catholics had taken the lead in creating the earliest CPCs in the late 1960s and early 1970s, evangelicals took a more active role in forming CPCs in the 1990s and afterward. The three largest national networks of CPCs in the early 2020s were either explicitly evangelical or generically "Christian," with both Catholics and evangelicals serving on their boards.[48]

Although supporters of reproductive rights accused CPCs of misleading their clients and offering misinformation about abortion, many pro-life evangelicals disputed that charge. In their view, CPCs were a way to provide material assistance and help to pregnant women in need, and to reduce the abortion rate and save unborn lives. CPCs often provided free ultrasounds, diapers, and sometimes parenting classes or more substantial material benefits to low-income women who were not sure how they could afford another baby. The evangelical Christians who supported CPCs sometimes touted these centers as a way to extend the social safety net through the private sector. They were pursuing the type of compassionate approach that many pro-life Catholics had long championed, they thought, but they were doing so in a way that put churches, families, and private citizens instead of the federal government at the forefront of charitable efforts. In 2002, for instance, when the evangelical Family Research Council joined with Southern Baptist leaders and other leading evangelicals and conservative Catholic laypeople to draw up an ecumenical document calling for specific steps to create a "culture of life," they called for tax cuts for families and emphasized the role of CPCs in decreasing the abortion rate, but did not say anything about expanding the social welfare state.[49]

At the same time, some pro-life evangelicals—though by no means all—decided in the early 2020s that CPCs and even abortion bans were not enough; they needed the law to treat abortion as murder by applying the full penalties for homicide. Pro-life evangelicals had always wanted abortion to be illegal, but until the 2020s, the idea that the law should treat those who obtained abortions as murderers was not very widespread. But in the early 2020s, this position began rapidly gaining ground among a minority of evangelicals who called themselves "abolitionists" in honor of the radical antislavery activists of the mid-nineteenth century who opposed all compromises on the matter. Demanding an immediate end to all abortions, they insisted that the law could accomplish this by adopting a zero-tolerance policy toward the procedure. In 2021, the SBC seemed to endorse their point of view when it passed the resolution "On Abolishing Abortion," which "state[d] unequivocally that abortion is murder." "We reject any position that allows for any exceptions to the legal protection of our preborn neighbors," the SBC said, in an apparent repeal of its long-standing acceptance of an exemption in cases in which an abortion was necessary to save a pregnant woman's life. "We humbly confess and lament any complicity in recognizing exceptions that legitimize or regulate abortion." Furthermore, the SBC said, "We will not embrace an incremental approach alone to ending abortion because it challenges God's Lordship over the heart and the conscience, and rejects His call to repent of sin completely and immediately." The resolution also repeatedly spoke of civil "punishment" for those who participated in abortion: "We affirm that the murder of preborn children is a crime against humanity that must be punished equally under the law." After all, "God establishes all governing authorities as His avenging servants to carry out His wrath on the evildoer," the SBC resolution said, in a reference to Romans 13.[50]

Immediately after the SBC adopted the resolution, some of the denomination's most respected conservative pro-life voices, including former Ethics and Religious Liberty Commission president Richard Land, accused it of going too far. Wouldn't a total opposition to incrementalism make it more difficult to save unborn lives by preventing Southern Baptists from supporting legislation, such as a ban on partial-birth abortion, that might pass even when it was impossible to enact a full ban? he asked. And wasn't the refusal to countenance an exception to save a woman's life a bit too extreme?[51]

The debate over the resolution indicated that even if Southern Baptists and other evangelicals were united in the aim of banning abortion, they might be divided about how to reach that goal. Nearly all of them wanted antiabortion laws, but how stringent those laws should be was a matter of disagreement. This debate spilled over into the secular political sphere only a year after the SBC adopted its no-exceptions resolution, when the Supreme Court finally did what pro-life activists had spent decades praying for. It overturned *Roe v. Wade*.

DOBBS AND THE POST-ROE FUTURE OF CHRISTIAN DISCUSSIONS OF ABORTION

In June 2022, the Supreme Court said in *Dobbs v. Jackson Women's Health* that the Constitution did not protect the right to an abortion. This meant that states or the federal government could make abortion policies as strict or as lenient as they chose. More than a dozen states responded to the ruling with immediate bans (or at least substantial restrictions) on abortion. On the other hand, some of the most politically liberal states, such as California, instead enacted policies that expanded both abortion access and abortion funding. The nation's political polarization on the issue closely echoed a religious polarization that had been building for decades.

The nation's religious polarization was reflected even in the Supreme Court opinion itself. Four of the five Supreme Court justices who voted to overturn *Roe* were Catholic, and the fifth, Neil Gorsuch, had been raised Catholic before moving into the Episcopal Church.[52] All five were conservatives who subscribed to some form of "originalism" when interpreting the Constitution. The author of the majority opinion, Samuel Alito, was a social conservative who had previously dissented from the Supreme Court's ruling in favor of a constitutional right to same-sex marriage in 2015. Alito did not mention Catholic doctrine in either his declaration that the Constitution did not guarantee a right to same-sex marriage or in his landmark majority opinion overturning *Roe v. Wade*, but in each case he made an argument that probably reflected decades of experience with social conservatives who opposed abortion and same-sex marriage. He argued that, contra Harry Blackmun's assumption in *Roe v. Wade* a half century earlier, the Supreme Court could not solve societal debates over either abortion or same-sex marriage by imposing a culturally liberal norm on those who disagreed; this would only contribute to further polarization, he believed. In keeping with his conservative "originalist" approach to constitutional interpretation, he also argued that the Constitution did not allow the Court to impose this norm, since the Fourteenth Amendment's framers did not intend to protect either same-sex marriage or abortion rights.[53]

For socially conservative Catholics, both of these arguments were obvious. *Roe* had clearly failed to end the debate over abortion; forty-nine years after Harry Blackmun delivered the Court's majority opinion in *Roe*, the nation was even more polarized over abortion than it had been in the 1970s. And if it was obvious to many conservative Catholics that the Court could not solve the abortion debate by imposing a culturally liberal norm with which they and many others disagreed, it was equally obvious to them that the Constitution's framers—those who drafted the original document in Philadelphia in 1787 and those who created the Fourteenth Amendment shortly after the Civil War—did not intend to protect abortion rights. To prove this point, Alito cited historical evidence that a majority of states had restrictive abortion laws in the 1860s and that several were in the process of tightening their abortion restrictions, which to an originalist such as Alito was sufficient proof that the congressional representatives who created the Fourteenth Amendment and the state legislatures that ratified it believed that the Fourteenth Amendment was perfectly compatible with abortion bans. But beyond that, for many pro-life Christians—whether Catholic or evangelical Protestant—it was inconceivable that the Constitution's framers would have ever intended to protect abortion rights. Francis Schaeffer had argued—and many other pro-life Christians, including those who were Catholic, had long believed—that *Roe* was a subversive decision that upended the historic relationship between Christian moral values and the U.S. government. If the nation was founded on Christian-based moral principles, its founding documents could not have included protection for abortion rights, pro-life conservative Christians believed.

All three of the dissenting justices—Steven Breyer, Sonia Sotomayor, and Elena Kagan—subscribed to a very different understanding of the Constitution that did not restrict rights to the original intentions of the framers. Although none of these justices were liberal Protestants (Breyer and Kagan were Jewish and Sotomayor was a liberal Catholic), their view of the Constitution as a living document that the Court could use to protect equality and minority rights in ways that went beyond the limited imagination of the document's original authors fit perfectly with the view that liberal Protestants had generally held for the previous half century or more. Alito's majority opinion in *Dobbs* was a direct assault on that constitutional understanding and a sign that the liberal view of the Constitution that had held sway on the Court for seventy-five years—and that liberal Protestants had long championed—no longer governed the country. The loss of this framework was about more than abortion, as important as that was; it was about a larger understanding of the nation's identity and foundational values. In the wake of *Dobbs*, some progressives called not only for federal protection for abortion rights but also for changes in the Supreme Court itself in order to ensure that the liberal principles of equality they cherished would not be further eviscerated.

Dobbs thus set in motion a battle that was every bit as polarizing as the half-century-long fight over *Roe*, because for many progressives what was at stake in this new battle was not only access to abortion but also the identity of the country and the meaning of the Constitution. The Democratic Party made abortion rights its central campaign issue in both the midterm elections in 2022 and the presidential election of 2024. Likewise, liberal Protestant denominations issued stronger declarations of support for abortion rights than they ever had before. They abandoned their long-standing reticence about the moral ambiguity of abortion and instead began defending abortion rights in the strongest terms, claiming that this was central to the message of Jesus—because in the new political climate after *Dobbs*, reproductive rights were the cornerstone of a larger agenda of gender equality, pluralism, and individual choice, and they believed these were foundational values for both liberal Christianity and democracy. "The court's decision betrays the nature of our society," Reggie Williams, a professor of Christian ethics at McCormick Theological Seminary, wrote in the *Christian Century* immediately after *Dobbs*, "and our response to it speaks to the kind of society that we want to live in. This moment is about women losing rights but also about the belief within our society that it's OK, even good, to take away those rights. It stems from a history of human hierarchy that always targets multiple groups of people and degrades everyone's quality of life. . . . I'm angry at injustice. I'd hoped that we'd be further along than this as a society." He now felt like his children were "entering a society that is moving in reverse," because to progressive Christians such as Williams, *Dobbs* represented a reversal of all the egalitarian principles that liberal Protestants had been advocating for more than half a century.[54]

But even the mostly liberal Jesuit magazine *America* pointed out that the supposed societal consensus whose demise Williams lamented was never as widespread as he imagined, because *Roe* imposed by judicial fiat an idea that had not been ratified through the democratic process. *Roe*, the editors of *America* said, "invented a right with no basis in the text of the Constitution and assigned a complex moral question on which Americans disagree passionately to judges unanswerable to voters."[55] Now at last voters would have the right to debate what sort of abortion law—and, by extension, what type of society—they really wanted.

The ideological fault lines in this debate fell largely along religious lines, but this time, the divisions were not quite what they had been half a century earlier. Liberal Protestants, though more united than ever in favor of abortion rights, would play a less politically influential role in this debate, because after experiencing steep membership declines for the previous half century, they no longer had the societal influence they had enjoyed in the 1960s and early 1970s. Catholics represented a larger share of the electorate than liberal Protestants did, but because two-thirds of Catholics rarely went to church—and because the majority of nonchurchgoing Catholics were pro-choice and liberal on most other cultural issues—the most heavily Catholic regions of the country were, paradoxically, the most culturally liberal and least likely to be aligned with the magisterium's view of abortion politics. This was a far cry from the political situation in the early 1970s, when the heavily Catholic New England states of Massachusetts and Rhode Island had been some of the nation's strongest opponents of abortion. But if the political influence of both liberal Protestants and Catholics was weaker than it had been in the early 1970s, the political power of evangelicals was stronger, largely because of evangelicals' near monolithic opposition to abortion and because of their regional concentration in the southern and midwestern Bible Belt, where they had the votes to push restrictive abortion laws through state legislatures. In fact, white evangelical Protestants were now the largest and most politically influential contingent of churchgoers in the United States, with 53 percent of them regularly attending church in 2022 (at a time when only 30 percent of white Catholics and only 17 percent of white mainline Protestants did). White evangelicals were also overwhelmingly opposed to abortion; in the spring of 2022, 74 percent said that abortion should be mostly or entirely illegal, and 86 percent said that a fetus was a "person with rights."[56]

With only a few exceptions, the states that enacted abortion bans in the wake of *Dobbs* were evangelical-dominated states with high church attendance rates. The three evangelical states with the highest church attendance rates—Alabama, Mississippi, and Tennessee—led the nation with near-total bans on abortion, while most of the other states in the Bible Belt and evangelical areas of the Midwest likewise adopted partial or near-total abortion bans. Conversely, most of the states that moved quickly to protect or even expand abortion access were states that in the recent past had had large Catholic or mainline Protestant populations, but that were currently experiencing rapidly declining church attendance rates. States such as Massachusetts, Rhode Island, California, New York, and Illinois—all of which had historically had large Catholic (but very low evangelical) populations—expanded abortion access, since the contingent of Catholics who were socially conservative, pro-life churchgoers in those states was too small to affect abortion legislation. This was especially evident in New England. In the early 1970s, Catholic New England had been a center of antiabortion opinion, which was why no New England state voluntarily legalized abortion before *Roe*. But by the 2020s, after the Catholic Church's sex abuse crisis and a decades-long decline in Catholic church attendance, the historically Catholic New England states had the lowest weekly church attendance rates in the nation, and their rapidly secularizing populations were strongly supportive of abortion rights.[57]

It was therefore easy for pro-life activists to envision the battle over abortion as a battle against secularism, which is how they had long portrayed it. Liberal Protestants reminded the public that not all Christians opposed abortion, and some Jews went even further in insisting that their religious views *mandated* abortion in certain cases, which was why they argued that abortion bans were a violation of the First Amendment's free exercise clause.[58] There were also a small number of nonreligious people who opposed abortion, the organization Secular Pro-Life pointed out. But these were exceptions to the general trend. Only 11 percent of atheists said that abortion should be illegal in most or all circumstances; 87 percent said that it should be generally legal.[59] Conversely, those who attended church weekly were overwhelmingly supportive of abortion restrictions.

In the early 2020s, before *Dobbs*, 78 percent of Americans who attended church weekly wanted abortion to be illegal in most or all cases.[60] Support for abortion restrictions might have been lower among churchgoing Black Protestants and white liberal Protestants, but because the overwhelming majority of regular churchgoers were now affiliated with conservative evangelical and Catholic traditions, weekly churchgoers were now more socially conservative than ever on abortion and related matters.

But although they could agree on the need to restrict abortion, pro-life Christians were divided about what type of society they wanted to create in the aftermath of *Dobbs*. Some Catholics still wanted to create the type of society that Vatican II and John Paul II's encyclicals had envisioned: a society whose laws valued all human life and human dignity. To a certain extent, this was still the dream of the USCCB. As soon as the *Dobbs* decision was released, the USCCB issued a communiqué exhorting pro-lifers to work with others to "build a society and economy that supports marriages and families, and where every woman has the support and resources to bring her child into this world in love." In keeping with Vatican II's affirmation of the value of representative democracy, *America* magazine warned pro-lifers not to make an end run around the democratic process by using the courts to impose abortion restrictions that voters did not support. The USCCB did not directly warn against short-circuiting the democratic process, but it did call for "civil dialogue," and said that it was "time for healing wounds and repairing social divisions" that had been strained during the years of debate over abortion.[61]

Some evangelicals said the same, but in keeping with their long-standing suspicion of government social welfare programs, many looked to churches rather than the government to help women facing crisis pregnancies. "Laws are critical, but they cannot change the fact that tomorrow there will still be many women who will face an unplanned pregnancy—afraid, unprepared and unsure of what to do and where to turn," Elizabeth Graham, vice president for life initiatives at the SBC's Ethics and Religious Liberty Commission, told her fellow Southern Baptists in June 2022. "The Church has a significant opportunity to serve and support these women in crisis and their preborn children in their time of need."

But though abortion legislation could not necessarily provide for all of the material needs of low-income women and their families, it could reduce the number of fetal deaths, pro-life evangelicals predicted. "Thousands of lives will now be saved," Graham said. *Christianity Today* predicted that the number of abortions would likely decline by 10 to 15 percent. And perhaps most importantly, *Dobbs* could provide an important stepping stone to pro-life Christians' "ultimate goal," which Graham said was for "every person, born and preborn to be protected and seen with inherent dignity and value."[62]

CHRISTIANS AND ABORTION IN A PLURALISTIC SOCIETY

Two years after *Dobbs*, many pro-life advocates wondered what had happened to this dream. They were dismayed to find that the number of abortions after *Dobbs* actually increased, perhaps partly because in the aftermath of *Dobbs*, several Blue states expanded funding for abortions and made abortion easier to access than ever.[63] The abortion bans that were implemented apparently did not create the "culture of life" that pro-life advocates had envisioned. The "civil dialogue" that the USCCB had called for was nowhere in sight. And pro-lifers themselves were divided. Some wanted to work for a national abortion ban, even if it included substantial exceptions that still allowed for many abortions. Others—especially the self-described "abolitionists"—did not support any exceptions. The division was especially strong in the SBC, where President Bart Barber denounced the abolitionists' tactics, claiming that they were a betrayal of a longstanding mainstream pro-life strategy that had united Southern Baptists and other evangelicals and conservative Catholics for decades.[64] "Chaos and confusion have followed the end of *Roe* as much as victory and celebration," said Karen Swallow Prior, an evangelical Christian writer and former Southeastern Baptist Theological Seminary professor, in January 2024. "The reality of a post-*Dobbs* world is that there is no longer one big political goal. There are 50 or 500 or 5,000 smaller goals." She still held out hope that pro-lifers could work incrementally to "promote a whole-life, pro-life ethic through a variety of policies," but she acknowledged that the task would be challenging. In the summer of 2024, when the Republican Party removed language from its platform calling for a pro-life constitutional amendment—and when the Democratic Party doubled down on its promise to repeal the Hyde Amendment and protect abortion rights nationwide—it appeared that the pro-life society that evangelicals and conservative Catholics sought was more elusive than ever.

The political challenges reflected the difficulties of applying theological visions to a divided, pluralistic society. In the early 1970s, liberal Protestants had attempted to solve the abortion debate by applying the principles of their ecumenical theology to create a national standard that preserved individual liberty while also acknowledging the moral ambiguities of at least some forms of abortion. But the results did not live up to liberal Protestants' expectations. *Roe v. Wade* galvanized a much larger opposition than liberal Protestants had ever expected, because it relied on liberal theological assumptions about human life and a view of church–state relations that most Catholics and evangelical Protestants did not share. Instead of lowering the temperature of the abortion debate, *Roe v. Wade* became a political lightning rod. For many evangelicals and conservative Catholics, it became the symbol of everything that was wrong with the United States, and it prompted them to increase their opposition to abortion and their commitment to a larger Christian political vision. Liberal Protestants, by contrast, doubled down on their commitment to abortion rights even as they came to believe that *Roe*'s principle of individual privacy might be an inadequate foundation for those rights. By 2022, liberal Protestants were committed to defending the results of *Roe*, but not necessarily the legal reasoning behind it, while evangelicals and conservative Catholics were committed to overturning *Roe* even though they could not win support for their pro-life vision from a majority of the population. In an era of declining church attendance and widespread disregard for traditional Christian sexual ethics, a majority of Americans wanted abortion to remain legal, at least in some circumstances. But among the minority who did attend church, most believed that abortion was wrong, and they remained committed to legally restricting it.

In such a polarized climate, the middle ground on the abortion question largely disappeared. In an earlier era, liberal Protestants had shaped national abortion policy around the assumption that abortion was both a fundamental right and a morally ambiguous choice that should therefore be "rare" but "legal." Pro-life Catholics had rejected those assumptions, but had sometimes found common ground with their opponents by arguing that restrictive abortion laws should be accompanied by expansions in the health care system and in antipoverty initiatives. And pro-life Anabaptists and mainline Protestants had sometimes argued that the church's moral stances on abortion should not necessarily be enshrined in law in a pluralistic society.

But the fusion of the pro-life movement with a campaign to return the country to Christian principles turned the abortion debate into a referendum on the religious identity of the nation. Would the United States be a secular, pluralistic nation, or would it be a nation whose legal framework was guided by Christian moral principles? This was not what the abortion debate had been about in the early 1970s, but it was the framework for discussions of abortion in the 2020s. Pro-life Christians were divided about what exactly they meant by a "Christian nation," with some preferring a pluralistic nation guided by the Christocentric humanism of Vatican II and others preferring a less pluralistic, more hardline Christian nationalism. But for most, a revulsion at the moral relativism of a secular society that disregarded the value of unborn human life guided their thinking. And in turn, for most advocates of abortion rights, a commitment to a pluralistic social vision in which people had the freedom to follow their own intuitions as the highest moral authority instead of enshrining the fixed dictates of a particular religious tradition in civil law was central to their campaign.

For the most part, the pro-life side won the debate in the churches. To be sure, there were still plenty of liberal denominations that championed abortion rights, and many of those that did so became even more strongly supportive of reproductive freedom after *Dobbs*. But most of those denominations were rapidly losing members, and they occupied an increasingly marginalized space in American Christianity. The majority of regular churchgoers held pro-life views, and in many cases they were also drawn to the fixed, transcendent standards of moral authority that undergirded pro-life Christianity. Pro-life Catholics were disproportionately respectful of the authority of the church's magisterium, and pro-life Protestants were disproportionately likely to affiliate with churches that stressed the inerrant, unchanging standard of biblical truth.

But if the pro-life side won the debate in the churches, it did not fare so well in the political realm. Its political victories were confined almost entirely to states that were generally socially conservative and, in most cases, largely evangelical, which meant that pro-life advocates had very little political power in most of the rest of the country.

Yet that did not mean that the abortion rights campaign could win national political victories either. The failure of *Roe v. Wade* offered a cautionary note for those who wanted to pass a national law protecting abortion rights. Because the pro-life cause in the churches was associated so closely with a political mandate, it seemed certain that any national legislation that required states to allow abortion would be met with a strong backlash from pro-life Christians.

There was no easy way to resolve this debate. All sides in the conflict had deep ethical commitments that reflected their religious assumptions and their political views. There was no way to separate religion from the abortion question. And there seemed to be no way to find a compromise that would satisfy all sides as long as one side remained convinced that abortion was murder and the other was convinced that abortion rights were essential for the protection of gender equality, personal liberty, and foundational American values. Both of these assumptions were shaped by religious views. If there was a path forward, it would come only through a genuine quest to understand these views and the theologies behind them. But in the politically polarized environment that the country faced after *Dobbs*, genuine quests for understanding were in short supply.

UNDERSTANDING THE THEOLOGICAL ASSUMPTIONS BEHIND "PRO-CHOICE" AND "PRO-LIFE"

The religious campaign for reproductive rights is grounded in a theology that emphasizes individual choice as central to what it means to be human, which is a reflection of liberal Protestant views in the postwar era. This theology has had greatest appeal to those who believe that personal moral intuition is a better guide to moral truth than fixed ecclesiastical or scriptural standards of authority. Those who subscribe to this view have been suspicious of government coercion in areas of personal moral decision-making. And because they believe that choice is central to human personhood, they have tended to be skeptical about claims that an embryo or first-trimester fetus that lacks any capability to think or make choices could have the same value as an adult woman. They view the denial of choice to women as dehumanizing, which is why they view their campaign for abortion rights primarily as a campaign to defend the personhood and equality of women. But secondarily, this campaign is also a campaign for the right of everyone to make choices that are free of state or religious coercion. In the view of many of its proponents, the right to an abortion is so central to the preservation of a pluralistic democratic society free of theocratic controls that they have even been willing to risk subverting the religious freedom of some of their opponents (such as CPCs that do not want to post notices of abortion availability or companies that do not want to offer insurance plans that include coverage of contraceptives that they believe are abortion-inducing) in order to preserve abortion rights for society as a whole.

Though these principles are grounded in historical values of liberal Protestantism, they have had widespread appeal to nonreligious and post-Christian Americans, so as the number of liberal Protestants has declined and the number of religious "nones" has expanded, support for abortion rights has remained strong. But as both religious and nonreligious supporters have become ideologically removed from the mid-twentieth-century Protestant framework for valuing fetuses as at least *potential* human beings, the historic mainline Protestant moderation on abortion that has long influenced mainstream U.S. politics has begun to rapidly disappear. Fewer pro-choice Americans now express moral reservations about abortion. The Democratic Party no longer promises to make abortion "safe, legal, and rare." Though Americans may not yet support abortion itself as a positive good, those who support abortion rights are nevertheless far less likely than liberal Protestants of the previous generation to view abortion as morally problematic. In the 1970s, many religious supporters of abortion rights said that the law should allow women to make their own decisions about pregnancy termination even if the abortion decisions they made were morally wrong. Now abortion rights supporters are more likely to say that if an individual makes a decision for abortion, it must be the morally right choice for them, which is a consistent application of the principle that the highest form of moral authority is individual moral intuition.

As a result, there is now a very close correlation between Americans' views of abortion's morality and their views of whether it should be legal. Thus, for instance, a 2022 Pew survey showed that among those who thought that abortion should always be legal, only 7 percent viewed abortion as morally wrong in all or most cases, and among those who said that abortion should mostly be legal but with some exceptions, only 28 percent viewed abortion as morally wrong in all or most cases. By contrast, 94 percent of those who thought abortion should always be illegal viewed abortion as wrong in most or all cases, as did 86 percent of those who thought abortion should be mostly illegal but with some exceptions.[65]

For several decades, liberal Protestants who wanted abortion to remain legal were still willing to question its morality, but now this attempt to differentiate between the morality and legality of abortion has become increasingly rare. When liberal Presbyterian minister Rebecca Todd Peters insisted that she was not sinning when she had two abortions — and that her denomination should remove any suggestion that abortion was morally shameful from its official statements on abortion — it was a sign that many liberal Protestants were ready to abandon the moral reservations with which they had generally tempered their abortion rights campaigns. And when Kamala Harris became the first vice president to tour an abortion clinic, it was a similar sign that the Democratic Party was ready to quit moderating its abortion rights advocacy with any hint that abortion rates needed to be lowered and that the party now intended to treat abortion not merely as a choice but as necessary health care, just as liberal Protestant churches were doing.

The liberal Christian campaign for reproductive justice is thus becoming less moderate and less predominantly Christian than it has been in the past. And if liberal pro-choice Christians failed to find a way in the early 1970s to reconcile an affirmation of abortion rights with a commitment to a religiously pluralistic society that included people with a wide variety of views on abortion, they are even less likely to do so today, especially if they do not have an answer for how people with alternative sources of moral authority on the issue of abortion can work together in the same political space.

In contrast to the pro-choice cause, the religious campaign against abortion is grounded in a theology that emphasizes fixed, transcendent moral standards and God's sovereignty in creating life. Pro-life Christians define the value of human beings not in terms of their relationship to other people or in terms of their ability to make rational choices or enjoy a certain quality of life, but rather in their relationship to their Creator. People are eternally valuable because they are made in the image of God, a principle that applies to all people at every stage of development, regardless of whether others around them recognize their value or welcome their existence. That is why a zygote created in the image of God has just as much value as a full-grown adult, because it is part of God's eternal plan. The biblical prohibition against taking human life is not merely a useful social principle but is rather an unchangeable divine mandate based on the recognition that human beings exist only because of God's will and that God has created them for an eternal purpose and has given them infinite worth. Pro-life Christians therefore see abortion not only as an attack on human beings but as a direct affront to God. They also believe that unless the value of human life is grounded in theistic principles, no human rights or human lives are secure. To live in a society stripped of all theistic underpinnings or divinely grounded fixed moral principles is deeply frightening to them.

Pro-life Christians have not always agreed on what a pro-life society would look like. Some have imagined a liberal democratic, pluralistic society that is nevertheless grounded in Christian humanism, as Vatican II envisioned. Others have imagined a society of limited government but with a strong tradition of religious liberty and parental rights. Still others in recent years have imagined some sort of postliberal society that emphasizes community values at the local level.[66] But nearly all pro-life Christians have been alarmed at the prospect of a secular society that has no framework for valuing human life.

Pro-life Christians have often hoped that their cause might appeal to those outside of their own religious tradition, and on occasion they have found a few nonreligious people and even atheists who were willing to champion the pro-life cause on secular philosophical grounds. But because the pro-life cause is grounded in an understanding of the value of fetal life that is difficult for many people who lack a theistic framework to fully embrace—and because the pro-life ethic requires many people to sacrifice their own interests and well-being when preserving fetal life and bringing a child into the world is inconvenient—the majority of people who lack a theistic framework for understanding the value of human life have not sided with the pro-life campaign. To sustain its numbers, the pro-life cause has instead had to deepen its support among religious Americans, becoming more overtly Christian and more theologically and socially conservative over time. During the past half century, Christians who believe in a fixed standard of moral authority—whether scripture alone or the moral authority of the church—have united across the Protestant/Catholic divide to support the pro-life cause, even as others who do not share this moral framework have abandoned it. And in turn, the pro-life campaign has itself become less secular and pluralistic. Pro-life advocates are more willing than ever before to ground their campaign in explicitly theistic claims and to link their campaign for unborn human life to a campaign for a Christian nation.

Because the Christian framework for opposition to abortion is not based on the primacy of individual choice, pro-lifers have generally been far less concerned than pro-choice advocates about restricting people's right to make choices that are evil. They have been much more interested in building a humane or rightly ordered, God-honoring society than in empowering people to make choices that they think will destroy themselves and others. They believe that expanding abortion availability will not ultimately advance women's well-being, because giving people the power to destroy others' lives will never lead to ultimate happiness. What appears to their opponents to be misogyny or opposition to feminism is in reality a reflection of a very different understanding of what a good and humane society looks like. Pregnant women are not liberated by being given the tools to destroy the children they are carrying in their wombs, pro-lifers believe; instead, they are given true freedom when they are empowered to care for their children and pursue the calling that God has given them, a calling of genuine love for others.

Is there any room for common ground between these competing views? Perhaps one can start by acknowledging the different frames of moral reference that each side has embraced. If advocates of reproductive rights acknowledge that the pro-life campaign is not based on opposition to women's rights but instead is grounded in a concern for human life and a belief in divinely ordained transcendent moral principles, they could at least understand where their opponents are coming from. And similarly, if pro-life Christians recognize that advocates of reproductive rights are motivated by a commitment to a religiously pluralistic society that values free choice and gender equality, they might be able to take the first step toward a meaningful dialogue with those who disagree with their position.

The two sides do not necessarily have equal claims to validity. When it comes to Christian theology, the pro-life position is grounded in claims that have much deeper roots in the Christian tradition than the pro-choice position, which is why most contemporary advocates of abortion rights, even while citing some scriptures or Christian theologians that might provide some support for their interpretations, concede that their ultimate source of moral authority is not a direct scriptural mandate or church tradition but rather the right of individuals to make moral choices for themselves. But when it comes to matters of politics, the pro-choice side is probably on much firmer ground, because its emphasis on gender equality and the primacy of individual choice accords well with the values that most Americans outside of conservative religious circles generally share. It is difficult to see how the pro-life side can prevail at a moment when only a minority of Americans are churchgoing Christians. Regular church attenders may be becoming more strongly pro-life than ever, but if the rest of society is not, it's difficult to see how the pro-life side can win lasting political victories in a culture that generally rejects their assumptions about God, human life, and transcendent sources of moral authority. If the pro-life ethic demands self-sacrifice and a commitment to marriage, sexual chastity, and care for others that is largely foreign to the values of an individualistic society, an ethic of "choice" and reproductive rights will probably seem more appealing to a majority of voters in all but the most heavily churchgoing states.

Faced with this conundrum, some pro-life Christians will likely be tempted to abandon the concept of a pluralistic democracy altogether and double down on efforts to impose Christian values on society, even when they are in the political minority. If they attempt to do this by short-circuiting the democratic process through the courts, it will only exacerbate political polarization and invite a greater backlash from those who view Christian politics as a threat to their own values.

But likewise, pro-choicers who are outraged at the rescinding of *Roe v. Wade* and the rise of abortion bans across much of the Bible Belt will be tempted to overlook the ways in which their own assumptions have blinded them to the reasons why a majority of churchgoing Christians view the pro-choice agenda as a grave threat to human rights and an attack on fundamental American values. They have failed to understand why their opponents cannot in good conscience simply retreat to their churches and make their own moral decisions for themselves without interfering with anyone else's right to do the same. Both sides in the conflict have failed to understand their opponents and have instead viewed their own political platform as an axiomatic way to preserve the foundational values of the nation and of their own religious faith.

That is why this debate is so intractable. But if we're ever going to make headway, it will come not from trying to crush one's opponents, but by dialoguing with them. And when we do that, we may find that despite deep disagreements, all of us want to live out the values of our own consciences, honor the principles of God as we understand them, and champion foundational human rights that are the basis for a humane and just society. Yet we have different understandings of what those values are and how they should be applied, and that's where the challenge lies. More than fifty years after *Roe*, we are still left with the questions that the Supreme Court could not resolve in that decision. As a result, the debate continues, both in our churches and in our national life.

NOTES

Introduction

1. Charles Carroll, "Abortion without Ethics? The Legal Becomes Moral," n.d. [ca. 1972], folder 7, box 15, George Huntston Williams Papers, Harvard Divinity School; Patrick Joyce, "'Choose Life,' Speakers Singers Tell Youth Rally," National Catholic News Service, September 5, 1972, Folder: "Series 7.2: 1972 Campaign Subject File—Health: Abortion [Ahmann] (2 of 3)," R. Sargent Shriver Papers, John F. Kennedy Library, Boston, MA.

2. Germain Grisez, *Abortion: The Myths, the Realities, and the Arguments* (New York: Corpus Books, 1970), 259–60; Daniel Callahan, *Abortion: Law, Choice and Morality* (New York: Macmillan, 1970), 436; Raymond A. Schroth, *Bob Drinan: The Controversial Life of the First Catholic Priest Elected to Congress* (New York: Fordham University Press, 2011).

3. For an exposition of this view, see Randall Balmer, "The Religious Right and the Abortion Myth," *Politico*, May 10, 2022, https://www.politico.com/news/magazine/2022/05/10/abortion-history-right-white-evangelical-1970s-00031480. For a refutation of some of Balmer's arguments, see Gillian Frank and Neil J. Young, "What Everyone Gets Wrong about Evangelicals and Abortion," *Washington Post*, May 16, 2022.

4. For an overview of the formation of twentieth-century liberal Protestant theology and politics, see Gene Zubovich, *Before the Religious Right: Liberal Protestants, Human Rights, and the Polarization of the United States* (Philadelphia: University of Pennsylvania Press, 2022); David A. Hollinger, *Christianity's American Fate: How Religion Became More Conservative and Society More Secular* (Princeton, NJ: Princeton University Press, 2022); Gary Dorrien, *The Spirit of American Liberal Theology: A History* (Louisville, KY: Westminster John Knox Press, 2023).

5. For histories of the formation of American evangelicalism, see George M. Marsden, *Fundamentalism and American Culture*, 3rd ed. (New York: Oxford

University Press, 2022); Thomas S. Kidd, *Who Is an Evangelical? A History of a Movement in Crisis* (New Haven, CT: Yale University Press, 2019).

6. For more on the LDS Church's position on abortion and its relationship to the larger Religious Right, see Neil J. Young, *We Gather Together: The Religious Right and the Problem of Interfaith Politics* (New York: Oxford University Press, 2015).

7. For a more broadly focused study of religion and abortion that includes some non-Christian religious traditions, see Rebecca Todd Peters and Margaret D. Kamitsuka, eds., *T&T Clark Reader in Abortion and Religion: Jewish, Christian, and Muslim Perspectives* (New York: Bloomsbury Academic, 2023).

8. For studies of abortion politics, see Mary Ziegler, *After Roe: The Lost History of the Abortion Debate* (Cambridge, MA: Harvard University Press, 2015); Ziegler, *Abortion and the Law in America: Roe v. Wade to the Present* (New York: Cambridge University Press, 2020); Jennifer L. Holland, *Tiny You: A Western History of the Anti-Abortion Movement* (Oakland: University of California Press, 2020); David J. Garrow, *Liberty and Sexuality: The Right to Privacy and the Making of Roe v. Wade* (Berkeley: University of California Press, 1994). For sociological studies of the motivations of activists on both sides of the political debate over abortion, see Kristin Luker, *Abortion and the Politics of Motherhood* (Berkeley: University of California Press, 1984); Ziad W. Munson, *The Making of Pro-Life Activists: How Social Movement Mobilization Works* (Chicago: University of Chicago Press, 2008).

9. For evidence of the close connection between denominational identity, regular church attendance, and adherence to a particular denomination's views on abortion, see the polling data presented in the Pew Research Center's Religious Landscape Study of 2014; for example, Pew Research Center, "Religious Landscape Study: Views about Abortion among Members of the Southern Baptist Convention" (2014), https://www.pewresearch.org/religious-landscape-study/database/religious-denomination/southern-baptist-convention/views-about-abortion/; Pew Research Center, "Religious Landscape Study: Views about Abortion among Members of the United Church of Christ" (2014), https://www.pewresearch.org/religious-landscape-study/database/religious-denomination/united-church-of-christ/views-about-abortion/.

10. See, for instance, Michele F. Margolis, *From Politics to the Pews: How Partisanship and the Political Environment Shape Religious Identity* (Chicago: University of Chicago Press, 2018).

CHAPTER 1. Liberal Protestants before *Roe*

1. Douglas Martin, "Howard Moody, Who Led a Historic Church, Dies at 91," *New York Times*, September 13, 2012. For an estimate on the annual number of illegal abortions in New York during the mid-twentieth century, see "Huge Profit Laid to Abortion Ring," *New York Times*, October 16, 1941.

2. John Calvin, "Commentary on Exodus 21," quoted in Dennis Di Mauro, *A Love for Life: Christianity's Consistent Protection of the Unborn* (Eugene, OR: Wipf and Stock, 2008), 26.

3. David Albert Jones, *The Soul of the Embryo: An Enquiry into the Status of the Human Embryo in the Christian Tradition* (London: Continuum, 2004), 141–50.

4. James C. Mohr, *Abortion in America: The Origins and Evolution of National Policy, 1800–1900* (New York: Oxford University Press, 1978); Marvin Olasky and Leah Savas, *The Story of Abortion in America: A Street-Level History, 1652–2022* (Wheaton, IL: Crossway, 2023), 45–47.

5. Cornelia Hughes Dayton, "Taking the Trade: Abortion and Gender Relations in an Eighteenth-Century New England Village," *William and Mary Quarterly* 48 (1991): 23.

6. Mohr, *Abortion in America*; Leslie J. Reagan, *When Abortion Was a Crime: Women, Medicine, and Law in the United States, 1867–1973* (Berkeley: University of California Press, 1997); Frederick N. Dyer, *The Physicians' Crusade against Abortion* (Sagamore Beach, MA: Science History Publications, 2005).

7. Dyer, *Physicians' Crusade against Abortion*, 121–26.

8. Dyer, *Physicians' Crusade against Abortion*, 126.

9. Quoted in Sabrina Danielsen, "Creating the Litmus Test: Abortion, Mainline Protestants, and the Rise of the Religious Right" (PhD diss., University of Pennsylvania, 2014), 62.

10. Joanna N. Lahey, "The Effect of Anti-Abortion Legislation on Nineteenth Century Fertility," *Demography* 51 (2014): 939–48. For antivice legislative campaigns of the post–Civil War era, see Gaines M. Foster, *Moral Reconstruction: Christian Lobbyists and the Federal Legislation of Morality, 1865–1920* (Chapel Hill: University of North Carolina Press, 2002). The text of the Comstock Act can be found at https://www.congress.gov/42/llsb/S.1572v3.pdf.

11. For the Social Gospel, see Christopher H. Evans, *The Social Gospel in American Religion: A History* (New York: New York University Press, 2017).

12. Federal Council of Churches, "The Social Creed of the Churches" (1908), https://nationalcouncilofchurches.us/common-witness-ncc/the-social-creed-of-the-churches/.

13. For the history of Protestant attitudes toward birth control before and after the 1920s, see Kathleen A. Tobin, *The American Religious Debate over Birth Control, 1907–1937* (Jefferson, NC: McFarland and Co., 2001); Allan Carlson, *Godly Seed: American Evangelicals Confront Birth Control, 1873–1973* (New Brunswick, NJ: Transaction, 2012).

14. Melissa J. Wilde, *Birth Control Battles: How Race and Class Divided American Religion* (Oakland: University of California Press, 2020). For the larger social context of birth control discussions among Protestants, see Simone M. Caron, *Who Chooses? American Reproductive History since 1830* (Gainesville: University Press of Florida, 2008).

15. "Dr. Fosdick Urges Birth Rate Control," *New York Times*, December 5, 1927.

16. Wilde, *Birth Control Battles*, 101.

17. Wilde, *Birth Control Battles*, 8. For liberal Protestant ministers' support for birth control in the 1920s, see also R. Marie Griffith, *Moral Combat: How Sex Divided American Christians and Fractured American Politics* (New York: Basic Books, 2017), 1–48.

18. Tom Davis, *Sacred Work: Planned Parenthood and Its Clergy Alliances* (New Brunswick, NJ: Rutgers University Press, 2005), 55–56.

19. Wilde, *Birth Control Battles*; Davis, *Sacred Work*, 56–61.

20. Joseph Fletcher, *Situation Ethics: The New Morality* (Philadelphia: Westminster Press, 1966).

21. Daniel K. Williams, *Defenders of the Unborn: The Pro-Life Movement before Roe v. Wade* (New York: Oxford University Press, 2016), 20–35.

22. Fletcher, *Morals and Medicine* (1954), as quoted in Kerry N. Jacoby, *Souls, Bodies, Spirits: The Drive to Abolish Abortion since 1973* (Westport, CT: Praeger, 1998), 3; "Abortion Laws Should Be Revised," *Christian Century*, January 11, 1961, 37; "Abortion by Consent?," *Christian Century*, February 1, 1967, 132.

23. "Abortion by Consent?," 132; Lawrence Lader, *Abortion* (Indianapolis: Bobbs-Merrill, 1966), 99; "Abortion Laws Should Be Revised."

24. National Council of Churches of Christ in the USA, "Responsible Parenthood," February 28, 1961, https://nationalcouncilofchurches.us/common-witness-ncc/responsible-parenthood/.

25. Frank J. Curran, "Religious Implications," in *Abortion in America: Medical, Psychiatric, Legal, Anthropological, and Religious Considerations*, ed. Harold Rosen (Boston: Beacon Press, 1967), 157, 160.

26. Langdon Gilkey, "Dissolution and Reconstruction in Theology," *Christian Century*, February 3, 1965, 135. For the role of civil rights and antiwar activism in shaping liberal Protestantism during the 1960s, see Michael B. Friedland, *Lift Up Your Voice Like a Trumpet: White Clergy and the Civil Rights and Antiwar Movements, 1954–1973* (Chapel Hill: University of North Carolina Press, 1998).

27. Margaret Lamberts Bendroth, *A School for the Church: Andover Newton across Two Centuries* (Grand Rapids, MI: William B. Eerdmans, 2008), 165–66.

28. Harvey Cox, *The Secular City: Secularization and Urbanization in Theological Perspective* (New York: Macmillan, 1965), 30–31, 214.

29. Tom Davis, *Sacred Work: Planned Parenthood and Its Clergy Alliances* (New Brunswick, NJ: Rutgers University Press, 2005), 129–31; Doris Andrea Dirks and Patricia A. Relf, *To Offer Compassion: A History of the Clergy Consultation Service on Abortion* (Madison: University of Wisconsin Press, 2017).

30. This analysis is based in part on information in Dirks and Relf, *To Offer Compassion*; Alan Petigny, *The Permissive Society: America, 1945–1960* (New York: Cambridge University Press, 2009); Beth Bailey, *Sex in the Heartland* (Cambridge, MA: Harvard University Press, 1999).

31. Sabrina Danielsen, "Creating the Litmus Test: Abortion, Mainline Protestants, and the Rise of the Religious Right" (PhD diss., University of Pennsylvania, 2014), 72–74.

32. Eunice Kennedy Shriver and Alan F. Guttmacher, "When Pregnancy Means Heartbreak," *McCall's*, April 1968, 133.

33. Letter to the editor on abortion, *Christian Century*, August 12, 1970, 972–73.

34. Karl Barth, *Church Dogmatics*, trans. G. T. Thomson (Edinburgh: T&T Clark, 1962), 3:4, sec. 55.2.

35. Letter to the editor on abortion, *Christian Century*, August 12, 1970, 972–73; J. Claude Evans, "The Abortion Decision: A Balance of Competing Rights," *Christian Century*, February 14, 1973, 197.

36. David R. Mace, *Abortion: The Agonizing Decision* (Nashville: Abingdon Press, 1972).

37. John Moore and John Pamperin, "Abortion and the Church," *Christian Century*, May 20, 1970, 629.

38. Charles H. Bayer, "Confessions of an Abortion Counselor," *Christian Century*, May 20, 1970, 626.

39. J. Robert Nelson, "What Does Theology Say about Abortion?," *Christian Century*, January 31, 1973, 128.

40. Resolution of the UMC Board of Christian Social Concerns, October 8, 1969, in "Background Statement for the Vote of the United Church Board for Homeland Ministries on Abortion," April 1970, Folder: "Post, A.D.—Current Projects, Abortion," box 7, Office of the President—Avery D. Post Papers, United Church of Christ (UCC) Archives, Cleveland, OH.

41. Paul Ramsey, "Feticide/Infanticide upon Request," *Religion in Life*, Summer 1970.

42. Religious Coalition for Abortion Rights, "The Abortion Rights Issue: How We Stand," February 15, 1974.

43. Lutheran Church in America, "Resolution on Abortion Passed at the Fifth Biennial Convention," June 1970, in Massachusetts Commission on Christian Unity, "Abortion: Positions Taken by Religious Bodies," n.d. [ca. 1970 or 1971], Folder: "Moss—Subject Files—Abortion Issues," box 3, Office of the President—Robert V. Moss Papers, UCC Archives.

44. Reproduced in Religious Coalition for Abortion Rights, "The Abortion Rights Issue: How We Stand," February 15, 1974, Folder: Moss—Subject Files—Abortion Issues," box 3, Office of the President—Robert V. Moss Papers, UCC Archives.

45. "Resolution of the 62nd General Convention of the Episcopal Church (1967)," quoted in Episcopal Church, Resolution 1976-D095, "Reaffirm the 1967 General Convention Statement on Abortion" (1976), https://episcopalarchives.org/cgi-bin/acts/acts_resolution.pl?resolution=1976-D095.

46. Episcopal Church Women, "Resolution on Abortion," October 1970, in Massachusetts Commission on Christian Unity, "Abortion: Positions Taken by Religious Bodies."

47. "Summit Conference on Abortion," *Christian Century*, March 25, 1970, 348.

48. Quoted in Mary S. Melcher, *Pregnancy, Motherhood, and Choice in Twentieth-Century Arizona* (Tucson: University of Arizona Press, 2012), 145.

49. "Pornography and Court Presuppositions," *Christian Century*, July 18, 1973, 748. For liberal Protestants' emphasis on personal moral decision-making in the 1950s, see George M. Marsden, *The Twilight of the American Enlightenment: The 1950s and the Crisis of Liberal Belief* (New York: Basic Books, 2014).

For the effects that the Vietnam War and the civil rights movement had on liberal Protestant ministers' ethical and political views, see Michael B. Friedland, *Lift up Your Voice Like a Trumpet: White Clergy and the Civil Rights and Antiwar Movements, 1954–1973* (Chapel Hill: University of North Carolina Press, 1998).

50. "UCC Synod Narrows Behavior-Belief Gap," *Christian Century*, July 14, 1971, 850.

51. American Baptist Convention, "Resolution on Abortion," June 1968, Baylor University, https://digitalcollections-baylor.quartexcollections.com/Documents/Detail/resolution-on-abortion-from-the-american-baptist-convention/809704.

52. United Methodist Church, "Statement of Social Principles" (1972), in *Before Roe v. Wade: Voices That Shaped the Abortion Debate before the Supreme Court's Ruling*, ed. Linda Greenhouse and Reva B. Siegel (New York: Kaplan, 2010), 70.

53. "Physician Statistics Summary (1970–1999)," Pinnacle Health Group, http://www.phg.com/2000/01/physician-statistics-summary/; Ethan Michelson, "Women in the Legal Profession, 1970–2010: A Study of the Global Supply of Lawyers," *Indiana Journal of Global Legal Studies* 20 (2013): 1082; Rita G. Burnett, "The Evolution of Women Pastors in Mainline Protestant Denominations" (PhD diss., Western Kentucky University, 2017), 6.

54. Betty Friedan, "Abortion: A Woman's Right," speech at the First National Conference on Abortion Laws, Chicago, February 16, 1969, https://awpc.cattcenter.iastate.edu/2022/02/23/abortion-a-womans-civil-right-feb-16-1969/. For a history of the abortion rights movement in the late 1960s and early 1970s, see David J. Garrow, *Liberty and Sexuality: The Right to Privacy and the Making of Roe v. Wade*, 2nd ed. (Berkeley: University of California Press, 1998).

55. Williams, *Defenders of the Unborn*, 149.

56. Editor's response to letter to the editor on abortion, *Christian Century*, August 12, 1970, 973.

57. For second-wave feminism and reproductive rights in the early 1970s, see Sara M. Evans, *Tidal Wave: How Women Changed America at Century's End* (New York: Free Press, 2003).

58. Church Women United, Resolution on Abortion, March 19, 1970, Folder: "Subject Files: Abortion, 1969–1971," box 12, Council for Christian Social Action, 1957–1975, UCC Archives.

59. Friedan, "Abortion: A Woman's Right."

60. Church Women United, Resolution on Abortion, March 19, 1970, Folder: "Subject Files: Abortion, 1969–1971," box 12, Council for Christian Social Action, 1957–1975, UCC Archives. Cleveland, OH.

61. Quoted in Religious Coalition for Abortion Rights brochure, "We Affirm . . .," 1982, Folder: "Post, A.D.—Current Projects, Abortion," Office of the President—Avery D. Post Papers, UCC Archives.

62. Rachel Conrad Wahlberg, "An Author's Response," *Christian Century*, March 1, 1972, 264.

63. Judith Jarvis Thomson, "A Defense of Abortion," *Philosophy and Public Affairs* 1 (Fall 1971), https://spot.colorado.edu/~heathwoo/Phil160,Fall02/thomson.htm.

64. Glenda Adams Hess, "Biological Personhood," *Christian Century*, December 8, 1971, 1450–51.

65. J. Claude Evans, "Defusing the Abortion Debate," *Christian Century*, January 31, 1973, 118.

66. Howard Moody, "Church, State and the Rights of Conscience," *Christianity and Crisis*, January 8, 1973, 293.

67. Dena S. Davis, "Moral Ambition: The Sermons of Harry A. Blackmun," *Brooklyn Law Review* 72 (2006): 211–35.

68. *Roe v. Wade*, 410 U.S. 113 (1973), https://supreme.justia.com/cases/federal/us/410/113/.

69. *Roe v. Wade*, 410 U.S. 113 (1973), https://supreme.justia.com/cases/federal/us/410/113/.

70. Mary Ellen Haines and Helen Webber, "Reflections on the Supreme Court's Ruling on Abortion," *A.D.*, April 1973, 60.

71. Harry Blackmun to conference of Supreme Court justices, December 11, 1972, and December 15, 1972, folder 4, box 151, Harry Blackmun Papers, Library of Congress, Washington, DC; Lewis Powell to Harry Blackmun, November 29, 1972, folder 8, box 151, Blackmun Papers; Thurgood Marshall to Harry Blackmun, December 12, 1972, folder 4, box 151, Blackmun Papers; Harry Blackmun to Lewis Powell, December 4, 1972, folder 4, box 151, Blackmun Papers; Harry Blackmun to conference of Supreme Court justices, November 21, 1972, folder 8, box 151, Blackmun Papers.

72. Harry A. Blackmun, "Statement from the bench re: *Roe v. Wade* and *Doe v. Bolton*," January 1973, folder 3, box 151, Blackmun Papers.

73. Harry Blackmun to Joseph H. Pratt, January 31, 1973, folder 1, box 68, Blackmun Papers.

74. Barbara Campbell, "Mrs. Abzug Spurs Bill to End All Abortion Laws," *New York Times*, January 27, 1973.

75. Lee Gidding to Robert H. Tamis, April 17, 1973, Folder: "AZ, 1969–75," carton 2, NARAL Records, 1968–1976, Schlesinger Library, Harvard University.

76. Planned Parenthood, "Could the Supreme Court 'Abortion' Decisions Be Lost? Yes!," April 1973, folder 12, box 11, Wilma Scott Heide Papers, Schlesinger Library, Harvard University.

77. For the process by which this happened, see Mary Ziegler, *After Roe: The Lost History of the Abortion Debate* (Cambridge, MA: Harvard University Press, 2015); Ziegler, *Roe: The History of a National Obsession* (New Haven, CT: Yale University Press, 2023).

CHAPTER 2. Catholics before *Roe*

1. Grace Burns to Harry Blackmun, January 30, 1973, Folder 4: "Supreme Court—Correspondence—Abortion Mail—Unanswered—Reviewed—Critical, Jan. 28–31, 1973," box 71, Harry Blackmun Papers, Library of Congress, Washington, DC.

2. Most of the biographical information about Burns and her family comes from her husband's obituary: Obituary for Paul Francis Burns, *Tecumseh (MI) Herald*, September 11, 2014, https://www.tecumsehherald.com/content/paul-francis-burns.

3. These assessments are based on a survey of letters to Blackmun that are included in box 71 of the Blackmun Papers, Library of Congress.

4. *Didache*, trans. G. C. Allen (London: Astolat Press, 1903), 2.2. Other translations quoted come from Alexander Roberts and James Donaldson (1886), Tony Jones (2009), and Cyril C. Richardson (1953).

5. Athenagoras, *A Plea for the Christians*, trans. B. P. Pratten (Buffalo, NY: Christian Literature Publishing, 1885), chap. 35.

6. Tertullian, *A Treatise on the Soul*, trans. Peter Holmes (Buffalo, NY: Christian Literature Publishing, 1885), chap. 27.

7. Tertullian, *Apology*, trans. S. Thelwall (Buffalo, NY: Christian Literature Publishing, 1885), chap. 9.

8. Council of Ancyra (314), canon 21, https://www.newadvent.org/fathers/3802.htm; Basil, "First Canonical Epistle," canon 2, https://orthodoxchurchfathers.com/fathers/npnf214/npnf2284.htm.

9. John Connery, *Abortion: The Development of the Roman Catholic Perspective* (Chicago: Loyola University Press, 1977), 50.

10. Connery, *Abortion*, 51–59; David Jones, *The Soul of the Embryo: An Enquiry into the Status of the Human Embryo in the Christian Tradition* (London: Continuum, 2004), 109–24.

11. Jones, *Soul of the Embryo*, 133–34.

12. Connery, *Abortion*, 168–224; Jones, *Soul of the Embryo*, 166–70.

13. Connery, *Abortion*, 146–49, 212; Jones, *Soul of the Embryo*, 178–85.

14. Quoted in John T. McGreevy, *Catholicism and American Freedom: A History* (New York: W. W. Norton, 2003), 222.

15. For an example of the early twentieth-century debate between Protestants and Catholics over abortions that were necessary to save a pregnant woman's life, see Hector Treub et al., *The Right to Life of the Unborn Child* (New York: Joseph F. Wagner, 1903). For a historical study of this debate, see Connery, *Abortion*, 225–303.

16. National Catholic Welfare Conference, "Pastoral Letter of 1919," https://www.ewtn.com/catholicism/library/pastoral-letter-of-1919-3819.

17. "Cheapening Human Life," *America*, January 5, 1924, 283. For a study of the Protestant liberalization on birth control in the 1920s and 1930s, see Melissa J. Wilde, *Birth Control Battles: How Race and Class Divided American Religion* (Oakland: University of California Press, 2020).

18. Wilfrid Parsons, "A Crisis in Birth Control," *America*, May 4, 1935, 80.

19. Pius XI, *Casti Connubii* (1930), sec. 64, https://www.vatican.va/content/pius-xi/en/encyclicals/documents/hf_p-xi_enc_19301231_casti-connubii.html.

20. Quoted in McGreevy, *Catholicism and American Freedom*, 230.

21. Parsons, "A Crisis in Birth Control," 79–80; John LaFarge, "The Soviet Law concerning Legal Abortions," *America*, January 30, 1937, 388–89; J. Gerard Mears, "In Fear and in Secret They Do Damnable Deeds," *America*, May 2, 1942, 96–97; Harold C. Gardiner, "Hucksters in Death," *America*, January 25, 1947, 462–64.

22. See, for instance, lesson 35 in the third edition of the *Baltimore Catechism* (1949). For rates of Catholic compliance with the Church's teaching on contraception, see Leslie Woodcock Tentler, *Catholics and Contraception: An American History* (Ithaca, NY: Cornell University Press, 2004), 133–34.

23. Quoted in McGreevy, *Catholicism and American Freedom*, 258.

24. *Baltimore Catechism*, 3rd ed. (New York: Benziger Brothers, 1949), lesson 5.

25. *Baltimore Catechism*, 3rd ed., lesson 5.

26. "Therapeutic Abortion Is Wrong Morally and Medically Both," *Catholic Transcript*, July 31, 1958.

27. "A Pretty Bad Companion," *Catholic Standard and Times*, October 14, 1955.

28. McGreevy, *Catholicism and American Freedom*, 226–28.

29. "Dr. Moran Speaks against So-Called 'Abortion' Bill," *Nashua (NH) Telegraph*, February 23, 1961; "Nashua Area Ministers See Merit in New Therapeutic Abortion Bill," *Nashua (NH) Telegraph*, March 1, 1961.

30. Quoted in "Looming Moral Thunderheads," *America*, January 16, 1960, 444.

31. "Slaughter of the Innocent," *America*, June 2, 1962, 339.

32. "Slaughter of the Innocent," 339.

33. "Arizona Abortion Case," *America*, August 11, 1962, 582.

34. Gallup poll on abortion, August 23–28, 1962, in Gallup Organization, *America's Opinion on Abortion, 1962–1992* (Princeton, NJ: Gallup Organization, 1992); George Gallup, "Public Gives Its Views on Finkbine Case," *Los Angeles Times*, September 20, 1962.

35. For a historical study of Vatican II, see John W. O'Malley, *What Happened at Vatican II* (Cambridge, MA: Harvard University Press, 2008).

36. Vatican II, *Dignitatis Humanae*, sec. 2, https://www.vatican.va/archive/hist_councils/ii_vatican_council/documents/vat-ii_decl_19651207_dignitatis-humanae_en.html.

37. For liberal Catholics' emphasis on the moral authority of the individual conscience in the 1960s and afterward, see Peter Cajka, *Follow Your Conscience: The Catholic Church and the Spirit of the Sixties* (Chicago: University of Chicago Press, 2021).

38. George Weigel, *To Sanctify the World: The Vital Legacy of Vatican II* (New York: Basic Books, 2022).

39. Quoted in McGreevy, *Catholicism and American Freedom*, 238.

40. Vatican II, *Gaudium et Spes*, sec. 51, https://www.vatican.va/archive/hist_councils/ii_vatican_council/documents/vat-ii_const_19651207_gaudium-et-spes_en.html.

41. *Gaudium et Spes*, sec. 27.

42. "Catholics Draft Human-Rights Aim," *New York Times*, February 2, 1947.

43. John XXIII, *Pacem in Terris* (1963), sec. 11, https://www.vatican.va/content/john-xxiii/en/encyclicals/documents/hf_j-xxiii_enc_11041963_pacem.html.

44. *Pacem in Terris*, sec. 16.

45. *Pacem in Terris*, sec. 36.

46. James T. McHugh, "Abortion—Background Material," August 25, 1966, Folder 7: "Social Action: Health & Medicine: Abortion, 1966," box 87, National Catholic Welfare Conference Papers, Catholic University, Washington, DC.

47. Philip Denvir, "Cardinal Asks Change in Birth Control Law," *Boston Globe*, June 23, 1965.

48. "Note: The Current Trend to Liberalize Abortion Laws—An Analysis and Criticism," *Catholic Lawyer* 10, no. 2 (1964): 173.

49. "Morality and Policy: I," *America*, February 27, 1965, 280.

50. "Abortion and Divorce Reform," *America*, February 11, 1967.

51. "Morality and Policy, IV," *America*, April 17, 1965.

52. "Direct Abortion Opposed to God's Law," *Catholic Bulletin*, March 3, 1967.

53. Robert M. Byrn, "The Abortion Question: A Nonsectarian Approach," *Catholic Lawyer* 11, no. 4 (1965): 316.

54. Paul V. Harrington to W. N. Bergin, July 21, 1966, Folder: "Abortion, 1965–1967," box 1, Rev. Paul V. Harrington Papers, Archdiocese of Boston.

55. Richard A. McCormick, "Abortion," *America*, June 19, 1965.

56. Richard McCormick, "The Silence since *Humanae Vitae*," *Linacre Quarterly*, February 1974, 28, https://epublications.marquette.edu/cgi/viewcontent.cgi?article=3223&context=lnq. For a history of American Catholic dissent on contraception, see Tentler, *Catholics and Contraception*.

57. Marvin R. O'Connell, "Abortion Rhetoric and Hypocrisy," *Catholic News*, November 19, 1970, 5.

58. Lawrence Lader, "Why Birth Control Fails," *McCall's*, October 1969, 164–65.

59. Germain Grisez, *Abortion: The Myths, the Realities, and the Arguments* (New York: Corpus Books, 1970), 424.

60. Paul F. Tanner to Albert J. Bell, June 25, 1966, Folder 7: "Social Action: Health & Medicine: Abortion, 1966," box 87, National Catholic Welfare Conference Papers, Catholic University Archives, Washington, DC.

61. James T. McHugh, Sermon Outline, [January 1969], Folder 1: "Abortion," box 1, Chancery Office Records, Diocese of Harrisburg, PA.

62. For the history of this argument in the 1960s, see Daniel K. Williams, *Defenders of the Unborn: The Pro-Life Movement before Roe v. Wade* (New York: Oxford University Press, 2016), 47–48.

63. National Conference of Catholic Bishops, Declaration on Abortion, November 18, 1970, https://www.priestsforlife.org/magisterium/bishops/70-11-18declarationonabortionnccb.htm.

64. William Willoughby, "O'Boyle Charges Genocide," *Washington Evening Star-News*, August 7, 1972.

65. Grisez, *Abortion*, 323–25, 337–39.

66. Hiley H. Ward, "Dearden Ties War Protest to Fight against Abortion," *Detroit Free Press*, September 29, 1972.

67. Edward M. Kennedy to Mrs. Edward J. Barshak, August 3, 1971, Folder 31: "MORAL (Mass. Organization to Repeal Abortion Laws), 1970–1974," box 2, Patricia Gold Papers, Schlesinger Library, Harvard University.

68. Williams, *Defenders of the Unborn*, 163–64.

69. For one of the many examples of these predictions, see Frank J. Ayd Jr., "Liberal Abortion Laws," *America*, February 1, 1969.

70. Patricia Miller, *Good Catholics: The Battle over Abortion in the Catholic Church* (Berkeley: University of California Press, 2014), 74–75; Kenneth Briggs, "Ousted Jesuit Floats in an Earthly Limbo," *New York Times*, October 14, 1975.

71. John Deedy, "Abortion," *New York Times*, February 18, 1973.

72. "Gallup Poll Finds Public Divided on Abortions in First 3 Months," *New York Times*, January 28, 1973.

73. Rachelle Patterson, "Citizens for Life Replace Catholic Church as Leader in Mass. Abortion Battle," *Boston Globe*, May 15, 1974; Hamilton F. Allen, "Abortion Law Ruled Illegal," *Providence Evening Bulletin*, June 10, 1975.

74. Gallup poll on abortion, January 1966, in Gallup Organization, *America's Opinion on Abortion*.

75. Gallup poll on abortion, November 1969; Gallup, "Public Evenly Divided on Abortion during Early Stage of Pregnancy," 1973; Gallup poll on abortion, March 1974; Gallup, "Public Attitudes Are Split over Court Abortion Ruling," 1973, all in Gallup Organization, *America's Opinion on Abortion*.

76. Ashley Montagu, unpublished letter to the editor of the *New York Times*, March 3, 1967, box 2, Lawrence Lader Papers, Countway Medical Library, Harvard University.

77. Robert M. Byrn, "The Abortion Amendments: Policy in the Light of Precedent," *Saint Louis University Law Journal* 18 (1974): 391.

78. James T. McHugh, "Poor Distribution of Americans, Yes; Overpopulation, No," *Catholic Witness*, September 10, 1970.

79. *Gaudium et Spes*, sec. 22; McHugh, Sermon Outline.

80. "Abortion: The Catholic Presentation," *America*, January 23, 1971, 62.

81. Nora Clare Sharkey, "Alliance Formed to Fight N.Y. Abortion Law," *Catholic News*, October 22, 1970, 1; "Women's First Sermons Preach Anti-Abortion," *Catholic News*, October 29, 1970, 3.

82. Williams, *Defenders of the Unborn*, 147–55; 225–29; Stacie Taranto, *Kitchen Table Politics: Conservative Women and Family Values in New York* (Philadelphia: University of Pennsylvania Press, 2017).

83. Sidney Callahan, "Feminist as Antiabortionist," *National Catholic Reporter*, April 7, 1972, 11; Callahan, "Abortion: Abandoning Women and Children," Minnesota Citizens Concerned for Life publication [1970], Folder: "Miscellaneous Information and Handouts, 1971–1972," box 5, North Dakota Right to Life Association Records, State Historical Society of North Dakota, Bismarck.

84. Mary Winter, "Abortion—The Abandonment of Women and Children," 1972, Mary Winter Papers, Schlesinger Library, Harvard University.

85. Mary Winter, speech, West Virginians for Life Annual Banquet, October 1982, Mary Winter Papers.

86. Winter, "Abortion—The Abandonment of Women and Children."

87. Winter, "Abortion—The Abandonment of Women and Children."

88. Mary Ann Knight, Editorial Rebuttal for KHJ radio station (Hollywood, CA), November 3, 1970, folder 12, box 509, Anthony C. Beilenson Papers, UCLA.

89. Eileen King to Anthony Beilenson, April 17, 1967, folder 4, box 520, Beilenson Papers; Rosa J. Belonzie to Anthony Beilenson, March 30, 1967, folder 4, box 520, Beilenson Papers; Mary Miani to Anthony Beilenson, April 24, 1967, folder 4, box 520, Beilenson Papers; Mary Dowd to Anthony Beilenson, April 21, 1967, folder 4, box 520, Beilenson Papers.

90. Mary Kay Rennard to Beilenson, March 21, 1967, folder 4, box 520, Beilenson Papers; Maria K. Wagner to Anthony Beilenson, April 2, 1967, folder 4, box 520, Beilenson Papers.

91. Eunice Kennedy Shriver and Alan F. Guttmacher, "When Pregnancy Means Heartbreak: Is Abortion the Answer?," *McCall's*, April 1968, 140.

92. Shriver and Guttmacher, "When Pregnancy Means Heartbreak," 140.

93. Robert E. O'Malley to Harry Blackmun, January 25, 1973, folder 3, box 71, Blackmun Papers; Nancy Fillion to Harry Blackmun, January 25, 1973, folder 3, box 71, Blackmun Papers; Maureen E. Tauer to Harry Blackmun, January 28, 1973, folder 4, box 71, Blackmun Papers; Mrs. Paul Niem-

halt to Harry Blackmun, 30 January 1973, folder 4, box 71, Blackmun Papers; Mr. and Mrs. Warren A. Murray to Harry Blackmun, January 30, 1973, folder 4, box 71, Blackmun Papers; "Abortion Decision Assailed as Tragedy," *Catholic Standard*, January 25, 1973.

CHAPTER 3. Evangelicals before *Roe*

1. L. Nelson Bell, "An Alternative to Abortion," *Christianity Today*, June 18, 1971, 17.

2. One of the best studies of the origins of twentieth-century evangelicalism is George M. Marsden, *Fundamentalism and American Culture*, 2nd ed. (New York: Oxford University Press, 2006). Other useful historical studies of twentieth-century evangelicalism include Matthew Avery Sutton, *American Apocalypse: A History of American Evangelicalism* (Cambridge, MA: Harvard University Press, 2014); Steven P. Miller, *The Age of Evangelicalism: America's Born-Again Years* (New York: Oxford University Press, 2014); Joel A. Carpenter, *Revive Us Again: The Reawakening of American Fundamentalism* (New York: Oxford University Press, 1997).

3. Robert Hill, "The Home, the Key to the Situation," *Moody Monthly*, November 1928, 104. For the centrality of gender and family-related concerns in the fundamentalist movement of the 1920s, see Margaret Lamberts Bendroth, *Fundamentalism and Gender, 1875 to the Present* (New Haven, CT: Yale University Press, 1993).

4. John Roach Straton, *The Menace of Immorality in Church and State* (New York: George H. Doran, 1920), 82, 115.

5. Bob Jones Sr., "Editor's Page," *Bob Jones Magazine*, January 1930, 1; John R. Rice, *The Home: Courtship, Marriage, and Children* (Wheaton, IL: Sword of the Lord, 1945), 156. For a history of fundamentalists' opposition to abortion, see Andrew R. Lewis, "Abortion," in *The Oxford Handbook of Christian Fundamentalism*, ed. Andrew Atherstone and David Ceri Jones (New York: Oxford University Press, 2023), 474–94.

6. Evelyn Millis Duvall, *Facts of Life and Love for Teen-agers*, rev. ed. (New York: Popular Library, 1957), 57.

7. "Evangelicals Face Up to Birth Control Issue," *Christianity Today*, December 21, 1959, 31. For a history of evangelical attitudes toward birth control, see Allan Carlson, *Godly Seed: American Evangelicals Confront Birth Control, 1873–1973* (New Brunswick, NJ: Transaction, 2012).

8. Irene Soekren, "The Ring and the Pill," *Eternity*, September 1966, 32.

9. Robert H. Meneilly, "How Important Is the Sex Drive in the Middle Years?," *Christian Life*, April 1964, 38.

10. "Dr. Graham's View on Birth Control," *The Age* (Melbourne, Australia), December 16, 1959.

11. Billy Graham, "The Home," *Hour of Decision* (radio program), 1956, Billy Graham Center Archives, Wheaton College, Wheaton, IL.

12. All of these numbers are based on keyword searches in the *New York Times* database. The one *New York Times* article that mentioned abortion in 1961 was "Queens Doctor Held in Abortion-Death," *New York Times*, January 24, 1961.

13. Alfred Martin Rehwinkel, *Planned Parenthood and Birth Control in the Light of Christian Ethics* (St. Louis, MO: Concordia, 1959), 14.

14. Rehwinkel, *Planned Parenthood and Birth Control*, 93.

15. See, for instance, Ralph A. Cannon, "Sex and Smut on the Newsstands," *Christianity Today*, February 17, 1958.

16. Clyde M. Narramore, *Life and Love: A Christian View of Sex* (Grand Rapids, MI: Zondervan, 1956), 127–33.

17. Narramore, *Life and Love*, 169.

18. Megan Brenan, "Gallup Vault: Public Supported Therapeutic Abortion in 1962," Gallup, June 12, 2018, https://news.gallup.com/vault/235496/gallup-vault-public-supported-therapeutic-abortion-1962.aspx.

19. Frank J. Curran, "Religious Implications," in *Abortion in America: Medical, Psychiatric, Legal, Anthropological, and Religious Considerations*, 2nd ed., ed. Harold Rosen (Boston: Beacon Press, 1967), 154.

20. Roy Faulstick, "The Case against Abortion," *Lutheran News*, March 20, 1967, 6.

21. "And Now . . . A Nation of Mass Murder," *Baptist Bible Tribune*, September 22, 1967, 6.

22. William D. Freeland, "Inter-Faith Debate on Easing Abortion Laws," *Christianity Today*, April 28, 1967, 43.

23. S. I. McMillen, "Abortion: Is It Moral?," *Christian Life*, September 1967, 50, 53.

24. G. Archer Weniger, *Blu-Print* newsletter (Oakland, CA), May 31, 1977, Bob Jones University Archives.

25. Frank Stagg, *Polarities of Man's Existence in Biblical Perspective* (Philadelphia: Westminster Press, 1973), 51–53.

26. John Warwick Montgomery, "The Christian View of the Fetus," in *Birth Control and the Christian: A Protestant Symposium on the Control of Human Reproduction*, eds. Walter O. Spitzer and Carlyle L. Saylor (Wheaton, IL: Tyndale, 1968), 75, 83, 87.

27. Paul K. Jewett, "The Relationship of the Soul to the Fetus," in Spitzer and Saylor, eds., *Birth Control and the Christian*, 59–60.

28. Kenneth Kantzer, "The Origin of the Soul as Related to the Abortion Question," in Spitzer and Saylor, eds., *Birth Control and the Christian*, 556–58.

29. "A Protestant Affirmation on the Control of Human Reproduction," *Christianity Today*, 8 November 1968, 18.

30. "Capital Consistency," *Christianity Today*, June 20, 1969, 21.

31. Robert D. Visscher, "Therapeutic Abortion: Blessing or Murder?," *Christianity Today*, September 27, 1968, 6–8.

32. For the involvement of conservative Lutherans in the campaign against the proposal to liberalize California's abortion law in 1967, see "Right to Life League: Abortion Foes Open Campaign Here," *San Francisco Chronicle*, April 20, 1967.

33. Shortly before the Civil War, the Methodist, Baptist, and Presbyterian denominations in the United States split into southern and northern denominations. The Baptists are still divided into two regionally concentrated denominations today: the Southern Baptist Convention and the American Baptist Churches USA (formerly known as the Northern Baptist Convention). The southern and northern branches of the Methodists reunited in 1939. The Presbyterians remained regionally divided until 1983, when the southern Presbyterian denomination merged with the northern Presbyterian Church (USA). Until then, most southern Presbyterian churches were part of the southern regional denomination Presbyterian Church in the United States, which tended to be somewhat more socially conservative than its northern counterpart.

34. Presbyterian Church US, Minutes of the General Assembly, in Presbyterian Church US, "The Nature and Value of Human Life" (1981), 295, https://www.pcusa.org/site_media/media/uploads/_resolutions/the-nature-and-value-of-human-life.pdf.

35. Phil Strickland, "Changes Needed in TX Abortion Bill," *Baptist Standard*, March 31, 1971, 3.

36. Paul L. Sadler, "The Abortion Issue within the Southern Baptist Convention" (PhD diss., Baylor University, 1991), 25–26.

37. SBC, Resolution on Abortion, 1971, https://www.sbc.net/resource-library/resolutions/resolution-on-abortion-2/.

38. *Annual of the 1971 Southern Baptist Convention* (St. Louis, MO, June 1971), 72, http://media2.sbhla.org.s3.amazonaws.com/annuals/SBC_Annual_1971.pdf.

39. "The War on the Womb," *Christianity Today*, June 5, 1970, 24–25.

40. Billy Graham, "Any Abortion Method Violation of God's Law," *Atlanta Constitution*, November 27, 1972.

41. National Association of Evangelicals, "Abortion 1971," January 1, 1971, https://www.nae.org/abortion-1971/.

42. Carl F. H. Henry, *Confessions of a Theologian* (Waco, TX: Word Books, 1986), 333–34.

43. Lutheran Church—Missouri Synod (LCMS), Resolution 2-39: "To State Position on Abortion" (1971), https://files.lcms.org/dl/f/life-ministry-convention-resolutions-1941-2019.

44. LCMS Commission on Theology and Church Relations, "Abortion: Theological, Legal, and Medical Aspects" (1971), https://ctsfw.net/media/pdfs/CTCRAbortionTheologicalLegalandMedicalAspects.pdf.

45. Orthodox Presbyterian Church, "Report of the Committee to Study the Matter of Abortion," Presented to the Thirty-Eighth General Assembly of the Orthodox Presbyterian Church (1971), https://www.opc.org/GA/abortion.html#Action.

46. Orthodox Presbyterian Church, "Report of the Committee to Study the Matter of Abortion"; John M. Frame, "Abortion from a Biblical Perspective," in *Thou Shalt Not Kill: The Christian Case against Abortion*, ed. Richard L. Ganz (New Rochelle, NY: Arlington House, 1978), 43–75.

47. Christian Reformed Church, *Acts of Synod* (1972), 64, https://library.calvin.edu/ld.php?content_id=71779531.

48. For the role that the belief in moral absolutes played in the culture wars, see James Davison Hunter, *Culture Wars: The Struggle to Define America* (New York: Basic Books, 1991).

49. "Everyone Needs Theology," *Voice* (Dallas Theological Seminary), Fall 2006, https://voice.dts.edu/article/everyone-needs-theology-catherine-claire/.

50. "Women at Fuller: A History," Fuller Seminary, https://www.fuller.edu/wp-content/uploads/2019/01/HistoryofWomenatFuller.pdf.

51. *The Princeton Seminary Bulletin*, 1968–1969, https://archive.org/details/princetonseminar6151prin/page/14/mode/2up?view=theater.

52. Jewett, "The Relationship of the Soul to the Fetus," 65.

53. Nancy Hardesty, "Should Anyone Who Wants an Abortion Have One?," *Eternity*, June 1967, 32–34. For progressive evangelical feminism and discussions of abortion among progressive evangelicals, see Brantley W. Gasaway, *Progressive Evangelicals and the Pursuit of Social Justice* (Chapel Hill: University of North Carolina Press, 2014). For conservative evangelicals' rejection of feminism, see Kristin Kobes Du Mez, *Jesus and John Wayne: How White Evangelicals Corrupted a Faith and Fractured a Nation* (New York: Liveright, 2020).

54. Christian Action for Life newsletter, June 1980, digitized copy in author's personal collection; "Committee Is Working on New Abortion Statement," *Presbyterian Journal*, December 6, 1972, 6.

55. "The Big Issue: Women on the Move," *Christianity Today*, July 20, 1973. The article identifies Nelda Walker only as "Mrs. Harold Walker," and says that she was a pastor's wife in her thirties from Fort Smith, Arkansas, but through additional online research, I was able to establish that this "Mrs. Harold Walker" was almost certainly Nelda Walker, who was born in 1939 and was the wife of the pastor of Unity Missionary Baptist Church in Fort Smith, Arkansas.

56. "Against Abortion: Human Life Is Sacred, or It Isn't," *Indianapolis News*, January 28, 1971.

57. Robert J. Terrey, "Liberalizing Abortion or Murder?," *Plymouth Crusader* (MN), February 1971.

58. John R. Rice, *The Murder of the Helpless Unborn—Abortion* (Murfreesboro, TN: Sword of the Lord, 1971).

59. Joan Loebker, "Abortion Misconceptions," *Plymouth Crusader*, October 1973.

60. Edwin H. Palmer, "Abortions: A Form of Infanticide," *Presbyterian Journal*, March 24, 1971; Russell Chandler, "Death Knell for Southern Presbyterians?" *Christianity Today*, July 2, 1971.

61. Thomas Miller, "The Bible and Abortion," *Acccent!!!* (American Council of Christian Churches), April 1970.

62. "Conference Resolutions," *Ohio Bible Fellowship Visitor*, December 1970–January 1971.

63. Don Bell, "The Healer Has Become the Murderer," *Christian News*, October 19, 1970, 6.

64. William Robert Johnston, "Historical Abortion Statistics, United States," https://www.johnstonsarchive.net/policy/abortion/ab-unitedstates.html.

318   Notes to Pages 130–138

65. Assemblies of God, "Resolution on Abortion Adopted by the Thirty-Fourth General Council" (1971), in *Abortion, the Bible and the Church*, rev. ed., ed. T. J. Bosgra (Honolulu: Hawaii Right to Life Educational Foundation, 1980), 39.

66. Neel J. Price, "Abortion: Right? Wrong?," *Herald of Holiness*, July 31, 1974, 12. For discussions of abortion among Nazarenes in the mid-1970s, see James Dobson, *Family under Fire: A Conference Book* (Kansas City, MO: Beacon Hill Press, 1976). In the mid-1970s, James Dobson and his father, Reverend James Dobson Sr. (a Nazarene pastor), strongly opposed abortion, but some of their fellow Nazarenes accepted the legitimacy of abortion in at least some therapeutic cases.

67. Daniel K. Williams, *God's Own Party: The Making of the Christian Right* (New York: Oxford University Press, 2010), 19; J. Edgar Hoover, "The Faith of Our Fathers," *Christianity Today*, September 11, 1964, 6–7; Lerone A. Martin, *The Gospel of J. Edgar Hoover: How the FBI Aided and Abetted the Rise of White Christian Nationalism* (Princeton, NJ: Princeton University Press, 2023).

68. For evangelicals' culturally conservative campaigns of the 1960s and 1970s, see Williams, *God's Own Party*, 69–158; Axel R. Schäfer, ed., *American Evangelicals and the 1960s* (Madison: University of Wisconsin Press, 2013).

69. Williams, *God's Own Party*, 102.

70. "Abortion and the Court," *Christianity Today*, February 16, 1973.

CHAPTER 4.   Catholics and Evangelicals after *Roe*

1. National Conference of Catholic Bishops, Statement of the Committee for Pro-Life Affairs, January 24, 1973, https://www.usccb.org/issues-and-action/human-life-and-dignity/abortion/upload/Statement-of-the-Committee-for-ProLife-Affairs.pdf.

2. John Deedy, "Abortion: Counter-attack by the Bishops," *New York Times*, February 18, 1973.

3. "Abortion and the Court," *Christianity Today*, February 16, 1973.

4. "Abortion and the Court."

5. Patricia Miller, *Good Catholics: The Battle over Abortion in the Catholic Church* (Berkeley: University of California Press, 2014), 73.

6. Robert N. Lynch, "The National Committee for a Human Life Amendment, Inc.: Its Goals and Origins," *Catholic Lawyer* 20 (1974): 305.

7. John Krol, Testimony before the Subcommittee on Constitutional Amendments of the Senate Committee of the Judiciary, March 7, 1974, https://www.usccb.org/issues-and-action/human-life-and-dignity/abortion/upload/Testimony-of-Cardinal-John-Krol.pdf.

8. Sacred Congregation for the Doctrine of the Faith, *Declaration on Procured Abortion*, November 18, 1974, https://www.vatican.va/roman_curia/congregations/cfaith/documents/rc_con_cfaith_doc_19741118_declaration-abortion_en.html.

9. National Conference of Catholic Bishops, "Pastoral Plan for Pro-Life Activities," November 20, 1975, https://curate.nd.edu/articles/educational_resource/Pastoral_plan_for_pro-life_activities_November_20_1975_National_Conference_of_Catholic_Bishops_/24861489.

10. Joseph Bernardin, "Statement on the Fourth Anniversary of *Roe v. Wade*," January 22, 1977, Folder: "Department of Pastoral Services—Family Life Office—Abortion, 1978-82," box 47, Archbishop Joseph Bernardin Papers, Archives of the Archdiocese of Cincinnati.

11. Southern Baptist Convention, "Resolution on Beverage Alcohol as a Hazard," June 1, 1971, https://www.sbc.net/resource-library/resolutions/resolution-on-beverage-alcohol-as-a-hazard/; SBC, "Resolution on Voluntary Prayer," June 1, 1971, https://www.sbc.net/resource-library/resolutions/resolution-on-voluntary-prayer/.

12. SBC, "Resolution on Beverage Alcohol as a Hazard."

13. NCCB Committee for Pro-Life Activities, "A Human Life Amendment: The Time Is Now," 1981, Folder: "Pro-Life, 1976–1982," box 54, Bernardin Papers.

14. Joseph Bernardin to Emalie Smith, December 19, 1975, Folder: "Department of Pastoral Services—Pro-Life Activities, 1973-1975," box 53, Bernardin Papers.

15. Elizabeth Miller, "Religious Liberty and Abortion," speech delivered at the New England Conference of the Religious Coalition for Abortion Rights, North Andover, MA, November 4, 1976, Folder: "Abortion: Dialogue on Perspectives, by Yvonne V. Delk, 1989," box 4, Office for Church in Society, 1969–2000, UCC Archives.

16. Paul L. Sadler, "The Abortion Issue within the Southern Baptist Convention, 1969–1988" (PhD diss., Baylor University, 1991), 86–87; *Religious Herald*, February 22, 1973; W. Barry Garrett, "High Court Holds Abortion to Be 'A Right of Privacy,'" *Baptist Press*, January 31, 1973.

17. Stan Hastey, "Senate Panel Rejects Abortion Amendments," *Baptist Press*, September 18, 1975.

18. Floyd A. Craig, "Abortion Issue Has Shifted to Churches, Theologian Says," *Baptist Press*, August 30, 1976; David Sapp, "Foy Dan Valentine (1923–2006): Helping Changed People Change the World," in *Twentieth-Century Shapers of Baptist Social Ethics*, ed. Larry L. McSwain (Macon, GA: Mercer University Press, 2008), 309.

19. For the division between conservatives and moderates in the SBC, see Barry Hankins, *Uneasy in Babylon: Southern Baptist Conservatives and American Culture* (Tuscaloosa: University of Alabama Press, 2002); Nancy Tatom Ammerman, *Baptist Battles: Social Change and Religious Conflict in the Southern Baptist Convention* (New Brunswick, NJ: Rutgers University Press, 1990).

20. Robert Holbrook, "Court Ruling Forces Issue," *Baptist Standard*, May 16, 1973.

21. *Annual of the Southern Baptist Convention, 1974* (Nashville, TN: Southern Baptist Convention, 1974), 73, https://digitalcollections-baylor.quartexcollections.com/Documents/Detail/annual-of-the-southern-baptist-convention-1974/623540.

22. *Annual of the Southern Baptist Convention, 1974*, 75–76.

23. "Reaffirm Abortion Stand," *Baptist Standard*, June 19, 1974, 4; Bob Adams, "Abortion: A Look at a Life or Death Question," *Baptist Standard*, July 31, 1974, 4.

24. *Annual of the Southern Baptist Convention, 1975* (Nashville, TN: Southern Baptist Convention, 1975), 80, http://media2.sbhla.org.s3.amazonaws.com/annuals/SBC_Annual_1975.pdf.

25. SBC, "Resolution on Abortion," June 1976, https://www.sbc.net/resource-library/resolutions/resolution-on-abortion-3/.

26. Baptist Press, "President Ford's Visit Was High Hour of SBC Annual Meeting in Norfolk," *Alabama Baptist*, June 24, 1976; SBC, "Resolution on Abortion," June 1976.

27. Hankins, *Uneasy in Babylon*, 17.

28. SBC, "Resolution on Family Relationships," June 1, 1975, https://www.sbc.net/resource-library/resolutions/resolution-on-family-relationships/; SBC, "Resolution on Violence," June 1, 1975, https://www.sbc.net/resource-library/resolutions/resolution-on-violence/; SBC, "Resolution on Homosexuality," June 1, 1976, https://www.sbc.net/resource-library/resolutions/resolution-on-homosexuality/; SBC, "Resolution on Beveraged Alcohol and Pornography," June 1, 1976, https://www.sbc.net/resource-library/resolutions/resolution-on-beveraged-alcohol-and-pornography/.

29. Billie Cheney Speed, "Ex-Jesuit Now Editing Fundamentalist Weekly," *Atlanta Journal*, January 24, 1976.

30. Norman Pyle, "When Is Life?," *Faith for the Family*, November/December 1975, 3–9.

31. General Association of Regular Baptist Churches, "Resolution on Abortion," June 27, 1973, Folder: "Abortion: 1974–1975," 79-1, CLC AR 138-2, Southern Baptist Historical Library and Archives (SBHLA), Nashville, TN.

32. RNS, "Aids 'Defense of Life,'" *Baptist Standard*, September 3, 1975, 4; RNS, "Protestants v. Abortion," *Catholic Voice*, August 18, 1975, 7; Daniel K. Williams, *God's Own Party: The Making of the Christian Right* (New York: Oxford University Press, 2010), 119.

33. Susan Wunderink, "Theologian Harold O. J. Brown Dies at 74," *Christianity Today*, July 9, 2007; "Is Abortion a Catholic Issue?," *Christianity Today*, January 16, 1976.

34. Harold O. J. Brown, *Death before Birth* (Nashville: Thomas Nelson, 1977), 41.

35. Harold O. J. Brown, "An Evangelical Looks at the Abortion Phenomenon," *America*, September 25, 1976, 162–63.

36. "A License to Live," *Christianity Today*, July 26, 1974, 23.

37. "Is Abortion a Catholic Issue?"

38. For Schaeffer's biographical background, see Barry Hankins, *Francis Schaeffer and the Shaping of Evangelical America* (Grand Rapids, MI: Eerdmans, 2008).

39. Francis A. Schaeffer, *How Should We Then Live? The Rise and Decline of Western Thought and Culture* (Old Tappan, NJ: Fleming H. Revell, 1976), 222–23.

40. For Schaeffer's influence on Terry, Falwell, and other evangelicals, see Williams, *God's Own Party*, 155–56.

41. C. Everett Koop and Francis A. Schaeffer, *Whatever Happened to the Human Race?* (Old Tappan, NJ: Fleming H. Revell, 1979), 20.

42. Gallup poll on constitutional amendment prohibiting abortions, March 1976, in Gallup Organization, *America's Opinion on Abortion, 1962–1992* (Princeton, NJ: Gallup Organization, 1992).

43. For Democratic presidential aspirants' positions on abortion in 1976, see Daniel K. Williams, *The Election of the Evangelical: Jimmy Carter, Gerald Ford, and the Presidential Contest of 1976* (Lawrence: University Press of Kansas, 2020), 129–34.

44. Stephen Wermiel, "Kennedy Leads Defeat of Anti-Abortion Provision," *Boston Globe*, April 11, 1975.

45. For Shriver, see Daniel K. Williams, *Defenders of the Unborn: The Pro-Life Movement before Roe v. Wade* (New York: Oxford University Press, 2016), 221–23.

46. Administrative Board of the United States Catholic Conference, "Political Responsibility: Reflections on an Election Year (1976)," United States Conference of Catholic Bishops, February 12, 1976, https://www.usccb.org/offices/justice-peace-human-development/political-responsibility-reflections-election-year-1976. For the bishops' support of an antiabortion constitutional amendment in 1976, see also Timothy A. Byrnes, *Catholic Bishops in American Politics* (Princeton, NJ: Princeton University Press, 1991), 68–81.

47. Jane Gilroy, "Changing the Culture through Politics and Media: Ellen McCormack's 1976 Presidential Campaign," *Life and Learning* 15 (2005): 367; Alice Hartle, "What Made the Difference? A Tale of Three Cities," *National Right to Life News*, July 1976, 3.

48. Carter Campaign, press release, "Carter-Catholics," September 5, 1976, Folder: "Abortion, 9/76," box 1, Records of the 1976 Campaign Committee to Elect Jimmy Carter, Jimmy Carter Library, Atlanta, GA.

49. Williams, *The Election of the Evangelical*, 224–28.

50. "1976 Democratic Party Platform," The American Presidency Project, https://www.presidency.ucsb.edu/documents/1976-democratic-party-platform.

51. Andrew Mollison, "Do Catholics Cut Carter Chances?," *Atlanta Constitution*, July 13, 1976.

52. Gilroy, "Changing the Culture through Politics and Media," 367.

53. Kenneth A. Briggs, "Carter and the Bishops," *New York Times*, September 3, 1976.

54. James M. Naughton, "Bishops 'Encouraged' by Ford on Abortion," *New York Times*, September 11, 1976.

55. "Candidate Ford and the Catholics," *America*, September 25, 1976, 157.

56. Philip Shabecoff, "Archbishop Asserts Church Is Neutral in White House Race," *New York Times*, September 17, 1976.

57. George Gallup, "Most of Public for Abortion on Legal Basis," *Cincinnati Enquirer*, January 22, 1978.

58. Mary Reed to Joseph Bernardin, May 10, 1974; Mrs. Robert Meyer to Joseph Bernardin, January 14, 1974; Joseph Bernardin to Sisters of Saint Clare Convent, January 16, 1974; all in Folder: "Department of Pastoral Services—Pro-Life Activities, 1973–1975," box 53, Bernardin Papers.

59. Donald Granberg, "The Abortion Activists," *Family Planning Perspectives* 13 (1981): 158–60.

60. James A. Bramlage to Joseph Bernardin, July 24, 1974, Folder: "Department of Pastoral Services—Pro-Life Activities, 1973–1975," box 53, Bernardin papers.

61. Roger Griese, "'Free Choice' Farce," *Bulletin of Sacred Heart Church* (Dayton, OH), September 20, 1978; Griese, "Invocation at Ohio Congressional Breakfast," March for Life, Washington, DC, January 22, 1979; Joseph Bernardin to Roger Griese, February 9, 1979; all sources in Folder: "Department of Pastoral Services—Family Life Office—Abortion, Talk by Fr. Joseph O'Rourke, Jan. 1979—Abortion," box 47, Bernardin Papers.

62. Joseph Bernardin to Marge Kelly, April 24, 1978, Folder: Department of Pastoral Services—Pro-Life Activities, 1977–1979," box 53, Bernardin Papers.

63. Carl F. H. Henry, "An Open Letter to President Ford," *Eternity*, January 1976, 23.

64. Brown, "An Evangelical Looks at the Abortion Phenomenon," 163.

65. Brown, *Death before Birth*.

66. Religious Coalition on Abortion Rights, "A Call to Concern," 1977, Folder: "Abortion—Religious Coalition for Abortion Rights, 1975–1978, 97.18," CLC / ERLC Resource, AR 138-2, SBHLA; Foy Valentine to Harry N. Hollis Jr., December 18, 1978, Folder: "Abortion—Religious Coalition for Abortion Rights, 1975–1978, 97.18," CLC / ERLC Resource, AR 138-2, SBHLA.

67. Foy Valentine to Richard S. Sternberger, April 26, 1978, and Foy Valentine to Russell Kaemmerling, April 21, 1980, Folder: "Abortion—Religious Coalition for Abortion Rights, 1975–1978, 97.18," CLC / ERLC Resource, AR 138-2, Southern Baptist Historical Library and Archives, Nashville, TN.

68. Robert Holbrook, "Is the Southern Baptist Convention Pro-Abortion?" [1976], Folder: "Abortion: 1976," 79-2, CLC AR 138-2, SBHLA.

69. Presbyterian Church in America, "Report of the AD Interim Committee on Abortion at the 6th General Assembly" (1978), in Dennis R. Di Mauro, *A Love for Life: Christianity's Consistent Protection of the Unborn* (Eugene, OR: Wipf and Stock, 2008), 136–37.

70. Jerry Falwell, *How You Can Help Clean Up America* (Lynchburg, VA: Liberty Publishing Company, 1978), 59, 65.

71. Jerry Falwell, *Strength for the Journey: An Autobiography* (New York: Simon & Schuster, 1987), 361–62.

72. George Vecsey, "Militant Television Preachers Try to Weld Fundamentalist Christians' Political Power," *New York Times*, January 21, 1980.

73. Jerry Falwell, direct mail from the Moral Majority, August 22, 1979, folder 2, MOR 1-5, Liberty University Archives, Lynchburg, VA.

74. *Southern Baptist Journal*, May 1977, 4; SBC, "Resolution on Abortion," June 1, 1980, https://www.sbc.net/resource-library/resolutions/resolution-on-abortion-6/. For more on the conservative takeover of the SBC and the role of abortion in that effort, see Barry Hankins, *Uneasy in Babylon: Southern Baptist Conservatives and American Culture* (Tuscaloosa: University of Alabama Press, 2002).

75. Andrew R. Lewis, *The Rights Turn in Conservative Christian Politics: How Abortion Transformed the Culture Wars* (New York: Cambridge University Press, 2017), 21.

76. "Editorial: The St. Louis Convention," *Religious Herald*, June 19, 1980.

CHAPTER 5. The Rise and Fall of a Consistent Life Ethic

1. United States Catholic Conference, "Political Responsibility: Choices for the 1980s," October 1979, https://curate.nd.edu/articles/educational_resource/Political_responsibility_choices_for_the_1980_s_a_statement_of_the_Administrative_Board_/24740790/1.

2. "George C. Higgins, "The Prolife Movement and the New Right," *America*, September 13, 1980, 107.

3. "A Spokesman for Catholics: John Raphael Quinn," *New York Times*, November 16, 1977.

4. NCCB, "Bishops' Statement on Capital Punishment," 1980, https://www.usccb.org/resources/bishops-statement-capital-punishment-1980.

5. Juli Loesch Wiley, "Solidarity and Shalom," in *Confessing Conscience: Churched Women on Abortion*, ed. Phyllis Tickle (Nashville: Abingdon Press, 1990), 43–48.

6. Wiley, "Solidarity and Shalom," 49.

7. Consistent Life Network, "Special Memorial Issue: Daniel Berrigan," *Peace and Life Connections*, May 3, 2016, https://consistent-life.org/weekly160503.html.

8. For progressive evangelicals' conversion to the pro-life cause at the beginning of the 1980s, see Daniel K. Williams, "Pro-Lifers of the Left: Progressive Evangelicals' Campaign against Abortion," in *The New Evangelical*

Social Engagement, ed. Philip Goff and Brian Steensland (Oxford: Oxford University Press, 2014). For a history of progressive evangelicalism in the 1970s and 1980s, see David R. Swartz, *Moral Minority: The Evangelical Left in an Age of Conservatism* (Philadelphia: University of Pennsylvania Press, 2012).

9. NCCB, "The Challenge of Peace: God's Promise and Our Response," May 3, 1983, https://www.usccb.org/upload/challenge-peace-gods-promise-our-response-1983.pdf.

10. Mary E. Bendyna, "JustLife Action," in *Risky Business? PAC Decision-making in Congressional Elections*, ed. Robert Biersack et al. (New York: M. E. Sharpe, 1994), 195–96; Ronald J. Sider, *Completely Pro-Life: Building a Consistent Stance* (Downers Grove, IL: Intervarsity Press, 1987).

11. NCCB, "The Challenge of Peace."

12. Jane Perlez, "Mrs. Ferraro for Vice President," *New York Times*, December 23, 1983.

13. "Cuomo to Challenge Archbishop over Criticism of Abortion Stand," *New York Times*, August 3, 1984.

14. "O'Connor, in a Letter, Is Resolute," *New York Times*, February 6, 1984.

15. "Cuomo to Challenge Archbishop over Criticism of Abortion Stand," *New York Times*, August 3, 1984.

16. Joe Klein, "Abortion and the Archbishop," *New York Magazine*, October 1, 1984, 40.

17. "On Her Constituents, Arms, and Abortion," *New York Times*, July 13, 1984.

18. Alfred G. Boylan, letter to the editor, *New York Times*, August 30, 1984.

19. Jane Perlez, "Ferraro Acts to Still Abortion Dispute," *New York Times*, September 12, 1984.

20. Mario Cuomo, "Religious Belief and Public Morality: A Catholic Governor's Perspective," speech delivered at the University of Notre Dame, September 13, 1984, https://archives.nd.edu/research/texts/cuomo.htm.

21. Patricia Miller, *Good Catholics: The Battle over Abortion in the Catholic Church* (Berkeley: University of California Press, 2014), 110–13.

22. Miller, *Good Catholics*, 67.

23. Kenneth A. Briggs, "Young Adult Church Attendance Found Stabilized in a Gallup Poll," *New York Times*, January 4, 1976.

24. "Election Profile: Catholics," Roper Center, September/October 1991, https://ropercenter.cornell.edu/sites/default/files/2018-07/26093.pdf.

25. Daniel C. Maguire, *Sacred Choices: The Right to Contraception and Abortion in Ten World Religions* (Minneapolis: Fortress Press, 2001), 41.

26. Frances Kissling, "The Place for Individual Conscience," *Journal of Medical Ethics* 27 (2001): 24.

27. Quote from Jamie Manson originally appeared on Catholics for Choice website, https://www.catholicsforchoice.org/, but it can now be found on Alex Peek's blog, July 24, 2022, https://alexpeek.org/should-abortions-be-allowed.html.

28. Congregation for the Doctrine of the Faith, "Doctrinal Note on Some Questions Regarding the Participation of Catholics in Political Life," November 2002, https://www.vatican.va/roman_curia/congregations/cfaith/documents/rc_con_cfaith_doc_20021124_politica_en.html.

29. Miller, *Good Catholics*, 111–19.

30. "Election Profile: Catholics," *American Enterprise*, September/October 1991, 98, https://ropercenter.cornell.edu/sites/default/files/2018-07/26093.pdf.

31. Miller, *Good Catholics*, 113–14; "Campaign Notes; 23 Bishops See Nuclear War as Top Issue," *New York Times*, October 23, 1984; Kenneth A. Briggs, "Cardinal Presses Catholics to Attack Wide Range of Social Issues," *New York Times*, October 26, 1984.

32. Joe Klein, "Abortion and the Archbishop," *New York Magazine*, October 1, 1984, 38.

33. Klein, "Abortion and the Archbishop," 38–39.

34. Klein, "Abortion and the Archbishop."

35. Joseph Berger, "The Papal Visit; Catholics, in Poll, Admire Pope but Disagree," *New York Times*, September 10, 1987.

36. E. J. Dionne Jr., "Poll on Abortion Finds the Nation Is Sharply Divided," *New York Times*, April 26, 1989.

37. Colman McCarthy, "Catholic Bishops: Activists for Peace," *Washington Post*, December 13, 1981.

38. Onalee McGraw, *Secular Humanism and the Schools: The Issue Whose Time Has Come* (Washington, DC: Heritage Foundation, 1976); Connaught Coyne Marshner, *Blackboard Tyranny* (New Rochelle, NY: Arlington House, 1978); Tom McFadden, "A History of Christendom College: The First 35 Years (1977–2012)," Christendom College website, April 6, 2013, https://www.christendom.edu/about/a-history-of-christendom-college/.

39. Donald Granberg, "The Abortion Activists," *Family Planning Perspectives* 13 (1981): 162.

40. Granberg, "The Abortion Activists," 162.

41. "Transcript of Pontiff's Homily at Mass," *New York Times*, October 8, 1979; Kenneth A. Briggs, "In Philadelphia, Pope Condemns Sexual 'Laxity,'" *New York Times*, October 4, 1979.

42. A poll conducted in 1986 showed that 72 percent of Protestants supported the death penalty for murderers; see Davison M. Douglas, "God and the Executioner: The Influence of Western Religion on the Use of the Death Penalty," *William & Mary Bill of Rights Journal* 9 (2000): 141–42. Unfortunately, the surveys available from the 1980s do not differentiate between evangelical opinion and general Protestant opinion on this issue, but surveys from the twenty-first century indicate that more than 70 percent of white evangelicals approve of capital punishment. The SBC adopted a resolution in 2000 endorsing capital punishment for murder. For an analysis of the connection between evangelicals' support for capital punishment and their opposition to abortion, see Andrew R. Lewis, *The Rights Turn in Conservative Christian Politics: How Abortion Transformed the Culture Wars* (New York: Cambridge University Press, 2017), 121–47.

43. Cal Thomas, Moral Majority Radio Report, March 26, 1984, folder 2, MOR 1-3, Liberty University Archives.

44. Francis A. Schaeffer, *A Christian Manifesto* (Westchester, IL: Crossway Books, 1981), 120.

45. Charles E. Shepard, "Operation Rescue's Mission to Save Itself," *Washington Post*, November 24, 1991. For a history of Operation Rescue and the use of direct action and illegal activities to stop abortion, see James Risen and Judy L. Thomas, *Wrath of Angels: The American Abortion War* (New York: Basic Books, 1998).

46. Christopher White, "Pro-Life Activist and Trump Apologist Frank Pavone Dismissed from Catholic Priesthood," *National Catholic Reporter*, December 18, 2022.

47. "Enemy of Abortion Is Also Taking Issue with Protest Tactics," *New York Times*, August 31, 1988.

48. For more on the centrality of the antiabortion message in Christian music and evangelical youth culture in the 1980s, see Eileen Luhr, *Witnessing Suburbia: Conservatives and Christian Youth Culture* (Berkeley: University of California Press, 2009).

49. Tammi Ledbetter, "Franky Schaeffer Demands," *Southern Baptist Advocate*, July/August 1984, 8; "Pastors Hit Abortion, Pornography, Hear Encouraging Words," *Baptist Standard*, June 20, 1984, 13.

50. SBC resolutions on abortion, 1982 and 1984, https://www.johnstonsarchive.net/baptist/sbcabres.html.

51. Charles F. Stanley to Janet Price, October 2, 1985, folder 1-1, Charles F. Stanley Papers, Southern Baptist Historical Library and Archives (SBHLA), Nashville, TN.

52. Ray Waddle, "Southern Baptists Ban Speaker Holding 'Pro-Choice' Views," *Tennessean*, March 9, 1990. Also see Nancy Tatom Ammerman, *Baptist Battles: Social Change and Religious Conflict in the Southern Baptist Convention* (New Brunswick, NJ: Rutgers University Press, 1990).

53. SBC resolutions on abortion in 1987, 1988, 1989, 1991, 1992, 1993, and 1996, https://www.johnstonsarchive.net/baptist/sbcabres.html.

54. Marv Knox, "Abortion Becomes 'Benchmark' for CLC Conference Speakers," Baptist Press, March 5, 1990.

55. Kevin Perrotta, "Differences of Opinion?," *Eternity*, January 1986, 56.

56. Paul B. Fowler, *Abortion: Toward an Evangelical Consensus* (Portland, OR: Multnomah Press, 1987), 14.

CHAPTER 6. Liberal Protestants after *Roe*

1. American Baptist Churches USA, "Resolution concerning Abortion and Ministry in the Local Church," June 1988, https://www.abc-usa.org/wp-content/uploads/2019/02/Abortion-and-Ministry-in-the-Local-Church.pdf. For more on this resolution, see "American Baptists Maximize the Middle," *Christian Century*, July 20–27, 1988, 660–61.

2. Kenneth Vaux, "After 'Edelin': The Abortion Debate Goes On," *Christian Century*, March 5, 1975, 213.

3. J. Claude Evans, "The Abortion Debate: A Call for Civility," *Christian Century*, March 21, 1979, 300.

4. Religious Coalition for Abortion Rights, brochure, 1974, Folder: Moss—Subject Files—Abortion Issues," box 3, Office of the President—Robert V. Moss (1969–1976) papers, UCC Archives.

5. Religious Coalition for Abortion Rights, brochure, 1974; Michael J. Gorman and Ann Loar Brooks, *Holy Abortion? A Theological Critique of the Religious Coalition for Reproductive Choice* (Eugene, OR: Wipf and Stock, 2003).

6. Avery D. Post, statement at service of, Washington, DC, January 22, 1981, Folder: "Post, A.D.—Current Projects—Abortion Service: Washington, 1981," box 7, Avery D. Post Presidential Papers, UCC Archives; United

Church of Christ, press release, January 22, 1981, Folder: "Post, A.D. — Current Projects — Abortion Service: Washington, 1981," box 7, Post papers, UCC Archives.

7. Robert V. Moss and Howard E. Spragg, "Freedom of Choice concerning Abortion," testimony before the Senate Subcommittee on Constitutional Amendments, March 7, 1974, Folder: Moss — Subject Files — Abortion Issues," box 3, Moss papers, UCC Archives.

8. Walter H. Krebs to Helen Webber, February 25, 1981, Folder: "Post, A.D. — Current Projects, Abortion," box 7, Post papers, UCC Archives.

9. Religious Coalition for Abortion Rights, direct mail to members, January 22, 1979, Folder: "Abortion, 1978-1981," box 4, Office for Church in Society, 1969–2000, UCC Archives.

10. "Six Years Later: Where Does the Abortion Issue Stand Today?," *Cincinnati Post*, February 26, 1979.

11. Jim Castelli, "Is Medicaid Abortion Funding a 'Catholic' Issue?," NC News Service, December 9, 1977, Folder: "Department of Pastoral Services — Family Life Office — Abortion, 1978-82," box 47, Archbishop Joseph Bernardin Papers, Archdiocese of Cincinnati.

12. Frederick W. Schroeder, "Unwanted Babies," January 1981, Folder: "Post, A.D. — Current Projects, Abortion," box 7, Post Papers, UCC Archives.

13. Timothy Bayly, "Stand Fast; Defend the Faith," *Presbyterians Pro-Life News*, Winter 1990; James A. DeCamp, "The Presbyterian Church (USA) Needs Those Who Will Stay and Call the Denomination Back to Holiness," *Presbyterians Pro-Life News*, Summer 1990; Martin W. Radcliff, "Presbyterians Face a Pastoral Crisis: Loss of Both Christian Heritage and Church Discipline; The Church Needs Proper Discipline," *Presbyterians Pro-Life News*, Winter 1990.

14. Ari L. Goldman, "Presbyterians Consider Shift in Stand for Abortion Rights," *New York Times*, June 11, 1985.

15. "G.A. Commissioners Hear Mother Teresa, Vote for New Study of Abortion," *Presbyterians Pro-Life News*, July/August /September 1988.

16. General Assembly of the Presbyterian Church (USA), "Report of the Special Committee on Problem Pregnancies and Abortion," 1992, https://www.pcusa.org/site_media/media/uploads/oga/pdf/problem-pregnancies.pdf.

17. United Methodist Church, Decision 683, https://www.resourceumc.org/en/churchwide/judicial-council/judicial-council-decision-home/judicial-decisions/consistency-of-support-of-religious-coalition-for-abortion-rights-with-par-71.

18. Lifewatch, "Durham Declaration," 1990, https://lifewatch.org/the-durham-declaration/.

19. United Methodist Church, "Does the UMC Fund . . .?," July 1, 2021, https://www.umc.org/en/content/ask-the-umc-does-the-umc-fund.

20. Episcopal Church, Acts of Convention, Resolution 1988-C047: "Adopt a Statement on Childbirth and Abortion," 1988, https://episcopalarchives.org/cgi-bin/acts/acts_resolution.pl?resolution=1988-C047.

21. R. Kenneth Ostermiller to Verna Uthman, May 18, 1990, folder 28, box 4, Office for Church in Society (OCS) Records, UCC Archives; UCC Southern Conference, "Resolution concerning Abortion," June 1990, folder 28, box 4, OCS records, UCC Archives; Denise Long, "Dealing with Abortion: Southern Conference Success Story," *Southern Conference News* (UCC), June 1990, folder 28, box 4, OCS records, UCC Archives.

22. Evangelical Lutheran Church in America, "A Social Statement on Abortion," 1991, https://www.elca.org/Faith/Faith-and-Society/Social-Statements/Abortion.

23. Lutheran Church in America, "Statement on Abortion," 1970, in Religious Coalition for Abortion Rights, "The Abortion Rights Issue: How We Stand," February 15, 1974, Folder: Moss—Subject Files—Abortion Issues," box 3, Office of the President—Robert V. Moss papers, UCC Archives.

24. Evangelical Lutheran Church in America, "A Social Statement on Abortion," 1991.

25. General Assembly of the Presbyterian Church (USA), "Christian Obedience in a Nuclear Age, 1988, https://oga.pcusa.org/media/uploads/oga/pdf/nuclear_age.pdf; General Assembly of the Presbyterian Church (USA), "God Alone Is Lord of the Conscience," 1988, https://oga.pcusa.org/media/uploads/oga/pdf/god-alone-is-lord.pdf.

26. Julie Ray, "Gallup Brain: Opinions on Partial-Birth Abortions," Gallup, July 8, 2003, https://news.gallup.com/poll/8791/gallup-brain-opinions-partialbirth-abortions.aspx.

27. Abigail Rian Evans, *The Presbyterian Church (USA) Tradition: Religious Beliefs and Healthcare Decisions* (Park Ridge, IL: Park Ridge Center, 2002), 5–6, https://www.advocatehealth.com/-/media/Project/Health-System-Enterprise/AdvocateHealthCom/advocatehealth/documents/about-us/faith-at-advocate/spiritual-health/religious-beliefs-health-care-decisions/presbyterian-tradition.pdf.

28. Episcopal Church, Resolution 1997-D065: "Express Grave Concerns over Misuse of Partial Birth Abortion," 1997, https://episcopalarchives.org/cgi-bin/acts/acts_resolution.pl?resolution=1997-D065.

29. Richard B. Hays, *The Moral Vision of the New Testament: A Contemporary Introduction to New Testament Ethics* (New York: Harper One, 1996), 456–57.

30. Stanley Hauerwas, "Abortion, Theologically Understood," in *The Church and Abortion: In Search of New Ground for Response*, ed. Paul T. Stallsworth (Nashville: Abingdon Press, 1993), 49–50, 57–58, 62.

31. General Conference Mennonite Church, "Guidelines on Abortion," 1980, https://www.anabaptistwiki.org/mediawiki/index.php?title=Guidelines_on_Abortion_(General_Conference_Mennonite_Church,_1980).

32. Mennonite Church USA, "Statement on Abortion," 2003, https://www.supremecourt.gov/opinions/URLs_Cited/OT2013/13-354/13-354-4.pdf.

33. Larry L. Petersen and Armand L. Mauss, "Religion and the 'Right to Life': Correlates of Opposition to Abortion," *Sociological Analysis* 37 (1976): 248.

34. Loretta J. Ross, "African-American Women and Abortion," in *Abortion Wars: A Half Century of Struggle, 1950–2000*, ed. Rickie Solinger (Berkeley: University of California Press, 1998), 168, 177.

35. Ross, "African-American Women and Abortion," 180.

36. For a history of forced sterilization of African American women living in poverty, see Johanna Schoen, *Choice and Coercion: Birth Control, Sterilization, and Abortion in Public Health and Welfare* (Chapel Hill: University of North Carolina Press, 2005).

37. Fannie Lou Hamer, "Is It Too Late?," speech at Tougaloo College, summer 1971, in *The Speeches of Fannie Lou Hamer: To Tell It Like It Is*, ed. Maegan Parker Brooks and Davis W. Houck (Jackson: University Press of Mississippi, 2011), 133.

38. "Black Churchmen Oppose Abortion as Genocide," *Jet*, July 26, 1973, 44.

39. Jesse L. Jackson, "How We Respect Life Is Over-riding Moral Issue," *National Right to Life News*, January 1977, 5.

40. African Methodist Episcopal Church, "Consideration of the Abortion Issue" (1977), in Dennis R. DiMauro, *A Love for Life: Christianity's Persistent Protection of the Unborn* (Eugene, OR: Wipf and Stock, 2008), 107.

41. Steve Kornacki, "1980: Carter vs. Kennedy Left African Americans Feeling Ignored," NBC News, July 29, 2019, https://www.nbcnews.com/politics/elections/1980-carter-vs-kennedy-left-african-americans-feeling-ignored-n1029591.

42. Jesse Jackson, 1984 Democratic National Convention Address, July 18, 1984, https://www.americanrhetoric.com/speeches/jessejackson1984dnc.htm.

43. Fay S. Joyce, "Presidential Decision Nears for Jackson," *New York Times*, September 22, 1983.

44. "The Democrats on the Issues: Military Budgets and Women as Running Mates," *New York Times*, January 16, 1984.

45. "Key Sections from Transcripts of Democrats' Debate in Iowa," *New York Times*, February 13, 1984.

46. Mark Weston, "Faith Abortion," *Washington Post*, January 23, 1990.

47. Leah MarieAnn Klett, "Tony Evans Urges Christian Voters on Life Issue: Don't Ignore 'Abortion' Outside the Womb," *Christian Post*, September 28, 2020, https://www.christianpost.com/news/tony-evans-urges-christian-voters-on-life-issue-dont-ignore-abortion-outside-the-womb.html.

48. Yolanda Baruch, "Dr. Alveda King Is Championing Civil Rights for the Unborn," *Forbes*, August 31, 2023, https://www.forbes.com/sites/yolandabaruch/2023/08/30/dr-alveda-king-is-championing-civil-rights-for-the-unborn/; "Alveda King: A Voice for the Voiceless," CBN, https://cbn.com/article/not-selected/alveda-king-voice-voiceless.

49. Church of God in Christ, "Resolution on the Sanctity of Life," November 2019, https://www.cogic.org/wp-content/uploads/2019/12/SOLife-Resolution-11_12_19-1.pdf.

50. "A Position Statement from the College of Bishops on Abortion," *Christian Index*, January 1, 1992, 4–5.

51. Yvonne V. Delk, "Dialogue on Abortion Perspectives," Kansas City, MO, November 17–19, 1989, Folder: "Abortion: Dialogue on Perspectives, by Yvonne V. Delk, 1989," box 4, Office for Church in Society, UCC Archives.

52. Beverly Wildung Harrison, *Our Right to Choose: Toward a New Ethic of Abortion* (Boston: Beacon Press, 1983).

53. Suzanne Staggenborg, *The Pro-Choice Movement: Organization and Activism in the Abortion Conflict* (New York: Oxford University Press, 1991), 102.

54. 2000 Democratic Party Platform, The American Presidency Project, https://www.presidency.ucsb.edu/documents/2000-democratic-party-platform.

55. "Safe, Legal and Rare," *Christian Century*, December 26, 2012.

56. Anglican Church in North America, "Celebrating 15 Years of the ACNA," March 25, 2024, https://anglicanchurch.net/celebrating-15-years-of-the-acna/.

57. Aaron Vriesman, "It Doesn't Work: Presbyterian Church USA," Abide Project, September 25, 2023, https://www.abideproject.org/p/it-doesnt-work-presbyterian-church.

58. Evangelical Lutheran Church in America, "A Social Statement on Human Sexuality: Gift and Trust," August 2009, https://download.elca.org/

ELCA%20Resource%20Repository/SexualitySS.pdf; North American Lutheran Church, History, https://thenalc.org/history/.

59. Kate Shellnutt and Daniel Silliman, "United Methodists Down 7,659 Churches as Exit Window Ends," *Christianity Today*, December 18, 2023.

60. David Paulsen, "Episcopal Church's Latest Parochial Reports Point to Denominational Decline, Hope for Future," Episcopal News Service, September 21, 2023, https://episcopalnewsservice.org/2023/09/21/episcopal-churchs-latest-parochial-reports-highlight-denominational-decline-hope-for-future/; Rick Jones, "PC(USA) Church Membership Still in Decline," May 1, 2023, https://www.pcusa.org/news/2023/5/1/pcusa-church-membership-still-in-decline/; Marc Ramirez, "A Quarter of Methodist Congregations Abandon the Church as Schism Grows over LGBTQ+ Issues," *USA Today*, December 20, 2023.

61. Mark Tooley, "What Might Come of the United Methodist Church's General Conference?," *Dispatch*, April 28, 2024, https://thedispatch.com/article/what-might-come-of-the-united-methodist-churchs-general-conference/; Shellnutt and Silliman, "United Methodists Down 7,659 Churches"; Ramirez, "A Quarter of Methodist Congregations Abandon the Church as Schism Grows over LGBTQ+ Issues."

62. Rebecca Todd Peters, *Trust Women: A Progressive Christian Argument for Reproductive Justice* (Boston: Beacon Press, 2018).

63. Peters, *Trust Women*, 166.

64. Eileen R. Campbell-Reed, "State of Clergywomen in the U.S.: A Statistical Update" (October 2018), https://eileencampbellreed.org/wp-content/uploads/Downloads/State-of-Clergywomen-US-2018-web.pdf.

65. Presbyterian Church (USA), "General Assembly Resolution on Reproductive Health (2012)," https://www.presbyterianmission.org/wp-content/uploads/1-res_on_reproductive_health_care_access-2012.pdf.

66. Episcopal Church Office of Government Relations, "Summary of General Convention Resolutions on Abortion and Women's Reproductive Health Care," February 23, 2024, https://www.episcopalchurch.org/ogr/summary-of-general-convention-resolutions-on-abortion-and-womens-reproductive-health/.

67. Chris Ratliff, "Shifts in Support for Abortion by Party and Religious Affiliation," PRRI, June 26, 2023, https://www.prri.org/spotlight/shifts-in-support-for-abortion-by-party-and-religious-affiliation/.

68. Ratliff, "Shifts in Support for Abortion by Party and Religious Affiliation"; Pew Research Center, "Views about Abortion among Members of the

Presbyterian Church USA" [2014], https://www.pewresearch.org/religious-landscape-study/database/religious-denomination/presbyterian-church-usa/views-about-abortion/.

69. North American Lutheran Church Joint Commission on Theology and Doctrine, "'The Lord Is with You': A Word of Counsel to the Church: The Sanctity of Nascent Life," December 2012.

70. Anglican Church in North America, "Anglican Laity, Clergy and Bishops March for Life," February 1, 2013, https://anglicanchurch.net/anglican-laity-clergy-and-bishops-march-for-life/.

71. Global Methodist Church, *Transitional Book of Doctrines and Discipline*, April 2024, 202.3, https://globalmethodist.org/wp-content/uploads/2024/05/Transitional-Discipline.pdf.

72. "EPC Statement on Recent Abortion Laws, February 2019," https://wrf.global/blog/blog-2/society/evangelical-presbyterian-church-speaks-about-abortion.

73. Jim Wallis, "My Personal 'Faith Priorities' for This Election," *Sojourners*, October 23, 2008.

74. Julie Polter, "Outrage over the Abortion Veto," *Sojourners*, July-August 1996.

75. Jim Wallis, "Pro-Life Democrats?" *Sojourners*, June 2004; Ron Sider, "Ron Sider: Why I Am Voting for Hillary Clinton," *Christianity Today*, September 23, 2016.

76. Stephanie Russell-Kraft, "Biden Is a Pro-Choice Catholic. Will He Expand Reproductive Health Care?," *Sojourners*, December 10, 2020.

77. Robin Toner, "The 2000 Campaign: Focus on the Issues; Both Sides on Abortion Issue Step up Fight," *New York Times*, October 27, 2000.

78. For the role of fear in influencing evangelical Christians' political choices, see John Fea, *Believe Me: The Evangelical Road to Donald Trump* (Grand Rapids, MI: Eerdmans, 2018).

79. "More State Abortion Restrictions Were Enacted in 2011–2013 Than in the Entire Previous Decade," Guttmacher Institute, January 2014, https://www.guttmacher.org/article/2014/01/more-state-abortion-restrictions-were-enacted-2011-2013-entire-previous-decade.

CHAPTER 7. The Conservative Christian Coalition That Overturned *Roe*

1. "Evangelicals and Catholics Together: The Christian Mission in the Third Millennium," *First Things*, May 1994, https://www.firstthings.com/article

/1994/05/evangelicals-catholics-together-the-christian-mission-in-the-third-millennium.

2. NCCB, "Resolution on Abortion," November 7, 1989, https://www.usccb.org/issues-and-action/human-life-and-dignity/abortion/resolution-on-abortion.

3. John Paul II, *Evangelium Vitae* (1995), sec. 62, https://www.vatican.va/content/john-paul-ii/en/encyclicals/documents/hf_jp-ii_enc_25031995_evangelium-vitae.html.

4. *Catechism of the Catholic Church*, 2nd ed. (New York: Doubleday, 1997), 2271.

5. John Paul II, *Evangelium Vitae*, sec. 59.

6. Ruth Graham, "America's New Catholic Priests: Young, Confident and Conservative," *New York Times*, July 10, 2024.

7. Joseph Bernardin to John F. Messmer, December 5, 1975, Folder: "Department of Pastoral Services—Pro-Life Activities, 1973–1975," box 53, Bernardin Papers.

8. Barry M. Horstman, "Communion Ban Unleashes Backlash," *Los Angeles Times*, November 18, 1989.

9. Gustav Niebuhr, "Bishops Take Bolder Stand in Battle against Abortion," *New York Times*, November 19, 1998.

10. Laurie Goodstein, "Kerry, Candidate and Catholic, Creates Uneasiness for the Church," *New York Times*, April 2, 2004; Robin Toner, "Kerry Criticizes Bush's Definition of Values," *New York Times*, July 5, 2004.

11. Laurie Goodstein, "Kerry, Candidate and Catholic, Creates Uneasiness for the Church," *New York Times*, April 2, 2004.

12. Katharine Q. Seelye, "Kerry Ignores Reproaches of Some Bishops," *New York Times*, April 11, 2004.

13. David Kocieniewski, "McGreevey Won't Receive Communion," *New York Times*, May 6, 2004; Daniel J. Wakin, "The Nation: Abortion to Annulment; Communion Becomes a Test of Faith and Politics," *New York Times*, May 9, 2004.

14. Laurie Goodstein, "Bishop Would Deny Rite for Defiant Catholic Voters," *New York Times*, May 14, 2004. Both McCarrick and Mahony would later be disgraced by revelations of their cover-up of sexual abuse among priests in their diocese and, in the case of McCarrick, his own participation in sexual abuse. McCarrick would become the highest-ranking American prelate to be defrocked because of his sexual abuse of minors. In 2004, though, when he took a leading role in urging that bishops not deny Communion to pro-choice

politicians, he was still serving as archbishop of Washington, DC, and the accusations against him were not yet widely known. Bishops on both sides of the debate over how the church should respond to Catholics who support abortion rights were implicated in the sex abuse crisis. Of the conservatives involved in the cover-up of sexual abuse, the most prominent may have been Cardinal Bernard Law, archbishop of Boston, who wrote the bishops' statement in 1998 declaring that "no appeal to policy, procedure, majority will or pluralism ever excuses a public official from defending life to the greatest extent possible."

15. USCCB, "Catholics in Political Life," June 2004, https://www.usccb.org/issues-and-action/faithful-citizenship/church-teaching/catholics-in-political-life.

16. Cardinal Joseph Ratzinger, "Worthiness to Receive Holy Communion: General Principles," July 2004, https://www.ewtn.com/catholicism/library/worthiness-to-receive-holy-communion-general-principles-2153.

17. USCCB, "Forming Consciences for Faithful Citizenship: A Call to Political Responsibility from the Catholic Bishops of the United States," November 2007, https://www.usccb.org/issues-and-action/faithful-citizenship/upload/forming-consciences-for-faithful-citizenship-2007.pdf; Michael Paulson, "U.S. Cardinal Draws Line with Democratic Party," *New York Times*, November 15, 2007.

18. David D. Kirkpatrick, "Abortion Issue Again Dividing Catholic Votes," *New York Times*, September 17, 2008.

19. David M. Herszenhorn and Jackie Calmes, "Abortion Was at Heart of Wrangling," *New York Times*, November 7, 2009.

20. John Paul II, *Evangelium Vitae*, sec. 60.

21. Rachel Benson Gold, "The Implications of Defining When a Woman Is Pregnant," *Guttmacher Policy Review* 8, no. 2 (2005): 7, https://www.guttmacher.org/sites/default/files/article_files/gr080207.pdf.

22. *Burwell v. Hobby Lobby Stores, Inc.*, 573 U.S. 682 (2014).

23. For this shift, see Laurie Goodstein, "Bishops Open 'Religious Liberty' Drive," *New York Times*, November 14, 2011.

24. Thomas A. Glessner, "Supreme Court Sides with Pro-Life Pregnancy Centers in Victory for Free Speech," *USA Today*, June 26, 2018.

25. 2016 Democratic Party Platform, American Presidency Project, https://www.presidency.ucsb.edu/documents/2016-democratic-party-platform.

26. Pope Francis, *Evangelii Gaudium* (2013), sec. 213, https://www.vatican.va/content/francesco/en/apost_exhortations/documents/papa-francesco_esortazione-ap_20131124_evangelii-gaudium.html.

27. Pope Francis, *Laudato Si'* (2015), sec. 120, https://www.vatican.va/content/francesco/en/encyclicals/documents/papa-francesco_20150524_enciclica-laudato-si.html.

28. Jim Yardley, "Pope Francis Suggests Donald Trump Is 'Not Christian,'" *New York Times*, February 18, 2016; Pope Francis, *Laudato Si'*; and Pope Francis, *Fratelli Tutti* (2020), https://www.vatican.va/content/francesco/en/encyclicals/documents/papa-francesco_20201003_enciclica-fratelli-tutti.html.

29. Laurie Goodstein, "Pope Francis Names 17 New Cardinals, Including 3 Americans," *New York Times*, October 9, 2016; Brian Fraga, "Pope Francis Faces Chance to Radically Reshape US Catholic Hierarchy," *National Catholic Reporter*, March 20, 2023.

30. Charles Chaput, "Justice, Prudence and Immigration Reform," Catholic Philly.com, February 19, 2013, https://catholicphilly.com/2013/02/weekly-message-from-archbishop-chaput/justice-prudence-and-immigration-reform/.

31. Christopher White, "Bishop Laments Questioning of Biden's Faith Due to Abortion Policies," *National Catholic Reporter*, October 13, 2020.

32. Quoted in Daniel K. Williams, *Defenders of the Unborn: The Pro-Life Movement before Roe v. Wade* (New York: Oxford University Press, 2016), 267.

33. White, "Bishop Laments Questioning of Biden's Faith Due to Abortion Policies."

34. USCCB, Press release: "'We Are with You,' Say U.S. Bishops in Calling Elected Officials and Americans to Work Together to Welcome Refugees and Immigrants without Sacrificing Core Values, Security," November 17, 2016, https://www.usccb.org/news/2016/we-are-you-say-us-bishops-calling-elected-officials-and-americans-work-together-welcome.

35. Tom Roberts, "Bishops Pass 'Faithful Citizenship,' Some Call for New Document," *National Catholic Reporter*, November 17, 2015.

36. Stephen J. Fichter et al., *Catholic Bishops in the United States: Church Leadership in the Third Millennium* (New York: Oxford University Press, 2019), 136.

37. Michael J. O'Loughlin, "Bishops Chose Naumann over Cupich for Pro-Life Chair in Bellwether Vote," *America*, November 14, 2017; "US Bishops Reject Cardinal Cupich as Head of Pro-Life Committee," *Catholic Herald*, November 14, 2017.

38. USCCB, "Forming Consciences for Faithful Citizenship," November 2019, https://www.usccb.org/about/leadership/usccb-general-assembly/upload/usccb-forming-consciences-faithful-citizenship-introductory-letter-20191112.pdf.

39. Christopher White, "US Bishops Issue Warning to President-Elect Joe Biden on Abortion," *National Catholic Reporter*, November 17, 2020.

40. Brian Fraga and Joshua J. McElwee, "After Year of Divisive Debate, US Bishops Approve Tepid Document on Communion," *National Catholic Reporter*, November 17, 2021.

41. Michael Sean Winters, "US Bishops to Choose Culture War or Communion in Baltimore," *National Catholic Reporter*, November 3, 2021; Fraga and McElwee, "After Year of Divisive Debate."

42. Ruth Graham, "America's New Catholic Priests: Young, Confident and Conservative," *New York Times*, July 10, 2024.

43. Jeffrey M. Jones, "Church Attendance Has Declined in Most U.S. Religious Groups," Gallup, March 25, 2024, https://news.gallup.com/poll/642548/church-attendance-declined-religious-groups.aspx; Gregory A. Smith, "Like Americans Overall, Catholics Vary in Their Abortion Views, with Regular Mass Attenders Most Opposed," Pew Research Center, May 23, 2022, https://www.pewresearch.org/short-reads/2022/05/23/like-americans-overall-catholics-vary-in-their-abortion-views-with-regular-mass-attenders-most-opposed/.

44. Leslie Woodcock Tentler, *Catholics and Contraception: An American History* (Ithaca, NY: Cornell University Press, 2004), 133–34.

45. Pew Research Center, "Detailed Tables: Abortion Views of U.S. Catholics," March 2022, https://www.pewresearch.org/wp-content/uploads/2022/05/W104Catholics_Abortion-DetailedTables_MOE.pdf; Marina E. Franco, "Latinos Split on Abortion by Generation," *Axios*, June 28, 2022, https://www.axios.com/2022/06/28/abortion-views-latinos-supreme-court-roe-poll; "Among U.S. Latinos, Catholicism Continues to Decline but Is Still the Largest Faith," Pew Research Center, April 13, 2023, https://www.pewresearch.org/religion/2023/04/13/among-u-s-latinos-catholicism-continues-to-decline-but-is-still-the-largest-faith/; Joseph P. Bartkowski et al., "Faith, Race-Ethnicity, and Public Policy Preferences: Religious Schemas and Abortion Attitudes among U.S. Latinos," *Faculty Publications—Department of World Languages, Sociology, and Cultural Studies* 20 (2012), https://digitalcommons.georgefox.edu/cgi/viewcontent.cgi?referer=&httpsredir=1&article=1019&context=lang_fac.

46. Southern Baptist Convention, *2000 Baptist Faith and Message*, https://bfm.sbc.net/bfm2000/.

47. Southern Baptist Convention, "Resolution on Thirty Years of *Roe v. Wade*," June 2003, https://www.johnstonsarchive.net/baptist/sbcabres.html.

48. Melissa N. Montoya, Colleen Judge-Golden, and Jonas J. Swartz, "The Problems with Crisis Pregnancy Centers: Reviewing the Literature and Identifying New Directions for Research," *International Journal of Women's Health* 14 (2022): 757–63; Anna North, "The Anti-abortion 'Social Safety Net,'" *Vox*, June 28, 2022, https://www.vox.com/23184939/abortion-ban-roe-wade-crisis-pregnancy-centers; Kaylee Cameron, "The Truth: 'Fake' Crisis Pregnancy Centers," Focus on the Family, March 3, 2023, https://www.focusonthefamily.com/pro-life/the-truth-fake-crisis-pregnancy-centers/. Of the three largest national CPC networks, Care Net advertised itself as an evangelical organization, while Heartbeat International and the National Institute of Family and Life Advocates (NIFLA) described themselves as interdenominational, faith-based Christian groups that worked with both Catholics and evangelical Protestants. For histories of crisis pregnancy centers, see Karissa Haugeberg, *Women against Abortion: Inside the Largest Moral Reform Movement of the Twentieth Century* (Urbana: University of Illinois Press, 2017); Jennifer L. Holland, *Tiny You: A Western History of the Anti-Abortion Movement* (Oakland: University of California Press, 2020).

49. Tom Strode, "Call to Build 'Culture of Life' Draws SBC Leaders' Endorsement," Baptist Press, April 24, 2002.

50. Southern Baptist Convention resolution, "On Abolishing Abortion," June 21, 2021, https://www.sbc.net/resource-library/resolutions/on-abolishing-abortion/.

51. Denny Burk et al., "Why We Opposed an Anti-Abortion Resolution at the Southern Baptist Convention," *Public Discourse*, June 22, 2021, https://www.thepublicdiscourse.com/2021/06/76465/.

52. A sixth justice, Chief Justice John Roberts, issued a concurring opinion that upheld the Mississippi law and abandoned some of the stipulations of *Roe v. Wade*, but, unlike the majority opinion, suggested that the right to an abortion could remain intact. Like most of the justices who voted with the majority in *Dobbs*, Roberts was a Catholic.

53. Though I characterize *Dobbs* as an originalist decision, there are legal scholars who dispute this categorization. For more on this debate—and a defense of the use of the term "originalist" to describe Alito's majority opinion—see Stephen E. Sachs, "Dobbs and the Originalists," *Harvard Journal of Law and Public Policy*, May 15, 2024, https://papers.ssrn.com/sol3/papers.cfm?abstract_id=4829599.

54. Reggie Williams, "To My Daughter, after *Dobbs*," *Christian Century*, July 27, 2022.

55. "The Still-Elusive Path to Limiting Abortion," *America*, July/August 2024, 8–9.

56. Jennifer Benz, Lindsey Witt-Swanson, and Daniel A. Cox, "Faith after the Pandemic: How COVID-19 Changed American Religion," Survey Center on American Life (American Enterprise Institute), January 2023, https://www.aei.org/wp-content/uploads/2023/01/Faith-After-the-Pandemic.pdf?x85095; Pew Research Center, "America's Abortion Quandary," May 6, 2022, https://www.pewresearch.org/religion/2022/05/06/americas-abortion-quandary/; "Survey: White Evangelicals Oppose Abortion; All Other Religious Groups Support It," *National Catholic Reporter*, May 6, 2022.

57. Pew Research Center, "Religious Landscape Study: Attendance at Religious Services by State" [2014], https://www.pewresearch.org/religious-landscape-study/database/compare/attendance-at-religious-services/by/state/; Caroline Kitchener et al., "States Where Abortion Is Legal, Banned, or under Threat," *Washington Post*, July 29, 2024, https://www.washingtonpost.com/politics/2022/06/24/abortion-state-laws-criminalization-roe/.

58. Yonat Shimron, "Jewish Women Sue over Kentucky Abortion Laws, Citing Religious Freedom," *Washington Post*, October 14, 2022.

59. Pew Research Center, "Religious Landscape Study: Views about Abortion among Atheists" [2014], https://www.pewresearch.org/religious-landscape-study/database/religious-family/atheist/views-about-abortion/.

60. Frank Newport, "Personal Religiosity and Attitudes toward Abortion," Gallup, May 13, 2022, https://news.gallup.com/opinion/polling-matters/392648/personal-religiosity-attitudes-toward-abortion.aspx.

61. United States Conference of Catholic Bishops, Press release: "USCCB Statement on U.S. Supreme Court Ruling in Dobbs v. Jackson," June 24, 2022, https://www.usccb.org/news/2022/usccb-statement-us-supreme-court-ruling-dobbs-v-jackson; "Roe v. Wade: An End and a Beginning," *America*, June 2022, 8–9.

62. "Breaking: ERLC Calls SCOTUS Dobbs Ruling Significant Victory in the History of the Pro-Life Movement," Baptist Resource Network, June 24, 2022, https://www.brnunited.org/news/breaking-erlc-calls-scotus-dobbs-ruling-significant-victory-in-the-history-of-the-pro-life-movement/; Daniel Silliman, "Goodbye Roe v. Wade: Pro-Life Evangelicals Celebrate the Ruling They've Waited for," *Christianity Today*, June 24, 2022.

63. Isaac Maddow-Zinet and Candace Gibson, "Despite Bans, Number of Abortions in the United States Increased in 2023," Guttmacher Institute,

March 2024, https://www.guttmacher.org/2024/03/despite-bans-number-abortions-united-states-increased-2023.

64. Daniel Silliman, "Strategy Questions Divide Pro-Life Politics after 'Dobbs,'" *Christianity Today*, September 16, 2022; Bart Barber, "Working toward the End of Abortion: A Pro-Life Response to Abolitionism's Critiques," Southern Baptist Convention Ethics and Religious Liberty Commission, December 27, 2022, https://erlc.com/resource/working-toward-the-end-of-abortion/.

65. Pew Research Center, "America's Abortion Quandary," May 6, 2022, https://www.pewresearch.org/religion/2022/05/06/americas-abortion-quandary/.

66. For examples of this postliberal vision, see Patrick J. Deneen, *Why Liberalism Failed* (New Haven, CT: Yale University Press, 2018); Deneen, *Regime Change: Toward a Postliberal Future* (New York: Sentinel, 2023).

INDEX

A

abolitionists, 280, 288
abortifacients, 4, 5–6, 251, 266–68
abortion(s), 2–10
   accepted as medical necessity, 17
   access to, 282, 288
   as an individual moral crime, 7
   as a capital offense, 4
   elective (*see* elective abortion)
   as evil, 93
   funding, 282, 288
   as genocide, 228
   as homicides (*see* homicides)
   illegal (*see* illegal abortion)
   induced (*See* induced abortion)
   industrial era and, 5–6
   as infanticide (*see* infanticide)
   legal, 130–31
   medical definitions, 267
   physicians on, 6, 7
   Protestant Reformers and, 3–4, 12, 122–23
   restrictive law (*see* restrictive abortion laws)
   state legislators on, 6
   as taking of innocent human life, 197
   therapeutic (*see* therapeutic abortions)
   See also Catholics, and the Catholic Church; Protestants
Abortion Law Reform Association, 32
abortion rights, 38, 39, 42, 81, 282–96
   advocates of, 42, 62, 73, 189
   Black Protestants and, 230–31
   Catholics and, 259, 261–64, 268, 269, 274–77, 286
   conscience rights for women, 34
   Democratic Party, 160, 162, 164, 284, 293–94
   evangelicals and, 94
   late twentieth-century advocates, 3–4
   liberal Protestants and, 172, 211–14, 217, 220, 236–38, 241–45, 269, 285, 290, 292–93
   National Organization for Women, 32, 84, 126
   pro-choice feminists, 87–88
   religious supporters, 293
   Republican states, 246
   secular and Jewish advocates, 22
   Valentine on, 172
   women's denominational organizations, 34

abortion rings, 9
Abzug, Bella, 32, 42
accidental destruction, 121
Affordable Care Act. *See* Obamacare
African Methodist Episcopal (AME) Church, 231–32, 234
alcohol, 132
   advertisement of, 142
   legal restrictions on, 143
   moral campaigns against, 10
Alcoholics Anonymous, 268
Alito, Samuel, 267, 282, 283
America, 70, 85, 166, 284–85, 287
American Baptist Convention/Churches USA, 21, 27, 30, 31, 40
   abortion resolution of 1988, 209, 210, 220
American Citizens Concerned for Life, 166
American Council of Christian Churches (ACCC), 129
American Law Institute, 15–16, 30
Americans against Abortion, 152
Americans United for Life, 39
Anderson, Deborah, 218
Anglican Church in North America, 13, 239, 246
antiabortion laws, 9, 10, 16, 22, 36, 56, 59, 76, 97, 161, 173, 190, 231, 234, 281. *See also* restrictive abortion laws
antislavery movement, 11
Apology (Tertullian), 47
Aquinas, Thomas, 49, 50, 52, 193
Association for the Study of Abortion, 31–32
atheists, 286, 295

Athenagoras of Athens, 46–47
Augustine, 48–49
Ayres, Richard Flagg, 13

B
Balsamon, Theodore, 47–48
Baltimore Catechism, 57, 58
Baptist Bible Tribune, 107, 152
Baptist Joint Committee on Public Affairs (BJCPA), 144–45
Baptists. *See* American Baptist Convention/Churches USA; Progressive National Baptist Convention; Southern Baptist Convention
Baptists for Life, 147, 152, 206
Baptist Standard, 117, 147, 149
Baptist Viewpoint, 117
Barber, Bart, 288
Barth, Karl, 4, 23, 109
Basil, 47–48
Bayh, Birch, 160
Bayly, Timothy, 217
Beilenson, Anthony, 88, 89
Bell, L. Nelson, 93–94
Belonzie, Rosa, 88
Benedict XVI. *See* Ratzinger, Joseph
Bernardin, Joseph, 141, 143–44, 164–70, 182, 185–86, 196, 197, 259, 274
Berrigan, Daniel, 184
BFM. *See 2000 Baptist Faith and Message*
Bible, 99, 107–9, 113, 115, 144, 146, 149, 154–55, 216, 217
   authority and historicity, 95
   Christian Life on, 108–9
   colleges, 128

discussions of abortion, 94–95
individual ethics, 96
personal reading, 64
prenatal human life in, 121–22
as a source of divine wisdom, 95
Bible Belt, 225, 285, 297
Biden, Joe, 265, 275, 276
birth control, 12–14, 214
Blacks and, 227, 228
evangelical discussions on, 100
as genocide, 228
international campaigns, 99
Rehwinkel on, 101
as a vice, 12
Black Lives Matter, 244
Blackmun, Harry, 37–45, 91, 282
Burns's letter to, 43–44
Black Protestants, 226–35, 245–46
civil rights movement, 227
fundamentalist church members, 226
moral reservations, 227
Boston Women's Health Collective, 32
Bozell, L. Brent, 199, 200
Bramlage, James, 168
Brave New People (Jones), 207
Breyer, Steven, 283
Brown, Harold O. J., 152–53, 171, 173
Brown, Judie, 200
Buber, Martin, 14
Burke, Raymond, 261
Burns, Grace, 43–44, 45, 307n2
Burwell v. Hobby Lobby Stores, Inc., 267
Bush, George W., 250, 278
Byrn, Robert, 82

C
California, 268–69
Callaghan, Catherine, 200
Callahan, Sidney, 85–86
Calvin, John, 3
Calvinists, 3–4, 121, 123
Camp, Donald, 128
canon law, 50
Gregory XIV adjusting, 50
revision of, 258–59
sterilization as homicide, 51
Care Net, 339n48
Carroll, Charles, 23
Carter, Jimmy, 163–66, 171–73, 180
Casey, Bob, Jr., 265
Castelli, Jim, 215
Casti Connubii (Pius XI), 55, 74
Catechism of the Catholic Church, 256–57
Catholic Lawyer, 70
Catholics, and the Catholic Church, 43–91, 143–44
civil disobedience for moral causes, 135–36
crisis pregnancy centers (CPC) and, 279
criticism of pro-life position of, 81–84
decline in attendance, 286
immigration, 7
liberalization proposals of abortion, 60–63
liberal Protestants vs., 214–15
moral perspective, 45–52
New York Times/CBS News poll, 197–98
NRLC and, 168, 200

Catholics, and the Catholic Church (*cont.*)
  Pastoral Plan for Pro-Life Activities, 139–40, 141
  political influence, 285
  popular opinion, 78–81
  post-*Roe* abortion issue, 137–41
  probabilism, 194
  pro-choice politicians, 258–65
  pro-life campaign, 69–84
  sex abuse crisis, 286
  therapeutic abortion and, 116
  unborn human life and, 52–60
  Vatican II (*see* Vatican II)
  women, 84–91
  See also Protestants
Catholics for a Free Choice, 65, 191–95
Catholic Standard and Times, 59
Catholic Transcript, 59
"Challenge of Peace, The" (NCCB), 185–86
Chaput, Charles, 271–72
Chavez, Cesar, 23
Christendom College, 199
Christian Action Council, 152, 207
Christian Action for Life, 127
Christian Century, 16–17, 21, 23, 24, 28, 29, 32, 34, 36, 37, 40, 41, 102, 106, 211, 238, 284
Christianity Today, 100, 105, 106, 107, 108, 114, 115, 125, 130, 132, 142, 170, 220, 288
  abortion liberalization laws of late 1960s, 93
  antiabortion editorials, 119
  denunciating abortion, 93–94
  on issue of abortion, 153–55
  predicting decline in number of abortions, 288
  on *Roe v. Wade*, 133, 136, 153–54
Christian Life, 99, 108–9, 114
Christian Life Commission (CLC), 117, 145, 146, 206–7
Christian Methodist Episcopal Church, 235
Christian nationalism, 290
Christian News, 129
Christian Reformed Church, 122, 231
Christian Right, 185, 203, 222, 250
Christocentric humanism, 133
Church, Frank, 268
Church Amendments of 1973, 268
Church of God in Christ, 234, 235
Church of the Nazarene, 130–31
class-based frameworks, 10
Clergy Consultation Service on Abortion, 19–21, 24, 28, 30, 37, 146, 209
Clinton, Bill, 222, 238, 248, 265, 278
Clinton, Hillary, 248
Colson, Charles, 253–54
Commonweal, 79, 136
communism, 100, 132, 202
Completely Pro-Life (Sider), 186
Comstock Act, 8, 12, 53
Conscience, 194
consistent life-ethic, 180, 269–70
Constitution, 281–82
contraception, 8
  accepted forms, 267
  Black proponents, 227
  emergency, 267
  evangelicals' early views of, 94–105
  Graham on, 99–100

health care coverage for, 267–68
mainline Protestants, 17
contraceptives, 8, 12, 13, 54–55, 69, 73–74, 99, 101, 189, 251
　Ella and Plan B, 267
　employers' coverage for, 267–68
　insurance plans, 267–68, 292
Council of Ancyra, 47–48, 50, 51
Council of Trent, 64
Cox, Harvey, 19
Cox, Ignatius, 55
criminally-induced abortion, 104
crisis pregnancy centers (CPC), 268–69, 279–80, 292, 339n48
Criswell, W. A., 109
Cuomo, Mario, 187, 188, 189, 190, 195, 237, 247–48, 259–60, 263, 275
Cupich, Blase, 274
Cushing, Richard, 56, 66, 69

D

Dallas Theological Seminary, 125
Dayton, Cornelia Hughes, 5
Dearden, John, 77, 78
Death before Birth (Brown), 153
Declaration on Procured Abortion, 138–39
Deedy, John, 79
"Defense of Abortion, A" (Thomson), 35
deliberate destruction, 121
Delk, Yvonne, 235–36
Democratic Party, 269
　abortion rights and, 284, 293–94
　platform of 2016, 269
　pro-choice Catholic politicians, 260–62

pro-life views, 161
religious politics, 159–70
restrictive abortion laws, 161
Didache, 46
Dobbs v. Jackson Women's Health Organization, 246, 254–55, 281–82
　abortion bans, 286
　Alito's majority opinion, 282, 283
　progressives on, 284
　pro-life Christians divided on, 287–88
　USCCB on, 287
　Williams on, 284
Dobson, James, 216
Doerflinger, Richard, 272
Doe v. Bolton, 41, 135
Dolan, Timothy, 274
Dole, Bob, 249–50
Douglas, William O., 40
Dowd, Mary, 89
Dred Scott v. Sandford, 41
Dreisbach, Jeannette, 259
Drinan, Robert, 65
drunkenness, 11. *See also* temperance
Duncan, Robert, 246
Duvall, Evelyn Millis, 97

E

ECO: A Covenant Order of Evangelical Presbyterians, 240, 246
Eddy, Thomas Mears, 6
Edwards, Jonathan, 5
Eisenhower, Dwight, 132
elective abortion, 60, 104, 112, 192, 207, 221
　as a constitutional right, 133
　first trimester and, 40

elective abortion (*cont.*)
  legalization of, 18, 40, 79–80, 93, 115, 117–18
  Medicaid funding for, 163, 269
  moral ambiguity, 120
  as morally problematic, 172
Ella (morning-after pill), 267
embryo, 4, 22, 26, 38, 47–48, 62, 82, 89–90, 103–4, 110–12, 115, 122, 143, 144, 270, 292. *See also* fetus; zygote
embryological science/studies, 50, 52, 278
Engel, Randy, 74
Engel v. Vitale, 142
English common law, 4
ensoulment, 48–52, 57, 58, 103, 109–12, 114, 129, 144, 193
Episcopal Church, 27, 31, 241, 282
  inclusion of same-sex couples, 239
  membership declined, 240
  partial-birth abortion and, 223
  resolution on abortion, 27, 219–20, 223
  women's reproductive health, 245
Episcopal Church Women, 27, 34
Equal Rights Amendment (ERA), 169, 200
Eternity, 98–99, 114, 119, 126
Evangelical Lutheran Church in America (ELCA), 26, 220–21, 240, 241
Evangelical Presbyterian Church, 246–47
evangelicals, 10, 93–133
  abortion bans in states dominated by, 286
  and Catholics as fellow Christians, 253–54
  crisis pregnancy centers (CPC) and, 279–80
  early views of contraception and abortion, 94–105
  as minorities, 215
  moral campaigns, 10
  outside of Baptist circles opposing abortion, 152–55
  political power of, 285
  pro-life commitment, 278–81
  reproductive justice and, 247–51
  salvation for, 10
  social welfare programs and, 287
  See also Southern Baptist Convention
"Evangelicals and Catholics Together," 253–54
Evangelicals for Social Action, 186, 207, 247
Evangelii Gaudium (Francis), 270
Evangelium Vitae (Paul II), 255–56, 257, 261, 266–67
Evans, J. Claude, 37, 211
Evans, Tony, 234, 235
Exodus 21, 48, 108, 114, 121, 122, 129, 149

F
Facts of Life and Love for Teen-agers (Duvall), 97
Faggioli, Massimo, 275–76
Faith for the Family, 152
Falwell, Jerry, 107, 157, 174, 175–76, 178, 199, 202, 203
Family Research Council, 280

Feast of the Immaculate Conception, 58
Federal Council of Churches, 11–12
  "Social Creed of the Churches, The," 12
  Social Gospel, 12, 13–14
feminism/feminists, 200
  abortion rights campaign, 124–25
  evangelical discussions of abortion, 125–28
Ferraro, Geraldine, 187, 188–89, 190, 196, 260, 261, 265
fetal development, 6, 9
fetal life, 6, 8
  biological evidence, 6
fetus, 4, 40, 106, 129, 131, 156, 170, 180, 204, 223–24, 285
  Aristotle on, 49
  Barth on, 4
  Calvin on, 3
  as cellular mass, 26
  constitutionally protected rights, 38
  as a creation of God, 17
  Dayton on, 5
  diary of, 61
  first-trimester, 292
  formed, 48, 50, 53
  Frame on, 121
  humanity of, 7, 60
  as human life, 17, 22, 23, 37, 50, 51, 52–53, 60, 75, 81, 88, 97, 112–13, 122–23, 124, 144, 147, 220
  immeasurable value, 112
  injuries to, 108
  Jewish rabbinic tradition, 22, 48
  Kantzer on, 111–12
  Lutheran Church in America on, 26
  Maximus on, 48
  Mennonites' resolution, 225
  Montagu on, 82
  Moody on, 20
  Mosaic law, 48
  Narramore on, 103–4
  PCUS resolution, 116
  as a person in prenatal injury cases, 38
  physicians on, 6
  pro-life women on, 88
  Ramsey on, 25–26
  right to life of, 6, 75, 88
  second-trimester, 218
  Shriver on, 89–90
  soul (see ensoulment)
  as tissue, 25–26
  unformed, 48–49, 50, 53
  United Methodist Church (UMC), 25–26
  value of, 108–9, 242
  Wahlberg on, 34–35
  See also embryo; zygote
Fifth Amendment, 75
Fillion, Nancy, 91
Finkbine, Sherri Chessen, 62–63, 104–6
Finley, Sarah, 125
First Amendment, 286
First Things, 254
Fletcher, Joseph, 15, 16, 35
Focus on the Family, 216
foeticide, 6
Food and Drug Administration, 267
Ford, Gerald, 163, 165–66, 170, 180

Ford, John, 59–60
Forming Consciences for Faithful Citizenship (USCCB), 264, 273
Fosdick, Harry Emerson, 13
Fourteenth Amendment, 75, 283
Fowler, Paul B., 207–8
Frame, John, 121, 122
Francis (pope), 269–76
    on abortion, 270
    consistent life ethic, 269–70, 271
    Evangelii Gaudium, 270
    on immigrants' rights, 271
    Laudato Si', 270–71
    on Trump, 271
Franciscan Sisters of the Poor, 167
Freedom of Choice Coalition, 215
Friedan, Betty, 32, 33, 34, 85
fundamentalists, 95, 96, 128–29
Furman v. Georgia, 182

G
Garrett, W. Barry, 145
Gaudium et Spes, 66–67, 83
gender roles, 99–100
General Association of Regular Baptists, 152
General Conference Mennonite Church, 224–25
Genesis 1, 98
Genesis 2, 48
Genesis 2:7, 109, 111
genocide, 77, 228
Gilkey, Langdon, 19
Ginsburg, Ruth Bader, 267–68
Gladden, Washington, 11
Glendon, Mary Ann, 254
Global Methodist Church, 240, 246

God
    decision and purpose, 112
    eternal plan, 294
    image-bearer of, 112
    image of, 294
    personal relationship with, 95
    sovereignty, 3–4, 122–23
God Who Is There, The (Schaeffer), 156
Goltz, Pat, 200
Gomez, José, 275
Goodwin, Elizabeth, 85
Gospel of Luke, 48, 113
Graham, Billy, 93, 99–100, 119–20, 123, 132, 133, 152, 177, 185, 200
Graham, Elizabeth, 287–88
Graham, Ruth Bell, 152
Gregg v. Georgia, 182
Gregory XIV, 50
Griese, Roger, 168–69
Grisez, Germain, 74, 77
Griswold v. Connecticut, 69
Guttmacher, Alan F., 22, 89, 90
Guttmacher Institute, 267

H
Haines, Mary Ellen, 40
Hamer, Fannie Lou, 228
Hardesty, Nancy, 126–27
Hargis, Billy James, 152
Harrington, Paul, 71–72
Harris, Kamala, 293–94
Harrison, Beverly Wildung, 237, 243
Hartle, Alice, 85
Hauerwas, Stanley, 223–24
Hays, Richard, 223, 247–48

Heartbeat International, 339n48
Henry, Carl F. H., 119, 120, 123, 170–71, 177
Herbert Mekeel, 98
Heritage Foundation, 176, 198–99
Hess, Glenda Adams, 35–36
Higgins, George, 180
Hiroshima, atomic bombing of, 60
Hispanics
  abortion views of, 277–78
  Catholics, 277, 278
  evangelical, 277–78
  Gen-Zers, 277
Hobby Lobby, 267
Holbrook, Robert, 147–50, 152, 173, 174, 177
Holy Spirit, 48, 112–13, 121, 171
homicides, 50–51, 72, 100, 193, 280
  involuntary, 47
  penalties for, 48
  sterilization as, 51
homosexuality, 200
Hoover, J. Edgar, 132
How Should We Then Live? (Schaeffer), 156, 157, 158, 199
Hoyt, Robert, 60–61
Humanae Vitae (Paul VI), 72–73
human dignity, 179, 180
Human Life Amendment, 138–40, 144, 168, 177, 178, 180, 225, 232
Human Life Sunday, 206
human rights, 179–80, 298
  pro-choice agenda as threat to, 297
Hyde Amendment, 163, 236–37, 265, 266, 268, 269, 275, 289
hysterectomy, 228

I
illegal abortion, 1–2, 8–9, 10, 12, 15–16, 19–21, 90, 96, 100–102, 215
  availability of, 8
  dangerous, 83
  early-stage abortions as, 6
  Protestant ministers and, 2
  providers as a serious social menace, 56–57
  See also elective abortion
Incarnation, 48, 49
individualism, 95–96
induced abortion, 104, 114
  criminally-induced abortion, 104
  therapeutic (*see* therapeutic abortions)
infanticide, 6, 46, 66, 71, 72, 75, 82, 129, 136, 155, 157, 158
In His Steps (Sheldon), 11
interracial marriage, 19

J
Jackson, Jesse, 229–33
Jesuits, 59–60, 79
  divinity of, 95
Jesus, 11, 113
  substitutionary atoning death, 95
Jewett, Paul, 111, 126
Jews, 116, 286
John-Stevas, Norman St., 70
John the Baptist, 113
John XXIII, 64
  Pacem in Terris, 67–68, 75, 76, 78, 181
Jones, Bob, Sr., 97
Jones, D. Gareth, 207
JustLife PAC, 186

K

Kagan, Elena, 283
Kantzer, Kenneth, 111–12
Kelly, Gerald, 57–58
Kelly, Marge, 169–70
Kennedy, John F., 89, 132, 189
Kennedy, Ted, 77, 160, 161, 187
Kerry, John, 196, 260–61, 262, 264, 265, 271–72
Killea, Lucy, 259
King, Alveda, 234, 235
King, Eileen, 88
King, Martin Luther, Jr., 23, 227, 228, 229, 234
Kinsolving, Lester, 32
Kissling, Frances, 194
Koop, C. Everett, 152, 158
Krebs, Walter, 214
Kreeft, Peter, 254
Krol, John, 138, 140

L

Lader, Larry, 73
Land, Richard, 253–54, 281
Law, Bernard, 260, 335–36n14
LGBTQ+ rights, 240, 269
liberal Protestants. *See* mainline Protestants
Lieberman, Joe, 250
Life and Love (Narramore), 103
Life before Birth (Montagu), 82
Lifewatch, 216, 219. *See also* United Methodist Church
Light, 206
Lindquist, Hugo, 148
Living Church, 13
Luce, Clare Boothe, 84–85
Luther, Martin, 3

Lutheran Church—Missouri Synod (LCMS), 106, 116–17, 120
Lutheran News, 106–7
Lutherans, 100–101, 107, 119, 120, 122–23, 129, 130, 220–21
Lynch, Robert, 138

M

Mace, David R., 24
Maguire, Daniel, 193, 195
Maher, Leo, 259
Mahony, Roger, 262, 335n14
mainline Protestants, 2–10
  abortion law liberalization, 15–18
  abortion rights and, 284–85
  debating abortion among, 215–26
  fundamentalists vs., 96
  lack of clarity on abortion, 124
  liberal democracy, 3
  minority, 23–37
  moral decision-making, 216–17
  partial-birth abortion and, 222–23
  political influence, 285
  pro-choice advocates, 217
  pro-life advocates, 217
  rights consciousness, 18–23
  Roe v. Wade and, 211–15, 289
  sacredness of life, 22
  sanctity of life, 22
  sexual liberalization, 18–23
  theological change, 10–15
March for Life, 168–69, 246
Marshall, Thurgood, 40
Marshner, Connie, 199
Marshner, William, 199
Marx, Paul, 74
Maximus the Confessor, 48

McCain, John, 250
McCall's, 89
McCarrick, Theodore, 262, 263, 335n14
McCormack, Ellen, 85, 160, 162–63
McElroy, Robert, 272, 273
McGovern, George, 133
McGraw, Onalee, 198–99
McGreevey, James, 261–62
McHugh, James, 69, 74–75, 78, 83–84
McQuillan, Patricia, 191–92
Medicaid funding for abortion, 160, 163, 172, 233, 268, 269
Mennonite Church USA, 225–26
Methodists. *See* African Methodist Episcopal (AME) Church; Christian Methodist Episcopal Church; Global Methodist Church; United Methodist Church
Meyer, Robert, 167
Miani, Mary, 88
Miller, Elizabeth, 145
Minnick, Liz, 207
miscarriage, 108, 121, 122
model abortion law, 15–16
Mohr, James, 4, 6
Mondale, Walter, 187
Montagu, Ashley, 82
Montgomery, John Warwick, 110–11, 112, 119
Moody, Howard, 2, 19–21, 30, 36–37, 38, 146, 209
Moody Monthly, 96, 207
Moore, Barbara, 237
Moore, John, 24

moral decision-making, 216–17
Moral Majority, 157, 176, 177–78, 199, 202, 203, 204–5, 207, 216
moral relativism, 217
Moral Vision of the New Testament, The (Hays), 223
Moss, Robert, 213
Murder of the Helpless Unborn, The (Rice), 128
Murray, John Courtney, 64, 66
Myers, John, 261, 264

N
NAACP, 227
Nagasaki, atomic bombing of, 60
Narramore, Clyde, 103–4
National Association of Evangelicals (NAE), 98, 119, 123, 129, 131–32, 202
National Catholic Reporter, 85, 276
National Committee for a Human Life Amendment, 137–38
National Conference of Catholics Bishops (NCCB), 76, 194–95, 255, 264
  "Challenge of Peace, The" (NCCB), 185–86
  Committee for Pro-Life Affairs, 135
  death penalty and, 182
  Human Life Amendment and, 139, 178
  nonpartisan consistent life ethic, 181
  See also United States Conference of Catholic Bishops
National Council of Churches of Christ, 17

National Institute of Family and Life Advocates (NIFLA), 268, 339n48
National Organization for Women (NOW), 32, 84, 125, 126, 169, 191, 200
National Right to Life Committee (NRLC), 74, 77, 138, 162, 166, 167–68, 200, 232
National Right to Life News, 229, 232
Nation of Islam, 227
Naumann, Joseph, 274
Negro Project, 227
Neuhaus, Richard John, 254
New American Standard Bible, 113, 122
New Revised Standard Version, 122
New Right, 175–76, 185, 198, 199, 201
New Testament, 46, 108, 110, 202
New York Times, 100, 182, 188, 218, 233
New York Times/CBS News poll, 197–98
Nixon, Richard, 132, 133, 185
Noonan, John, 74
North American Lutheran Church, 246
Northwestern Christian Advocate, 6–7
NOW. *See* National Organization for Women
NRLC. *See* National Right to Life Committee

O
Obama, Barack, 265–68
Obamacare, 266–68
Obergefell v. Hodges, 269

O'Boyle, Patrick, 73, 76–77, 91
Ockenga, Harold J., 98
O'Connell, Marvin, 73
O'Connor, John, 187–88, 196–98, 202, 254, 258, 274
Ohio Baptist Fellowship Churches, 129
Olasky, Marvin, 4, 5
Old Testament, 108, 202
O'Malley, Robert, 91
O'Malley, Sean, 261, 264, 265
Operation Rescue, 157, 169, 204–5, 250, 327n45
organized crime syndicates, 1
O'Rourke, Joseph, 78–79
Orthodox Presbyterian Church (OPC), 121, 231
Other Side, The, 184
Our Bodies, Ourselves, 32
Our Right to Choose (Harrison), 237
out-of-wedlock sex/pregnancy, 21, 103, 239

P
Pacem in Terris (John XXIII), 67–68, 75, 76, 78, 181
Partial-Birth Abortion Ban Act, 248, 265, 278
Pastoral Plan for Pro-Life Activities, 139–40, 141
Paul, John, II, 193, 197, 255–58, 260, 271, 274, 287
  on abortion, 201, 255–56
  Evangelium Vitae, 255–56, 257, 261, 266–67
  on marriage and sexuality, 201–2
  social teachings of, 201
  in the United States, 201–2

Paul VI, 186
  Humanae Vitae, 72–73
Pavone, Frank, 204
Pax Christi, 196
Peters, Rebecca Todd, 241–43, 244, 293
Pius IX, 51
Pius XI, 66
  Casti Connubii, 55, 74
  Quadragesimo Anno, 67
Pius XII, 66
Plan B, 267
Planned Parenthood, 14, 22, 42, 168–69, 218, 227
Playboy, 125
pluralistic society, 288–91
Plymouth Crusader, 128
Polter, Julie, 248
popular opinion of Catholics, 78–81
pornography, 8, 29, 100, 102, 132, 148–49, 151, 155, 158, 174, 176, 203, 279
Post, Avery, 213
poverty, 11, 14, 54, 77, 83, 145, 178, 180–81, 201, 202, 229, 231, 236, 237, 243, 247, 249, 272–73
Powell, Adam Clayton, 227
Powell, Lewis, 40
pregnancy, 123
  Catholic understanding of, 266–67
  CPCs, 268–69, 279–80
  medical community on, 267
  as part of God's divine plan, 104
  quickening, 4, 5, 6, 8, 40, 50
pregnancy termination. *See* abortion(s)

Presbyterian Church (USA), 129, 210, 215
  abortion rights argument, 241–43
  "God Alone Is Lord of the Conscience," 222
  "On Providing Just Access to Reproductive Health Care," 244–45
  ordaining openly gay clergy, 240
  pro-choice stance, 218–19
  pro-life advocates, 218
  repealing fidelity and chastity clause, 239–40
  resolution on abortion, 7–8
  split over sexuality, 240
Presbyterian Church in America (PCA), 129, 174, 207, 215
Presbyterian Church in the United States (PCUS) (Southern Presbyterians), 116, 129, 174, 215
Presbyterian Journal, 129
Presbyterians Pro-Life, 216, 217–18
Presbyterians Pro-Life News, 217
presidential election of 1976, 159–70
presidential election of 2020, 275
Prior, Karen Swallow, 288–89
probabilism, 194
pro-choice campaign/movement, 87–88, 210, 217–19, 236, 258–65, 297
  Catholic politicians and, 258–65
  feminists' advocacy of abortion rights, 200
  theological assumptions, 292–98
  See also Catholics, and the Catholic Church; Protestants

Progressive National Baptist
  Convention, 228
pro-life campaign/movement,
  69–84, 81–84, 139–40, 141,
  161, 254–55, 287–88
  Catholics and, 255–58
  Christian nation and, 290
  crisis pregnancy centers (CPC),
    279–80
  evangelicals' commitment to,
    278–81
  feminists and, 200
  political right and, 180
  religious liberty and, 266–78
  theological assumptions, 292–98
  See also Catholics, and the
    Catholic Church; evangelicals
pro-life clinics, 268–69
Prolifers for Survival, 183, 186
prostitution, 9, 10, 67
Protestant Reformers, 3–4, 12,
  122–23
Protestants
  Black (*see* Black Protestants)
  as dominant religious group, 2
  evangelicals (*see* evangelicals)
  intradenominational fights, 11
  mainline or liberal (*See* mainline
    Protestants)
  sixteenth-century reformers, 3
  vices and, 8
Protestant Symposium on the Control
  of Human Reproduction, 114

Q
Quadragesimo Anno (Pius XI), 67
quickening, 4, 5, 6, 8, 40, 50
Quinn, John Raphael, 182

R
Ramsey, Paul, 23, 25–26
Ratzinger, Joseph, 263–64
Rauschenbusch, Walter, 11
Reagan, Ronald, 185, 186, 198, 199,
  201, 202, 222, 232–33
Reed, Mary, 167
Reformed Protestant. *See* Protestant
  Reformers
Rehwinkel, Alfred Martin, 100–102,
  103
Religious Coalition for Abortion
  Rights (RCAR), 209, 219, 236
  "Call to Concern," 172
  Hyde Amendment, 236
  pro-choice campaign, 236
  public relations materials, 212
  on *Roe v. Wade*, 212, 213
  United Methodists and, 212
religious politics, 159–70
Rennard, Mary Kay, 89
Reproductive FACT Act, 268
reproductive justice, 235–51
  evangelicals and, 247–51
  framework of, 235–47
reproductive rights, 214, 296, 297
  crisis pregnancy centers (CPC)
    and, 279–80
  post-*Dobbs* political climate, 284
  religious campaign for, 292
Response to the Silent Scream, 218
restrictive abortion laws, 19–20, 22,
  27, 34, 117–19, 123, 151, 161,
  190, 207, 221–22, 236, 246,
  269, 283, 285, 290
  advocacy for, 123
  as inhumane, 15
  physicians on, 15

state legislatures enacting, 6, 8
twentieth-century belief, 17
Revised Standard Version, 122
Rice, Charles E., 38, 77
Rice, John R., 97, 128
Rich Christians in an Age of Hunger (Sider), 186
right to life, 254
Robertson, Pat, 253–54
Rockwell, Eric, 215
Roe v. Wade, 2, 282, 291
   America on, 284–85
   Blackmun's opinion in, 37, 38–42, 45, 282
   Catholics and, 289
   Christian Century on, 211
   evangelical politics before, 131–33
   Jackson on, 230
   liberal theological assumptions, 289
   overturning, 254–98
   as political lightning rod, 289
   Protestant denominations resolutions before, 122–23
   RCAR on, 212, 213
   as subversive decision, 283
   Weddington as plaintiff attorney in, 39
   See also Catholics, and the Catholic Church; Protestants
Rogers, Adrian, 176
Romney, Mitt, 250
Ryan, Juan, 77

S
Sacred Congregation for Religious and Secular Institutes, 194–95
Sacred Congregation for the Doctrine of the Faith, 138–39
sacredness of life, 22
salvation, 10, 95
same-sex marriage, 238, 239–40, 249, 251, 269, 282
sanctity of life, 22
Sanger, Margaret, 14, 97, 227
Savas, Leah, 4, 5
Scanzoni, Letha, 126
Schaeffer, Francis, 155–59, 175, 185, 198–99, 204, 205, 283
   God Who Is There, The, 156
   How Should We Then Live?, 156, 157, 158, 199
   on *Roe v. Wade*, 156
   Whatever Happened to the Human Race? (with Koop), 158
Schlafly, Phyllis, 200
Schroeder, Frederick W., 217
secularism, 199
sex education, 18
sex trade, 10
sexual liberalization, 18–23
sexual revolution, 132, 199
   conservative evangelicals, 124–25
Sheldon, Charles, 11
Shinn, Roger, 213–14
Shriver, Eunice Kennedy, 89–90, 161
Shriver, Sargent, 160–61
Sider, Ronald, 186, 247, 248
Silent Scream, The, 218
Simmons, Paul D., 145
sin, 95
Situation Ethics (Fletcher), 15
Smith, Michael D., 28
Smith, Noel, 107, 152
"Social Creed of the Churches, The" (Federal Council of Churches), 12

Social Gospel, 11–14, 96, 124
"Social Report on Human Sexuality, A" (ELCA), 240
Soekren, Irene, 99
Sojourners, 184, 185, 207, 237, 247, 248
sola fide (faith alone), 96
sola scriptura (scripture alone), 96
Sotomayor, Sonia, 283
Southern Baptist Convention (SBC), 105–6
   abortion as a signature issue for, 216
   Baptists for Life, 147, 152, 206
   Christian Life Commission, 117, 145, 146, 206–7
   church-state separation, 146
   denominational administrators, 106
   Ethics and Religious Liberty Commission, 281, 287–88
   Human Life Sunday, 206
   legalization of abortion, 117–19
   membership, 241
   moderates, 146–47, 148
   "On Abolishing Abortion," 280–81
   Partial-Birth Abortion Ban Act and, 278
   political debates among, 142–51
   pro-choice position, 117
   pro-life position and campaign, 117–18, 205–7
   religious liberty and, 142, 143
   resolutions committee, 149–50
   Roe v. Wade and, 278–79
   school prayer and, 142, 143
   Social Service Commission, 106
   therapeutic abortion, 105–6, 117–18, 148
Stagg, Frank, 109–10
Stanley, Charles, 204–5, 206
sterilization, 50–51, 154, 227
STOP-ERA campaign, 200
Storer, Horatio, 6
Straton, John Roach, 96–97, 98
Stupak, Bart, 266
Sword of the Lord, 97, 128

T
Tauer, Maureen, 91
temperance
   advocacy, 11
   campaign/movement, 7, 10–11
Teresa, Mother, 218, 222
Terrey, Robert J., 128
Tertullian, 46, 47, 48
Theodoret of Cyrus, 48
therapeutic abortions, 21–22, 104, 146–47, 159, 172, 227
   American Baptist Convention and, 21
   Catholics and, 59, 63, 88–89
   evangelicals and, 105–18, 227
   laws, 27, 116–19, 129–31, 148–49, 278–79
   liberal Protestant ministers, 27
   national news story, 104–5
   Presbyterian Church on, 17–18
   Southern Baptist Convention (SBC) and, 148
Thomson, Judith Jarvis, 35
Todd, John, 7
Treatise on the Soul (Tertullian), 47

Triumph, 199
Trump, Donald, 248–50, 269, 271, 273
  Francis on, 271
Trust Women (Peters), 241
2000 Baptist Faith and Message (BFM), 278

U
Udall, Mo, 160
United Church of Christ (UCC), 40, 212
  abortion rights and, 30, 213–14, 220
  Eden Seminary, 217
  evangelical minorities, 215
  Friends for Life, 216
  Hyde Amendment and, 236
  regional conferences, 220
  Vietnam War and, 29–30
United Methodist Church (UMC), 231, 240–41
  Board of Christian Social Concerns, 25, 34
  Durham Declaration, 219
  Lifewatch, 216, 219
  ordaining women, 31
  pro-choice position, 210, 219
  Religious Coalition for Reproductive Choice and, 219
  resolution on abortion, 25–26, 31, 39
United Nations, 132
United Presbyterian Church. *See* Presbyterian Church (USA)
United States Conference of Catholic Bishops (USCCB), 264, 272–75, 287, 288. *See also* National Conference of Catholic Bishops
University of Chicago Divinity School, 19

V
Valentine, Foy, 145–47, 148, 151, 163, 172–74, 177, 206
Vatican I, 63–64
Vatican II, 63–69, 74–76, 78, 83, 87, 133, 140, 161, 165–66, 170, 180, 181, 191, 193, 197, 258, 287, 290, 295
Vaux, Kenneth, 211
vices, 8
  birth control, 12
  moral preaching on, 10
Vietnam War, 75, 228
  Catholics on, 76, 77, 181, 184
  evangelicals on, 132
  mainline Protestants on, 18, 19, 29, 36, 222
  United Church of Christ (UCC) on, 29–30
Viguerie, Richard, 175, 198, 201
Virgin Mary, 86
Visscher, Robert, 115

W
Wagner, Maria, 89
Wahlberg, Rachel Conrad, 34–35
Walker, Nelda, 127–28, 317n55
Wallace, George, 160
Wallis, Jim, 247, 248
Wanderer, 199, 200
Washington Post, 234

Webb, June, 127
Webber, Helen, 40
Weddington, Sarah, 39
Weigel, George, 66, 254
Weyrich, Paul, 175, 176, 198, 199, 200, 201
Whatever Happened to the Human Race? (Schaeffer and Koop), 158
Whole Woman's Health v. Hellerstedt, 269
Wilde, Melissa J., 12–13
Wilder, John, 176–77
Wiley, Juli Loesch, 183–86
Willard, Frances, 11
Williams, Reggie, 284
Williams, Roger, 142
Willimon, William H., 223
Willke, Jack, 168
Winter, Mary, 32, 85, 86–88
Woman's Home Companion, 59
women, 31
  Catholic, 84–91
  evangelicals, 125–28
  liberal Protestant, 33–36
  pregnancy (*see* pregnancy)
  See also abortion(s)
Women's Christian Temperance Union, 11
Women's Strike for Equality, 32
Wyszynski, Stefan, 61

Y
Yoder, John Howard, 224

Z
zygote, 58, 61–62, 103, 110–11, 140, 144, 266, 294
  genetic composition of, 81–82
  as a miniature person, 58
  See also embryo; fetus

DANIEL K. WILLIAMS is an associate professor of history at Ashland University. He is the author of several books on modern American religion and politics, including *The Politics of the Cross: A Christian Alternative to Partisanship* and *Defenders of the Unborn: The Pro-Life Movement before "Roe v. Wade."* His work has been published in the *New York Times*, *The Atlantic*, and *Christianity Today*.